Handbook of Food Science and Nutrition

Handbook of Food Science and Nutrition

Edited by Dorothy Green

SYRAWOOD
PUBLISHING HOUSE
New York

Published by Syrawood Publishing House,
750 Third Avenue, 9th Floor,
New York, NY 10017, USA
www.syrawoodpublishinghouse.com

Handbook of Food Science and Nutrition
Edited by Dorothy Green

International Standard Book Number: 978-1-68286-713-6 (Hardback)

Cataloging-in-Publication Data

Handbook of food science and nutrition / edited by Dorothy Green.
p. cm.
Includes bibliographical references and index.
ISBN 978-1-68286-713-6
1. Food. 2. Nutrition. 3. Diet. 4. Health. I. Green, Dorothy.
TX353 .H36 2019
641.3--dc23

Printed in China.

TABLE OF CONTENTS

PREFACE

The study of the nature of food, effects of nutrients, causes of deterioration and improvement is dealt by the sciences of nutrition and food science. Nutrition refers to the scientific study of nutrients and their functional role in the growth and development of a human being. Food science covers physical, chemical and biochemical study of food as well as processing techniques. Food science and nutrition are interrelated fields which directly impact the health of living organisms. Malnutrition often results in obesity, cardiovascular disease, fatigue, etc. Food science focuses on maintaining the nutritional value of packaged foods and preventing them from contamination. This book discusses the essential aspects of food science and explores the recent studies contributing to the progress of the field. It attempts to understand the multiple branches that fall under food science and nutrition and how such concepts have practical applications. It will be immensely beneficial to all students and researchers involved at various levels in this area of study.

Significant researches are present in this book. Intensive efforts have been employed by authors to make this book an outstanding discourse. This book contains the enlightening chapters which have been written on the basis of significant researches done by the experts.

Finally, I would also like to thank all the members involved in this book for being a team and meeting all the deadlines for the submission of their respective works. I would also like to thank my friends and family for being supportive in my efforts.

Editor

1

Optimization of production and quality evaluation of maize-based snack supplemented with soybean and tiger-nut (*Cyperus esculenta*) flour

Olugbenga O. Awolu[1], Olufunmilayo S. Omoba[1], Olumide Olawoye[1] & Modupe Dairo[2]

[1]Department of Food Science and Technology, Federal University of Technology, Akure, Nigeria
[2]Quintas Renewable Energy Solutions Ltd, Akure, Nigeria

Keywords
Amino acid profile, optimization, pasting, proximate, snack toasted maize

Correspondence
Olugbenga O. Awolu, Department of Food Science and Technology, Federal University of Technology, Akure, Nigeria.
E-mail: ooawolu@futa.edu.ng

Funding Information
No funding information provided.

Abstract

Optimization of the production and evaluation of the quality of maize-based snack supplemented with soy and tigernut flour was carried out. Experimental design for the composite flour was carried out using optimal design model of response surface methodology. The variables were toasted maize flour (75–85%), soy flour (10–20%), and tigernut flour (5–10%); while the responses were proximate composition and mineral contents. Three blends were selected from optimization results; runs 2, 7, and 11. The functional properties, pasting properties, antioxidant, antinutritional, and amino acid profile of the three blends were evaluated. In addition, sensory evaluation of the cookies produced from the three blends was determined. The results (75/100 g toasted maize flour, 20/100 g soy flour, and 5/100 g tigernut flour) had 16.4/100 g protein, 4.2/100 g ash, 3.5/100 g moisture, 58.5/100 g carbohydrate, 3.0/100 g crude fiber, 14.4/100 g fat, 30.20 ppm calcium, 38.90 ppm potassium, 0.25 ppm manganese, 1.91 ppm iron, 0.14 ppm copper, and 0.98 ppm zinc contents. It also had best overall acceptability.

Introduction

Cookies are widely consumed all over the world and they represent the largest category of snack foods in most parts of the world. Generally, they are high in carbohydrates, fat, and calorie, but low in fiber, vitamin, and mineral. Currently, fortification of snacks has evolved to enhancing their nutritional quality (Neha and Ramesh 2012; Awolu et al. 2015a,b).

Maize is the most important cereal in the world after wheat and rice with regard to cultivation areas and total production (Osagie and Eka 1998). It has been discovered that maize is nutritionally superior to other cereals in many ways, except in protein value. Maize is low in two essential amino acids, lysine and tryptophan. The addition of soybeans which are rich in lysine and tryptophan was meant to enhance the nutritional capacity of the composite flour.

Soybean is an important legume. It has been found that soybean is a very rich source of protein and fat, phytochemicals, and minerals such as copper, zinc, and manganese (Nwokolo 1996). Tigernut is an underutilized crop reputed to be very rich in minerals such as calcium, magnesium and iron (Omode et al. 1995; Oladele and Aina 2007). Tigernuts have good dietary fiber, carbohydrate contents, and it is a rich source of antioxidant (Umerie and Enebeli 1997). Currently, the use and acceptability of tigernut in food formulation is on the increase (Ade-Omowaye et al. 2008; Omoba et al. 2015).

This study aimed at utilizing these rich crops in order to develop composite flour that is maize (toasted) based. Toasting had been found to enhance energy value, antioxidant capacity and calcium, sodium, magnesium, and zinc contents of maize (Oboh et al. 2010). The effect of the composite flour composition on the dependent variables was evaluated. The functional properties, antioxidant properties, and amino acid profile of the chosen best blends were determined. Cookies were produced and the sensory properties of the cookies were evaluated in order to determine its sensory acceptability.

Materials and Methodology

Materials

Maize grains, soy beans, and tigernut tubers were obtained from Akure, Nigeria. All chemicals were of analytical grade.

Toasted maize (corn) flour production

Dried white-maize grains were properly sorted, toasted at 150–200°C until a uniform golden brown color was obtained. The toasted grains were allowed to cool and milled into fine powder. The powder was sieved using a 2-mm mesh sieve in order to obtain the toasted corn flour (A).

Soy flour production

Soy flour (B) was produced according to the method of IITA, 1990.

Tigernut flour production

Tigernut flour (C) was produced according to the method of Adejuyitan (2011).

Experimental design and statistical analyses

Optimal mixture design of response surface methodology (Design Expert 8.0.3.1., Stat-Ease Inc., Minneapolis, USA trial version) was used. The variables were toasted corn flour (75–85%), soy flour (10–20%), and tigernut flour (5–10%); which generated 16 experimental runs. The responses were proximate and minerals compositions. Three best samples obtained from the optimization result were used for further analyses; functional properties, pasting characteristics, antioxidant and antinutritional evaluations, amino acid profile, cookies production, and sensory evaluation.

Proximate analysis

The proximate composition of the flour blend samples was determined using AOAC 2005 methods. The samples were analyzed for moisture, ash, crude fiber, crude protein, and crude fat, whereas carbohydrate was calculated by difference.

Determination of crude protein

Protein content was determined using Kjeldahl method, according to the procedure of AOAC (2005). Concentrated H_2SO_4 (12 mL) and two tablets of selenium catalyst were put into a Kjeldahl digestion flask containing 1 g of the sample. The flask was placed in the digester in a fume cupboard, switched on and digested for 45 min to obtain a clear colorless solution. The digest was distilled with 4% boric acid, and 20% sodium hydroxide solution was automatically metered into it in the distillation equipment until distillation was completed. The distillate was then titrated with 0.1-mol/L HCl until a violet color was formed, indicating the end point. A blank was run under the same condition as with the sample. Total nitrogen content was then calculated using equation (1).

$$\text{Protein} = \frac{[\text{titre value of sample-blank}] \times 0.01 \times 14.007 \times 6.25}{1000 \times \text{weight of sample}} \times 100 \tag{1}$$

Determination of ash content

Two grams of samples were weighed into well incinerated crucibles and then ashed in a muffle furnace at 600 °C for 3 h. The ash content was calculated using equation (2).

$$\text{Ash content} = \frac{\text{weight of ash}}{\text{weight of sample}} \times 100 \tag{2}$$

Determination of moisture content

Moisture content was determined using AOAC (2005) method. About 5 g of each sample was weighed into petri dishes of a known weight. It was then dried in the oven at 105 ± 1°C for 4 h. The samples were cooled in a desiccator and weighed. The moisture content was calculated applying equation (3)

$$\text{Percentage moisture content} = \frac{\text{change in weight}}{\text{weight of food before drying}} \times 100 \tag{3}$$

Determination of crude fiber

Crude fiber was determined using the AOAC (2005) method. About 5 g of each sample was weighed into a 500-mL Erlenmeyer flask and 100 mL of trichloroacetic acid digestion reagent added. It was then brought to boiling and refluxed for exactly 40 min counting from the start of boiling. The flask was removed from the heater, cooled a little, and filtered through a 15.0-cm Whatman paper. The residue was washed with hot water stirred once with a spatula and transferred to a porcelain dish. The sample was dried overnight at 105 °C. After drying, it was transferred to a desiccator and weighed W_1 when cool. It was ashed in a muffle furnace at 500°C for 6 h, allowed to cool, and reweighed W_2. The percentage crude fiber was calculated as shown in equation (4)

$$\%\text{crude fibre} = \frac{W_1 - W_2}{W_0} \times 100 \quad (4)$$

W_2 = Weight of crucible + fiber + ash, W_1 = Weight of crucible + ash, W_0 = Dry weight of food sample.

Determination of fat content

Fat content was determined using AOAC (2005) method. About 2 g of each sample was weighed on a chemical balance and wrapped in a filter paper. It was then placed in an extraction thimble. Extractor was cleaned, dried in an oven, and cooled in the desiccators before weighing. Then, 25 mL of N-hexane was measured into the round bottom; the fat content was extracted with this solvent. After extraction, the solvent was evaporated by drying in the oven. The flask and its contents were then cooled in a desiccator and weighed fat content. The percentage fat content was calculated as shown in equation (5)

$$\text{Fat content}(\%) = \frac{\text{weight of fat extracted}}{\text{weight of food sample}} \times 100 \quad (5)$$

Analyses of mineral compositions

The method described by AOAC (2005) was used for minerals analysis. The ash was digested with 3 cm^3 of 3 mol/L HCl and made up to the mark in a 100 cm^3 standard flask with 0.36 mol/L HCl before the mineral elements were determined by atomic absorption spectrophotometer (Buck scientific 210 VGP, Bulk Scientific Inc., 06855 USA). The following elements were determined for each of the 16 samples; Calcium, Potassium, Manganese, Iron, Copper, and Zinc.

Determination of functional properties

The best three samples selected based on the proximate and mineral analyses of all the samples were subjected to functional properties analyses.

Bulk density (BD)

Bulk density was estimated as described by Maninder et al. (2007).

Swelling index

The method of Ukpabi and Ndimele (1990) was used.

Foaming capacity and foam stability

The method described by Narayana and Narasinga Rao (1982) was used.

Water and oil absorption capacities

Water absorption capacity of flours blends was measured according to the centrifugation method (AOAC 2005).

Least gelation concentration

The least gelation concentration (LGC) was evaluated by using the method of Coffman and Garcia (1977) with some modifications. Appropriate sample suspension of 0.1, 0.2, 0.3, 0.4, 0.5, 0.6, 0.7, and 0.8 g was weighed into 5-mL distilled water each to make 20% (w/v) suspension. The test tubes containing theses suspensions were heated at 90°C for 1 h in water bath. The contents were cooled under tap water and kept for 1 h at 10°C. The LGC was determined as that concentration when the sample from inverted tube did not slip equation (6)

$$\text{LGC}\% = \frac{\text{weight of sample}}{\text{5ml of water}} 1 \times 100 \quad (6)$$

Determination of pasting properties

The selected three flour blends were subjected to rapid visco-analysis. Xanthan gum (0.3 g) was added to each of the samples and properly mixed. The flour sample (3 g) was mixed with 25-mL distilled water in the canister of a rapid visco-analyzer (RVA, model 3D; Newport Scientific, Sydney, Australia) monitored with RVA control software and operated.

Antioxidant and antinutritional properties determination

Oxalate was determined by the method of Day and Underwood (1986), whereas phytate was determined by the method of Major et al. 1990. Total Phenol was determined by the method of AOAC (2005).

Amino acid profile

Samples were prepared for amino acid determination by acid hydrolysis. Hydrochloric acid (6 N) was used to hydrolyze the sample for 24 h at 110°C in a vial under vacuum and N_2 atmosphere. The sample solution was evaporated and dissolved in sodium citrate buffer (pH 2.2). The hydrolysates were analyzed by a post-column derivative method using a HPLC, which was combined with a Pickering PCX5200 derivatizer (Pickering Laboratories, Inc., USA) and ion exchange column (3.0 × 250 mm, 8 μm). The amino acids were spectrophotometrically identified by measuring at 570 nm.

Cookies production

Twenty grams of hydrogenated fat and 30 g of powdered sugar were creamed together at medium speed until light and fluffy appearance was formed. Then 100 g of the composite flour sample was added with 0.3 g of xanthan gum, 1.7 g of salt, and 1.7-g baking powder (ammonium bicarbonate) and mixed together until uniform smooth dough was obtained. The dough was allowed to rest for 20 min and then rolled out to 10 mm thickness on a board and cut into round shape about 75 cm diameter with a biscuit cutter. The cookies were placed in a greased baking tray and baked in a preheated oven at 180°C for 10 min.

Sensory evaluation

Sensory analysis was carried out on the cookies produced from each of the flour blends. Ten members trained panelists were involved. Quality attributes evaluated were color, texture, taste, flavor, appearance, crispiness, and overall acceptability using a 9-point Hedonic scale, where 9 is like extremely and 1 is dislike extremely.

Results and Discussion

Proximate composition

The result of proximate composition is shown in Table 1. The protein content of the composite blends ranged from 10.9/100 g to 16.4/100 g. The highest protein percentage is recorded for sample 2 (16.4/100 g). This can be attributed to the highest ratio of soy flour percentage (20/100 g) in the flour component. Studies have also shown similar increase in protein content in soy-composite flours (Singh et al. 2000; Mashayekh et al. 2008). It has been discovered that most leguminous plant seeds are rich in nutrients with good arrays of amino acids and minerals (Fagbemi et al. 2004). Soybean is an excellent source of protein and a complement to lysine-limited cereal protein. The analysis of variance (ANOVA) result for protein showed the model (quadratic), and model terms (linear mixture, AB, AC, BC, A^2BC, AB^2C, and ABC^2) are significant ($P \leq 0.05$). The R-squared and Adjusted R-squared values were 0.9503 and 0.8935, respectively, which showed that the model was good. The 3D plot showing the effect of the composite flour on protein content is shown in the Figure 1A. Soybean contributes to the protein content most. Toasted maize. probably because of its quantity, also contributes to protein content. Tigernut flour had the least contribution.

The Ash content ranged from 2.6/100 g to 4.7/100 g. Ash is an indication of mineral contents of foods and has been discovered to be abundant in soy-supplemented cereal meals (Alabi and Anuonye 2007). The ANOVA result of ash showed that the model (quadratic) and the model terms (linear mixture and AB) were significant ($P \leq 0.05$). The R-squared and adjusted R-squared values are 0.7531 and 0.6341, respectively.

The moisture content of the composite flour ranged from 3.3/100 g to 7.3/100 g. This is lower than the minimum limit of 10/100 g moisture content for flour (Ihekoronye and Ngoddy 1985), which indicated that the composite flour can be used to produce a shelf stable products (Akhtar et al. 2008; Elleuch et al. 2011). The moisture contents of flour should be less than 10% as

Table 1. Proximate composition (g/100 g) of the composite blends from toasted maize, soy, and tigernut flour.

Runs	A(%)	B(%)	C(%)	Protein	Ash	Moisture	CHO	Crude fiber	Fat
1	81.702	10.000	8.298	12.9	4.6	5.0	59.9	3.5	14.1
2	75.000	20.000	5.000	16.4	4.2	3.5	58.5	3.0	14.4
3	75.117	17.308	7.576	14.9	4.2	5.2	56.4	3.3	16.0
4	77.437	17.563	5.000	12.5	4.0	4.6	59.3	3.2	16.4
5	75.117	17.308	7.576	14.8	4.3	5.0	57.4	3.3	15.2
6	78.567	11.433	10.000	14.4	4.4	5.4	55.8	4.1	15.9
7	77.290	15.138	7.572	13.3	3.8	3.3	61.5	3.3	14.8
8	85.000	10.000	5.000	11.2	3.7	6.0	63.3	3.0	12.8
9	81.702	10.000	8.298	13.8	4.7	5.2	59.6	3.6	13.1
10	75.000	20.000	5.000	16.4	4.4	5.1	55.6	3.1	15.4
11	76.299	13.701	10.000	15.0	3.7	5.7	55.4	4.0	16.2
12	85.000	10.000	5.000	12.8	3.8	5.3	62.3	3.0	12.8
13	76.299	13.701	10.000	15.1	4.6	6.4	54.0	4.0	15.9
14	80.152	12.337	7.511	12.5	3.5	6.6	57.1	3.4	16.9
15	82.540	12.460	5.000	10.9	2.6	5.5	63.0	3.1	14.9
16	79.683	14.616	5.701	13.5	3.2	7.3	56.8	3.3	15.9

A, toasted maize flour; B, soy flour; C, tigernut flour; CHO, carbohydrate.

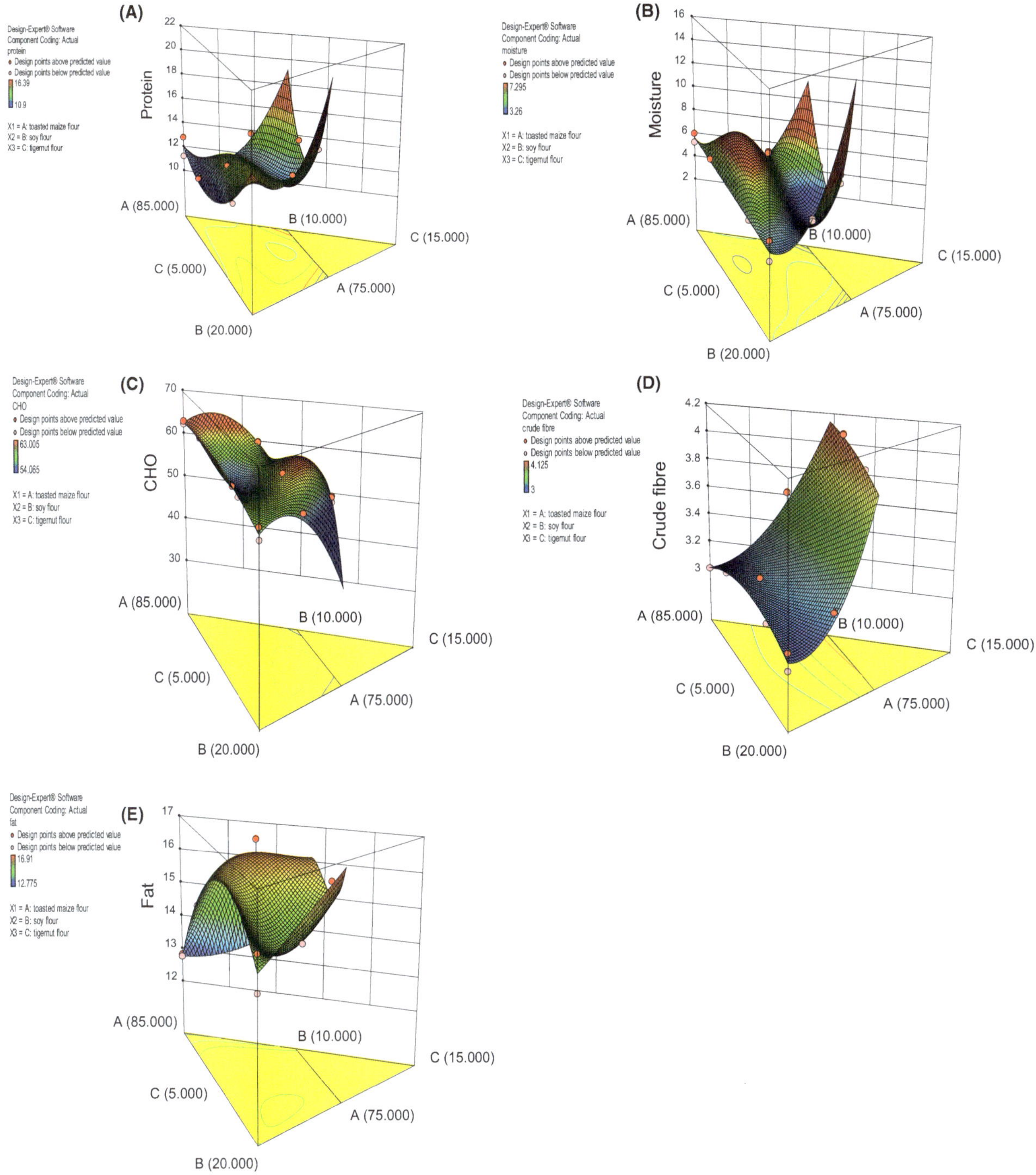

Figure 1. 3D plot showing the effect of variables on (A) protein content, (B) moisture content, (C) carbohydrate (CHO), (D) crude fiber, and (E) fat.

obtained in this work. The ANOVA result for moisture content showed that the model (quadratic) and model terms (AC, BC, A^2BC, and ABC^2) were significant ($P \leq 0.05$). The R-squared and adjusted R-squared values were 0.8301 and 0.6360, respectively. The 3D plot showing the effect of the variables on the moisture is shown in Figure 1B. The figure showed that toasted maize flour was responsible for the low value of the moisture content. This could be an additional advantage of using toasted maize in composite flour development.

The carbohydrate content of the composite flour blends ranged from 54.0/100 g to 63.3/100 g. The ANOVA result for the carbohydrate content showed that the model and model terms (linear mixture, AC, BC, A^2BC, and ABC^2) were significant ($P \leq 0.05$) indicating that all the samples are good sources of carbohydrate. The lack of fit is also not significant. The contribution of the variables to carbohydrate is high which might result in high energy content of the composite flour (Awolu et al. 2015a) as carbohydrate content and energy content of a food product are directly proportional. The R-squared and adjusted R-squared values are 0.9374 and 0.8658, respectively. The 3D plot as shown in the Figure 1C also buttressed the positive effects of the variables on the carbohydrate content.

Crude fiber content ranged from 3.1/100 g to 4.1/100 g; which increased as the quantity of tigernut flour in the composite sample increases. Total dietary fiber intake for adult men and women is 38 and 25 g/day, respectively (Neha and Ramesh 2012). Soluble fibers are effective in reducing total blood cholesterol, whereas insoluble fibers controls constipation and reduce the risk of colon cancer (Islam et al. 2007). Consumption of vegetable fiber has been shown to reduce serum cholesterol level, risk of coronary heart disease, colon and breast cancer, and hypertension; enhance glucose tolerance and increase insulin sensitivity (Hassan and Umar 2004a). The ANOVA result for crude fiber showed that the model (quadratic) and model terms (linear mixture, AB, AC, and BC) were significant ($P \leq 0.05$). The lack of fit F-value of 0.94 is not significant, whereas the R-squared and adjusted R-squared values were 0.9855 and 0.9783, respectively. The 3D plot showing the effect of the variables on the crude fiber as shown in Figure 1D showed that all the variables had positive effect on the fiber content.

The fat content of the composite blends ranged from 12.8/100 g to 16.9/100 g. High fat content could affect the shelf life of the composite flour due to oxidative activities (Awolu et al., 2015). The ANOVA result for the fat content showed that only the model (quadratic) and model terms (linear mixture and AB) were significant ($P \leq 0.05$). The R-squared and adjusted R-squared values are 0.9159 and 0.8198, respectively. The 3D plot showing the effect of the variables on the fat as shown in Figure 1E showed that soy flour and tigernut flour were the major contributors to fat contents.

Mineral composition

The result of the mineral compositions of the composite blends is shown in Table 2. Potassium and calcium were the most abundant elements in the samples. Potassium protects against arterial hypertension (Wardlaw 2004). Also, potassium is required to maintain osmotic balance of the body fluids, the pH of the body, to regulate muscle and nerve irritability, control glucose absorption, and enhance normal retention of protein during growth (Omoba et al. 2013). The values of calcium found in the composite flour are adequate for bone and teeth development (Oladele and Aina 2007). Inadequate intakes of Zinc and Iron have been associated with severe malnutrition, increased disease conditions, and mental impairment (Wardlaw 2004; Mannay and Shadaksharaswany 2005). The results from mineral analysis showed that the composite flour would contribute substantially to the recommended dietary requirements for minerals.

Considering the results of the protein content, crude fiber content, and mineral contents, the three best blends

Table 2. Mineral composition of composite blends of toasted maize, soy, and tigernut flour.

Runs	A(%)	B(%)	C(%)	Ca (ppm)	K (ppm)	Mn (ppm)	Fe (ppm)	Cu (ppm)	Zn (ppm)
1	81.702	10.000	8.298	40.80	50.00	0.17	1.52	0.11	1.09
2	75.000	20.000	5.000	30.20	38.90	0.25	1.91	0.14	0.98
3	75.117	17.308	7.576	30.80	40.60	0.26	1.73	0.14	1.12
4	77.437	17.563	5.000	43.50	54.60	0.21	1.83	0.19	0.83
5	75.117	17.308	7.576	30.50	40.50	0.30	1.76	0.14	1.11
6	78.567	11.433	10.000	55.70	60.30	0.16	1.61	0.16	0.85
7	77.290	15.138	7.572	30.10	64.70	0.30	2.44	0.18	1.41
8	85.000	10.000	5.000	49.60	59.30	0.20	2.06	0.26	0.77
9	81.702	10.000	8.298	40.70	50.30	0.17	1.53	0.11	1.09
10	75.000	20.000	5.000	30.10	39.00	0.24	1.90	0.14	0.95
11	76.299	13.701	10.000	48.40	51.10	0.28	2.60	0.11	1.20
12	85.000	10.000	5.000	49.60	59.30	0.21	2.05	0.27	0.80
13	76.299	13.701	10.000	47.90	50.90	0.26	2.59	0.10	1.21
14	80.152	12.337	7.511	51.40	40.70	0.18	1.75	0.24	0.88
15	82.540	12.460	5.000	49.60	41.30	0.26	2.02	0.22	1.18
16	79.683	14.616	5.701	47.30	39.80	0.22	2.01	0.16	1.05

A, toasted maize flour; B, soy flour; C, tigernut flour.

are run 2 (75.000/100 g of toasted maize flour, 20.000/100 g of soy flour, and 5.000/100 g of tigernut flour), run 7 (77.290/100 g of toasted maize flour, 15.138/100 g of soy flour, and 7.572/100 g of tigernut flour), and run 11 (76.299/100 g of toasted maize flour, 13.701/100 g of soy flour, and 10.000/100 g of tigernut flour).

Functional Properties

Functional properties determine the application and use of food materials for various food products. The results of functional properties of the best three blends of toasted maize, soy, and tigernut composite flour are presented in Table 3. The BD ranged from 0.77 to 0.82 g/mL. The BD is influenced by particle size and the density of the flour. It is important in determining the packaging requirement and material handling (Plaami 1997). It has been shown that high BD is desirable for greater ease of dispersibility and reduction of paste thickness (Amadinkwa 2012). It also determines the mixing quality of food materials (Lewis 1990). Low BD had been found to be an advantage in formulating complementary foods as it enhances nutrient and calorie density per feed of child (Akpata and Akubor 1999).

Sample 2 had the highest swelling power. Swelling index of flours depends on size of particles, type of variety, and types of processing methods or unit operation (Chandra and Samsher 2013). Also, sample 2 had the highest foam capacity. The high foam capacity of sample 2 could be as a result of its high protein content. Foaming ability has been related to the amount of solubilized protein (Narayana and Narasinga Rao 1982).

Sample 2 also had the highest water absorption capacity (4.00 g/sec). Water absorption characteristic represents the ability of a product to associate with water under conditions where water is limited. The result suggests that the composite flour samples would find application in cookies and biscuit (Oladele and Aina 2007). The LGC of the three samples was the same.

Pasting properties

The result of pasting properties of the three best blends is presented in the Table 4. Pasting property influences quality and esthetic considerations in the food industry as they affect texture and digestibility as well as the end use of starch-based food commodities (Adebowale et al. 2005). Sample 11 had the highest peak viscosity (222.08 RVU), whereas sample 2 had the least (199.00 RVU). The only reason that could account for the higher peak viscosity of sample 11 was the higher amount of tigernut flour in the sample blend. High peak viscosity is an indication of high starch content (Osungbaro 1990). Peak viscosity is an index of the ability of starch-based foods to swell freely before their physical breakdown (Sanni et al. 2006; Adebowale et al. 2008).

Sample 7 had highest peak time, closely followed by samples 11 and 2 in that order. Peak time is a measure of the cooking time. Pasting temperature ranged from 83.65 to 84.25°C. A high pasting temperature indicates high water-binding capacity, high gelatinization tendency, and low swelling property of starch-based flour due to high degree of association between starch granules (Adebowale et al. 2008). Sample 7 had highest pasting temperature followed by samples 11 and 2 in that order. Trough is the minimum viscosity value and it measures the ability of paste to withstand breakdown during cooling. The values ranged between 140.42 and 194.00 RVU with sample 2 having the highest and sample 11 lowest.

Table 3. Functional properties of toasted maize, soy, and tigernut flour composite blend.

Sample	BD (g/mL)	SI	FC(%)	FS(%)	WAC (gs^{-1})	(LGC)
2	0.77	0.80	31.37	19.61	4.00	0.40
7	0.81	0.70	17.65	9.80	3.70	0.40
11	0.82	0.70	21.57	5.88	3.70	0.40

BD, bulk density; SI, solubility index; FC, foaming capacity; FS, foaming stability; WAC, water absorption capacity; LGC, least gelation concentration.

Table 4. Pasting properties of toasted maize, soy, and tigernut flour composite blends values are mean of triplicate samples.

Sample	Peak viscosity (RVU)	Trough	Breakdown viscosity (RVU)	Final viscosity (RVU)	Set back viscosity (RVU)	Peak time (min)	Pasting temperature (°C)
2	199.00	194.00	5.00	235.58	41.58	6.54	83.65
7	221.42	157.00	64.42	237.08	80.08	6.74	84.25
11	222.08	140.42	81.67	233.00	92.58	6.66	82.58

Sample 11 had the highest set back and breakdown viscosities values while sample 2 had the lowest. Sample 2 is therefore more stable to heat and mechanical shear than samples 7 and 11(Oladele and Aina 2007). Retrogradation of the flour paste decreases with increasing setback viscosity; and the lower the staling rate of the product made from the flour (Adeyemi and Idowu 1990).

The final viscosity ranged from 233.00 to 237.08 RVU with sample 7 having the highest value, followed by sample 2 and sample 11, respectively. Final viscosity is commonly used to define the quality of particular starch-based flour, as it indicates the ability of the flour to form viscous paste after cooking and cooling. It also gives a measure of the resistance of paste to shear force during stirring (Adebowale et al. 2005, 2008).

Antioxidant and antinutritional properties

The result of oxalate, phytate, and total phenol constituent of the three choice blends is shown in Table 5. The total oxalate ranged from 3.53 mg ± 0.02/100 g to 3.79 mg ± 0.01/100 g. Sample 2 had the lowest value of total oxalate. The values were lower than a total oxalate of 366.6 mg/100 g and a soluble oxalate of 250 mg/100 g for a multimix diet reported by Okoro (1986). Raw and processed oxalate contents of grain amaranth were 91 mg/100 g and 57 mg/100 g, respectively. Large amounts of oxalate bind with calcium-forming calcium oxalate which is insoluble and not absorbed by the body. They are therefore considered poisonous at high concentration, but harmless when present in small amounts (Fox and Cameron 1986). High oxalate level in food has been implicated as the cause of kidney stones; it correlates with increase in calcium absorption in the kidney (Chai and Liebman 2004).

Phytates ranged from 5.78 mg ± 0.01/100 g to 6.07 mg ± 0.01/100 g. These antinutrients chelate divalent cations, such as calcium, magnesium, and iron, reducing their bioavailability (Sandberg 2002). Toxicity of oxalates and phytates for humans was set at 2–5 g/day and the consumption of diet rich in these antinutrients may result in kidney disease (Hassan and Umar 2004b; Hassan et al. 2007). The oxalate and phytate levels of the flour in this work are safe for human consumption.

Table 5. Result of oxalate, phytate, and total phenol constituent of the three best blends.

Sample	Oxalate (mg/100 g)	Total phenol (mg/100 g)	Phytate (mg/100 g)
2	3.53 ± 0.02	4.75 ± 0.02	5.95 ± 0.02
7	3.79 ± 0.01	4.63 ± 0.01	6.07 ± 0.01
11	3.54 ± 0.02	4.56 ± 0.02	5.78 ± 0.01

Total phenolic content in sample 2 (4.75 ± 0.02 mg/100 g) was the highest. This was followed by sample 7 (4.63 ± 0.01 mg/100 g) and then sample 11 (4.56 ± 0.02 mg/100 g). This result is similar to the values obtained for Marama-sorghum composite flours and porridges by Kayitesi et al. (2012). The high phenolic content could be attributed to the toasting of the maize grains before flour processing. Kayitesi et al. (2012) reported that dry heating Marama beans prior to its processing increased total phenolic content and antioxidant activity of the flours. Increase in total phenolic content and antioxidant activity following roasting peanuts was also reported by Talcott et al. (2005). Dewanto et al. (2002) reported that thermal processing may release bound phenolics from cellular constituents. In addition, heating induces production of Maillard reaction products, melanoidins, which have been reported to have antioxidant activity (Michalska et al. 2008). High phenolic content leads to high antioxidant activity. Free radicals and other reactive oxygen species contribute to the development of many diseases (Shahidi and Naczk 2004). Phenolic compounds scavenge free radicals by donating hydrogen atoms to free radicals; hence, may protect cell constituents against oxidative damage and limit the risk of various degenerative diseases associated with oxidative stress (Anderson and Wolf 1995).

Table 6. Amino acid profile of the three best blends.

Amino acid	Sample 2 (mg/100 g)	Sample 7 (mg/100 g)	Sample 11 (mg/100 g)
Valine	1889.22	1777.55	1669.25
Threonine	377.74	350.25	336.36
Isoleucine	557.35	525.28	562.25
Leucine	1126.25	1077.25	1114.25
Methionine	163.36	157.57	150.25
Phenylalanine	785.85	740.12	705.25
Lysine	1332.25	1263.36	1244.25
Histidine	444.25	420.25	433.36
Tryptophan	238.38	220.02	221.15
Essential AA	6914.65	6531.65	6436.37
Alanine	654.54	625.25	640.36
Aspartate	196.36	192.25	189.65
Glutamate	2244.25	2228.33	2202.25
Serine	1166.33	1144.22	1098.85
Glycine	667.67	650.42	625.58
Proline	666.33	642.25	635.35
Arginine	685.85	657.57	633.36
Tyrosine	374.22	340.45	355.58
Cysteine	119.63	112.25	109.65
Nonessential AA	6775.18	6592.99	5850.27
Total AA	3689.83	13124.64	12286.64

AA, Amino acid.

Table 7. Result of sensory evaluation of cookies produced from the three best blends.

Sample	Appearance	Color	Taste	Texture	Flavor	Crispiness	Overall acceptability
2	7.10^a	6.30^a	7.90^a	6.40^a	7.00^b	7.30^a	8.00^a
7	7.10^a	6.00^a	6.60^a	6.80^a	6.70^a	7.40^a	7.70^{ab}
11	6.50^a	5.60^a	6.50^a	7.50^a	6.00^{ab}	7.60^a	7.30^b

Amino acid profile

The amino acid profile of the three best blends is shown in Table 6. Essential and non-essential amino acid contents of the flour were determined. Sample 2 was the highest in all the amino acids. This could be as a result of soy protein influence on the composite. Sample 2 had the highest soy composition. Glutamic acid and valine were the most abundant amino acids in the three flour blends.

Lysine is a major limiting amino acid in maize. Lysine content in sample 2 (1332.24 ± 0.01 mg/100 g) was significantly higher than samples 7 and 11. The main role of lysine is to participate in protein synthesis, thus it is important for growth and maintenance of the body. All essential amino acids are considerably present in the three samples. Amino acids are important components for healing and protein synthesis; any deficiency in these essential amino acids will hinder recovery process (Zuraini et al. 2006). According to Witte et al. (2002), glycine together with other essential amino acids such as alanine, arginine, and phenylalanine forms a polypeptide that will promote growth and tissue healing.

Sensory evaluation of cookies

The sensory evaluation of cookies prepared from maize, soy, and tigernut flour presented in Table 7 showed that sample 2 was rated highest in terms of overall acceptability. The results also showed that increase in the level of tigernut flour in the composite improved crispiness and texture of the cookies. The incorporation of full fat soybean flour resulted in better taste and flavor. Sample 11 had the lowest values of 6.50 and 6.00 for taste and flavor, respectively; whereas sample 2 (20% soy flour) had the highest values of 7.90 and 7.00 for taste and flavor, respectively. There are no significant ($p \leq 0.05$) in appearance, color, taste, texture and crispiness. Significant differences ($p \leq 0.05$) however exist in flavour and overall acceptability.

Consumer quality is a major factor for selecting a product and among the main characteristics related to quality are texture, taste, and surface color of a biscuit (Omoba et al. 2013).

Conclusion

Composite flour from toasted maize, soybean, and tigernut could serve as a good substitute to a complete wheat flour in cookies production. The sensory evaluation was rated high which is an indication of high acceptability. In particular, composite flour with 75% toasted maize, 20% soybean, and 5% tigernut (sample 2) showed exceptional flour and nutritional quality. This blend had the overall best proximate composition, essential amino acid profile, antioxidant (total phenol), functional properties, and the least antinutritional content (precisely, oxalate content). However, blend with 76.3% toasted maize, 13.7% soybean, and 10% tigernut (sample 7) was next to sample 2 in terms of the properties mentioned. In addition, sample 7 had the best mineral composition and pasting properties. The samples could be used in the production of nutritionally rich cookies with strong antioxidant property which may be better alternatives to 100% wheat flour cookies.

Conflict of Interest

Authors declare that there is no conflict of interest.

References

Adebowale, A. A., L. O. Sanni, and S. O. Awonarin. 2005. Effect of texture modifies on the physicochemical and sensory properties of dried fufu. Food Sci. Technol. Int. 11:373–385.

Adebowale, A. A., S. A. Sanni, and F. O. Oladapo. 2008. Chemical, functional and sensory properties of instant yam-bread fruit flour. Niger. Food J. 26:2–12.

Adejuyitan, J. A. 2011. Tigernut processing: its food uses and health benefits. Am. J. Food Technol. 6:197–201.

Ade-Omowaye, B. I., B. A. Akinwande, I. F. Bolarinwa, and A. O. Adebiyi. 2008. Evaluation of tiger nut (Cyperusesculentus) - wheat composite flour and bread. Afr. J. Food Sci. 2:087–091.

Adeyemi, I. A., and M. A. Idowu. 1990. The evaluation of pregelatinized maize flour in the development of Maissa, a baked product. Niger. Food J. 26:2–12.

Akhtar, S., F. Anjum, S. Rehman, M. Sheikh, and K. Farzena. 2008. Effect of fortification on the physico-chemical and microbiological stability of whole wheat flour. Food Chem. 112:156–163.

Akpata, M. I., and P. I. Akubor. 1999. Chemical composition and selected functional properties of sweet orange (Citrus sinensis) seed flour. Plant Food Hum. Nutr. 54:353–362.

Alabi, M. O., and J. C. Anuonye. 2007. Nutritional sensory attributes of soy supplemented cereal meals. Niger. Food J. 25:100–110.

Amadinkwa, C. 2012. Proximate and functional properties of open air, solar and oven dried cocoyam flour. Int. J. Agric. Rural Dev. 15:988–994.

Anderson, L. R., and J. W. Wolf. 1995. Compositional changes in trypsin inhibitor, phytic acid, saponins and isoflavones related to soya bean processing. J. Nutr. 581S–588S.

AOAC. 2005. Official methods of analysis, association of official analytical chemists. 18th ed. Washington DC.

Awolu, O. O., and S. K. Layokun. 2013. Optimization of two-step transesterification production of biodiesel from neem (*Azadirachta indica*) oil. Int. J. Energy Environ. Eng. 4:1–9.

Awolu, O. O., R. O. Obafaye, and B. S. Ayodele. 2013. Optimization of solvent extraction of oil from 2 neem (*Azadirachta indica*) and its characterisations. J. Sci. Res. Rep. 2:304–314.

Awolu, O. O., P. M. Oluwaferanmi, O. I. Fafowora, and G. F. Oseyemi. 2015a. Optimization of the extrusion process for the production of ready-toeat snack from rice, cassava and kersting's groundnut composite flours. LWT Food Sci. Technol. 64:18–24.

Awolu, O. O., R. O. Osemeke, and B. O. T. Ifesan. 2015b. Antioxidant, functional and rheological properties of optimized composite flour, consisting wheat and amaranth seed, brewers' spent grain and apple pomace. J. Food Sci. Technol. 1–13.

Chai, W., and M. Liebman. 2004. Assessment of oxalate absorption from almonds and black beans with and without the use of extrinsic label. J. Urol. 172:953–957.

Chandra, S. and Samsher. 2013. Assessment of functional properties of different flours. Afr. J. Agric. Res. 8(38):4849–4852.

Coffman, C. W., and V. V. Garcia. 1977. Functional properties and amino acid content of protein isolate from mung bean flour. J. Food Technol. 12:473–484.

Day, R. A., Jr., and A. L. Underwood. 1986. 701. Quantitative analysis. 5th ed. Prentice-Hall Publication, London.

Dewanto, V., X. Wu, and T. H. Liu. 2002. Processed sweet corn has higher antioxidant activity. J. Agric. Food Chem. 50:4959–4964.

Elleuch, M., D. Bedigian, O. Roiseux, S. Besbes, C. Blecker, and H. Attia. 2011. Dietary fibre and fibre-rich by-products of food processing: characterisation, technological functionality and commercial applications. Rev. Food Chem. 124:411–421.

Fagbemi, T.N., A. A. Oshodi, and K. O. Ipinmoroti. 2004. Effect of processing and salt on some functional properties of some cashew nut (*Anarcadum occidentalis*) flour. J. Food Agric. Environ. 12:121–128.

Fox, B. A., and A. G. Cameron. 1986. Pp. 102. A chemical approach to food and nutrition. University of London Press Ltd, London.

Hassan, L. G., and K. J. Umar. 2004a. Proximate and mineral composition of seeds and pulp of Parkiabiglobosa. Niger. J. Basic Appl. Sci. 13:15–27.

Hassan, L. G., and K. J. Umar. 2004b. Anti-nutritive factors in African locust beans (*Parkiabiglobosa*). Proceedings of the 27th International Conference, Nigeria.

Hassan, L. G., K. J. Umar, and Z. Umar. 2007. Antinutritive factors in *Tribulus terrestris* (Linn) leaves and predicted calcium and zinc bioavailability. J. Trop. Biosci. 7:33–36.

Ihekoronye, A. I., and P.O. Ngoddy. 1985. Pp. 261–291. Integrated food science and technology for the tropics. 1st ed. McMillan publishers, London.

IITA. 1990. Soybeans for good health: how to grow and use soybeans in Nigeria. IITA publication, ISBN 97813101698. Pp. 23.

Islam, T., A. Chowdhury, M. Islam, and S. Islam. 2007. Standardization of bread preparation from soy flour. Int. J. Sustain. Crop Prod. 2:15–20.

Kayitesi, E., R. De Kock, A. Minnaar, and G. Duodu. 2012. Nutritional quality and antioxidant activity of marama-sorghum composite flours and porridges. Food Chem. 131:837–842.

Lewis, M. J. 1990. Physical properties of food and food processing systems. Hartnolls Limited, Bodman Cornwall, Great Britain.

Major, E. K., B. K. Simpson, J. S. Idowu, and O. L. Oke. 1990. Effects of local food processing on phytate levels in cassava, cocoyam and maize. J. Agric. Food Chem. 38:1580–1583.

Maninder, K., S. S. Kawaljit, and S. Narpinder. 2007. Comparative study of functional, thermal and pasting properties of flours from different field pea and pigeon pea cultivars. Food Chem. 104:259–267.

Mannay, S., and C. M. Shadaksharaswany. 2005. Foods: facts and principles. 2nd ed. New Age International Ltd. Publishers. New Delhi, India.

Mashayekh, M., M. R. Mahmoodi, and M. H. Enterazzi. 2008. Effect of fortification of defatted soy flour on sensory and rheological properties of wheat bread. Int. J. Food Sci. Technol. 43:1693–1698.

Michalska, A., M. Amigo-benaventb, H. Zielinski, and M. Dolores Del Castillo. 2008. Effect of bread making on formation of Maillard reaction products contributing to the overall antioxidant activity of rye bread. J. Cereal Sci. 48:123–132.

Narayana, K., and M. S. Narasinga Rao. 1982. Functional properties of raw and heat processed winged bean flour. J. Food Sci. 47:1534–1538.

Neha, Mishra, and Chandra Ramesh. 2012. Development of functional biscuit from soy flour and rice bran. Int. J. Agric. Food Sci. 2:14–20.

Nwokolo, E. 1996. Soybean [*Glycine max* (L.) Merr.]. Pp. 90–102 in S. E. Nwokolo, J. Smert, eds. Legume and oilseeds in nutrition. Chapman and Hull, UK.

Oboh, G., A. O. Ademiluyi, and A. A. Akindahunsi. 2010. The effect of roasting on the nutritional and antioxidant properties of white maize varieties. Int. J. Food Sci. Technol. 45:1236–1242.

Okoro, E. U. 1986. Chemical and biological evaluation of the nutritional value of a multimix weaning food formulated using local foodstuffs. M.Sc Thesis, University of Calabar, Nigeria.

Oladele, A. K., and J. O. Aina. 2007. Chemical composition and functional properties of flour produced from two varieties of tigernut (*Cyperus esculenta*). Afr. J. Biotechnol. 6:2473–2476.

Omoba, O. S., O. O. Awolu, A. I. Olagunju, and A. O. Akomolafe. 2013. Optimization of plantain-brewers spent grain biscuit using response surface methodology. J. Sci. Res. Rep. 2:665–681, Article no. JSRR.2013.015.

Omoba, O. S., O. O. Dada, and S. O. Salawu. 2015. Antioxidant properties and consumer acceptability of pearl millet – tigernut biscuit. Nutr. Food Sci. 45(6):818–828.

Omode, A., O. Fatoki, and K. A. Olaogun. 1995. Physicochemial properties of some underexploited and non-conventional oil seed. J. Agric. Food Chem. 11:50–53.

Osagie, A. U., and O. U. Eka. 1998. Pp. 246–249. Nutritional quality of plant foods. Post-harvest research unit, University of Benin, Nigeria.

Osungbaro, T. O. 1990. Effect of differences in variety and dry milling of maize on texture characteristics of ogi (fermented maize porridge) and Agidi (fermented maize meal). J. Sci. Food Agric. 52:1–11.

Plaami, S. P. 1997. Content of dietary fiber in foods and its physiological effects. Food Rev. Int. 13:27–76.

Sandberg, A. S. 2002. Bioavailability of minerals in legumes. Br. J. Nutr. 88:281–285.

Sanni, O. L., A. A. Adebowale, T. A. Filani, O. B. Oyewole, and A. Westby. 2006. Quality of flash and rotary dryer dried fufu flour. J. Food Agric. Environ. 4:74–78.

Shahidi, F., and M. Naczk. 2004. Phenolics in foods and nutraceuticals. CRC Press LLC, London.

Singh, R., G. Singh, and G. S. Chauhan. 2000. Nutritional evaluation of soy fortified biscuits. J. Food Sci. Technol. 37:162–164.

Talcott, S. T., S. Passeretti, C. E. Duncan, and D. W. Gorbet, . 2005. Polyphenolic content and sensory properties of normal and high oleic acid peanuts. Food Chem. 90:379–388.

Ukpabi, U. J., and C. Ndimele. 1990. Evaluation of garri production in Imo state, Nigeria. Niger. Food J. 8:105–110.

Umerie, S. C., and J. N. Enebeli. 1997. Malt caramel from the nut of *Cyperus esculentus*. J. Bioresour. Technol. 8:215–216.

Wardlaw, G. M. 2004. Perspectives in nutrition. 6th ed. McGram Hill Companies, New York, USA.

Witte, M. B., F. Thorton, U. Tantry, and A. Barbel. 2002. L-arginine supplementation enhances diabetic wound healing: involvement of the nitric oxide synthase and arginase pathways. Metabolism 51:1269–1273.

Zuraini, A., M. N. Somchit, M. H. Solihah, Y. M. Goh, A. K. Arifah, M. S. Zakaria, et al. 2006. Fatty acid and amino acid compositions of three local Malaysian Channa fish spicies. Food Chem. 4:674–678.

2

Effects of cranberry extracts on gene expression in THP-1 cells

Daniel B. Hannon[1], Jerry T. Thompson[1], Christina Khoo[2], Vijaya Juturu[3] & John P. Vanden Heuvel[1,4]

[1]Department of Veterinary and Biomedical Sciences and Center for Molecular Toxicology and Carcinogenesis, Penn State University, 325 Life Sciences Building, University Park, Pennsylvania 16802
[2]Ocean Spray Cranberries, Inc., One Ocean Spray Drive, Lakeville-Middleboro, Massachusetts 02349
[3]UnitedBio-Med Inc., 102 Hunters Run, Dobbs Ferry, New York 10502
[4]INDIGO Biosciences Inc., 1981 Pine Hall Road, State College, Pennsylvania 16801

Keywords
Gene expression, macrophage, nutrigenomics, proanthocyanidins, reactive oxygen species

Correspondence
Jack Vanden Heuvel, Penn State University, 325 Life Sciences Building, University Park, Pennsylvania 16802.
E-mail: jpv2@psu.edu

Funding Information
No funding information provided.

Abstract

Cranberry contains high levels of nutrients and bioactive molecules that have health-promoting properties. The purpose of the present studies was to determine if cranberry extracts (CEs) contain phytochemicals that exert anti-inflammatory effects. The human monocytic cell line THP-1 was treated with two CEs (CE and 90MX) and subsequently challenged with Lipopolysaccharides (LPS). Tumor necrosis factor α (TNFα) expression was decreased in the CE-treated cells, indicative of an anti-inflammatory effect. Gene expression microarrays identified several immune-related genes that were responsive to CEs including interferon-induced protein with tetratricopeptide repeats 1 and 3 (IFIT 1 and 3), macrophage scavenger receptor 1 (MSR1) and colony-stimulating factor 2 (CSF2). In addition, in the CE-treated cells, metallothionein 1F and other metal-responsive genes were induced. Taken together, this data indicates that CEs contain bioactive components that have anti-inflammatory effects and may protect cells from oxidative damage.

Introduction

Epidemiological, human intervention, and mechanistic trials have shown that polyphenol-rich foods, often found in a diet rich in fruits and vegetables, may have protective effects against chronic degenerative diseases linked to oxidative stress and reactive oxygen species (ROS)-mediated cell damage (Cassidy et al. 2011; Wedick et al. 2012; Del Rio et al. 2013). Flavonoids and other phenolic compounds in these foods are bioactive health components that are likely responsible for these effects. The North American cranberry (*Vaccinium macrocarpon* Ait. Ericaceae) is of growing public interest as a functional food because of potential health benefits linked to the high content of bioactive flavonoids in the fruit, including proanthocyanidins, flavonols such as quercetin and myricetin and anthocyanins. In fact, cranberry ranks high among fruit in both antioxidant quality and quantity (Vinson et al. 2001; Gu et al. 2004; Côté et al. 2010), and contain a higher amount of total phenols per serving (507–709 mg gallic acid equivalents/100 g) than other common fruits including blueberries (258–531 mg/100 g), apples (185–347 mg/100 g), and red grapes (175–370 mg/100 g) (Wu et al. 2004). Cranberries, in powder, extract or juice, have been reported to be beneficial for helping prevent urinary tract infections (Wang et al. 2012; Blumberg et al. 2013; Foxman et al. 2015), oxidative stress and cardiometabolic risk factors such as reducing C-reactive protein and lowering blood pressure (Basu et al. 2011; Dohadwala et al. 2011; Novotny et al. 2015). As cranberry is a natural food product and not a drug, the effect seen is often mild but that is consistent with the recommendation for a food with health components that is consumed as part of a healthy balanced lifestyle.

In vitro evidence has shown the antioxidant potential of cranberry phenolic compounds including protection of human microvascular endothelial cells against ROS, and HepG2 cells from inflammatory insults and reduced glycation (Caton et al. 2010; Crozier et al. 2010; Liu et al.

2011; Watson et al. 2014; Martín et al. 2015). A recent publication also showed the bioavailability and bioactivity of cranberry phenolics and metabolites from consuming cranberry juice beverage (McKay et al. 2015). The protective effect of these compounds may be related to their function in sequestering ROS and/or maintaining the cell components in their correct redox state, but emerging findings indicate that natural compounds may act by increasing the endogenous antioxidant defense potential through regulation of cell signaling pathways (Seeram et al. 2004; Stevenson and Hurst 2007; Martín et al. 2015). The objective of this study is to examine the anti-inflammatory activity of cranberry phenolic compounds in two different cranberry powders (90 MX and CE) by looking at changes in gene expression using human monocytic cells lines.

Material and Methods

Chemicals

Cranberry juice powder and extract were obtained from Ocean Spray Cranberries (Lakeville-Middleboro, MA; for chemical analysis see Table 1 and reference [Martín et al. 2015]). Cranberry juice powder (90MX) was prepared from the juice of mature berries of the commonly cultivated cranberry plant (*Vaccinium macrocarpon*). Cranberry juice processing consists of the milling and pressing of the berries after a hot (50°C for 1 h) commercial pectinase maceration. 90MX was then prepared by spray drying cranberry concentrate with magnesium hydroxide as the carrier and tri-calcium phosphate as an anti-caking agent. The powder is fine, free-flowing and rosy red in color, and contains approximately 90% cranberry solids. The cranberry extract (CE) powder is a water-soluble, phenolic-rich extract of cranberry utilizing a proprietary resin separation process. CE was standardized to 55% proanthocyanidin (PAC) content on a dry weight basis as analyzed by a modified 4-dimethylaminocinnamaldehyde (DMAC) method (Martín et al. 2015). Finally, 100 mg/mL stock solutions of 90MX and CE were prepared in Dimethylsulfoxide (DMSO) for cell treatment. All media components and fetal bovine serum (FBS) were purchased from Gibco BRL/Life Technologies (Carlsbad, CA). Phorbol 12-myristate 13-acetate (PMA), used to differentiate THP-1 cells, was purchased from Sigma Chemical Company (St. Louis, MO). All other chemicals and reagents were of highest quality available.

Cell culture and treatment

THP-1 (*Homo sapiens* monocyte) cells were obtained from the American Type Culture Collection (ATCC; Rockville, MD) and cultured in RPMI 1640 with 10% heat inactivated FBS, 50 μmol/L 2-mercaptoethanol, 1 mmol/L sodium pyruvate, 100 U/mL penicillin and 100 μg/mL streptomycin. These cells were seeded in 24-well plates at a density of 3×10^5/well and differentiated into macrophages with 100 nmol/L PMA (Sigma) for 48 h. For in vitro treatment experiments, THP-1 cells were grown to 75% confluency and treated with 90MX or CE (0, 25, 50, 100 μg dry weight/mL media, heretofore listed as μg/mL). Sixteen hrs after treatment, the cells will be stimulated with 10 ng/mL LPS for 6 h.

RNA extraction, reverse transcription, real-time PCR

Total RNA was isolated by Qiagen RNeasy Mini Kit (Qiagen, Valencia, CA) according to the manufacturer's instructions. The total RNA was reverse transcribed, using the ABI High Capacity cDNA archive kit (Applied Biosystems, Foster City, CA). Standard curves were made using serial dilutions from pooled cDNA samples. Real-time polymerase chain reaction (PCR) was performed with the use of the SYBR Green PCR Master Mix (Applied Biosystems) according to the manufacturer's protocol and amplified on the ABI Prism 7000 Sequence Detection System. Primers are listed in Table 2.

Microarray experiments and statistical analysis

THP-1 cells were treated with CE or 90MX at 100 μg/mL or control (DMSO, 0.1% v/v) for 16 h followed by stimulation with LPS for 6 h. RNA was extracted, using Qiagen RNeasy and quality assessed by RNA Nano Chips on the Agilent Bioanalyzer (Agilent Technologies, Santa Clara, CA). Each sample was labeled using the Affymetrix IVT Express Kit according to the manufacturer's protocol. The GeneChip Human Genome U133A 2.0 (Affymterix, Santa Clara, CA), representing 14,500 well-characterized genes, was hybridized with the labeled RNA using GeneChip Hybridization Wash and Stain Kit (#702232) in the Affymetrix GeneChip Hybridization Oven 640, according to the manufacturer's instructions. Following hybridization, the arrays were washed and stained using the Affymetrix GeneChip Fluidics Station 450 according to the manufacturer's protocol and scanned using the GeneChip Scanner 3000 7G. The scanned image file (DAT) and the intensity data (CEL) was imported into ArrayStar (DNASTAR, Inc., Madison, WI). The Robust Multi-array Average (RMA) was used to normalize the data. The nine slides were grouped based on treatment and Student t-test with asymptotic P-value and Benjamini–Hochberg multiple corrections was performed comparing CE versus DMSO and 90MX versus DMSO. At a P-value of 0.05 and a

Table 1. Content of phenolic compounds and other major components in cranberry juice and extract powders.

	Cranberry juice powder (90MX, mg/100 g)	Cranberry extract powder (CE, mg/100 g)	Enrichment (CE/90MX)[3]
Proanthocyanidins			
By OS-DMAC method[1]	2800	51,600	18.4
By BL-DMAC method[2]	653	15,000	23.0
Organic acids			
Citric acid	14,200	2850	0.2
Malic acid	8510	1660	0.2
Quinic acid	13,500	2040	0.2
Galacturonic acid	3300	78.4	0.0
Sugars			
Glucose	31,300	4700	0.2
Fructose	8120	1100	0.1
Anthocyanins			
Cyanidin-3-arabinoside	33.8	420	12.4
Cyanidin-3-galacoside	41.7	508	12.2
Cyanidin-3-glucose	1.3	25.4	19.5
Peonidin-3-arabinoside	17.3	239	13.8
Peonidin-3-galactose	41.9	530	12.6
Peonidin-3-glucoside	3.0	36.6	12.2
Phenolic acids			
Benzoic acid	84.5	2550	30.2
Salicylic acid	0.6	13.4	22.3
Protocatechuic acid	15.6	120	7.7
Gallic acid	4.2	25.8	6.1
Vanilic acid	4.9	85.4	17.4
t-Cinnamic acid	7.7	72.8	9.5
p-Coumaric acid (4-hydroxycinnamic acid)	30.2	436	14.4
Caffeic acid (3,4-dihydroxycinnamic acid)	3.0	50.5	16.8
Ferulic acid (3-methoxy-4-hydroxycinnamic acid	0.9	54.7	60.8
Chlorogenic acid	22.8	793	34.8
Ellagic acid	1.3	2.2	1.7
Flavon-3-ols			
Catechin	8.0	43.3	5.4
Epicatechin	31.7	2.2	0.1
Flavonols			
Quercetin	37.3	404	10.8
Quercitrin (quercetin-3-*O*-rhamnoside	20.8	527	25.3
Hyperoside (quercitin-3-*O*-galactoside)	53.1	2720	51.2
Myricetin	40.5	657	16.2
Myricetrin (myrocetin-3-*O*-rhamnoside)	7.6	125	16.4
Total phenolic by Folin-Ciocalteu method (GAE)	2600	45,000	17.3

From Martín et al. (2015).
[1]Expressed in milligram (mg) of cranberry-specific PACs equivalents per 100 g of powder.
[2]Expressed in milligram (mg) of procyanidine A-2 equivalents per 100 g of powder.
[3]Enrichment is the ratio of each component in the CE extract relative to that of 90MX.

twofold change, a total of 236 entities were significantly regulated by CE while there were no genes that met the criteria for 90MX. The group of genes was examined by hierarchical clustering using complete linkage analysis of the normalized data (JMP 7.0; SAS Institute, Cary, NC). Gene Ontology (GO) and pathway analysis was performed, using Ingenuity Pathway Analysis (Qiagen, Redwood City, CA).

Statistical analysis

One-way analysis of variance, followed by Dunnett's post hoc test, was used to test the difference between treatments ($P < 0.05$). The values were expressed as mean ± SEM. All data analyses were performed by JMP 7.0 (SAS Institute) and data plotted by Prism 5.01 (GraphPad Software, Inc., San Diego, CA).

Table 2. Primer sequences used for quantitative real-time PCR.

Gene	Forward primer	Reverse primer
18S	ACCCGTTGAACCCCATTCGTGA	GCCTCACTAAACCATCCAATCGG
ABCG2	ACGAACGGATTAACAGGGTCA	CTCCAGACACACCACGGAT
CAT	TGTTGCTGGAGAATCGGGTTC	TCCCAGTTACCATCTTCTGTGTA
CCNL2	GTACTCCGGGGTGCTCATC	GAGGTCGGTCTCTGTGTCG
COX2	CGGTGTTGAGCAGTTTTCTCC	AAGTGCGATTGTACCCGGAC
CSF2	TCCTGAACCTGAGTAGAGACAC	TGCTGCTTGTAGTGGCTGG
HERC5	GGTGAGCTTTTTGCCTGGG	TTCTCCGGCAGAAATCTGAGC
IFIT1	GCGCTGGGTATGCGATCTC	CAGCCTGCCTTAGGGGAAG
IFIT3	AGAAAAGGTGACCTAGACAAAGC	CCTTGTAGCAGCACCCAATCT
IL-1α	CTCCCAATCTCCATTCCCAA	CGTAAGGCCTCAGCCAGAAG
IL6	GCCACTCACCTCTTCAGAACG	CCGTCGAGGATGTACCGAATT
MSR1	GCAGTGGGATCACTTTCACAA	AGCTGTCATTGAGCGAGCATC
MT1F	TCCTGCAAGAAGAGCTGCTG	ACTTCTCTGACGCCCCTTTG
OAS1	TGTCCAAGGTGGTAAAGGGTG	CCGGCGATTTAACTGATCCTG
SLC7A11	TCTCCAAAGGAGGTTACCTGC	AGACTCCCCTCAGTAAAGTGAC
SOD1	GGTGTGGCCGATGTGTCTAT	CCTTTGCCCAAGTCATCTGC
TNFA	ATCAATCGGCCCGACTATCTC	TGGATGTTCGTCCTCCTCACA

Results

Regulation of inflammation-related genes in THP-1 cells

The ability of CEs to regulate proinflammatory gene expression in THP-1 cells was examined using an LPS-challenge model (Lee et al. 2009; Zhang et al. 2010). A single concentration of each extract (100 μg/mL) was examined; there was no sign of overt toxicity at this dose (data not shown). The 90MX powder had no effect on expression of interleukin-1α (IL-1α), interleukin-6 (IL6), tumor necrosis factor-α (TNFα), catalase (CAT), cyclooxygenase-2 (COX2) or superoxide dismutase 1 (SOD1) mRNA (Fig. 1). The CE extract at this dose resulted in a significant increase in IL-6 mRNA (2.5-fold) with decreased expression of TNFα, CAT and SOD1 mRNA (1.6, 1.5 and 1.8-fold, respectively) relative to the vehicle control. The pattern of gene expression, with several LPS-induced genes being repressed while others are either unaffected or augmented, suggests an atypical mechanism of action and prompted a more comprehensive examination of mRNA concentration.

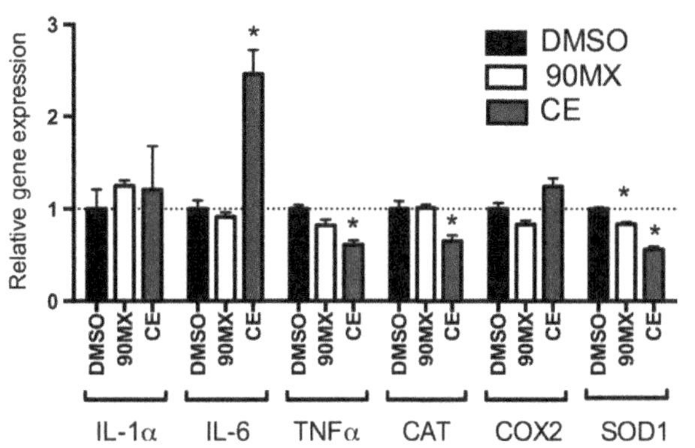

Figure 1. Regulation of inflammation-related genes by cranberry extracts in THP-1 cells. Cells were treated and RNA extracted as described in Materials and Methods. Gene expression following treatment with DMSO (0.1% v/v),CE or 90MX (100 μg/mL) is expressed relative to a housekeeping gene (18S) and normalized to vehicle control (DMSO). Asterisks denote significantly different than control ($P < 0.05$, $n = 3$, bars represent mean and SEM).

Comprehensive analysis of gene expression

The design of the present experiments was aimed to understand the anti-inflammatory effects of cranberry polyphenol extracts to identify sensitive biomarkers for subsequent studies and to begin understanding their potential mechanism of action. The THP-1 monocytes were treated with CE or 90MX at 100 μg/mL for 16 h, followed by stimulation with LPS and the RNA was used to examine gene expression by high-density microarray. A total of 236 genes were significantly regulated by CE with a two-fold change (Table S1 and Fig. 2) with 64 genes reaching a threefold threshold (Table 3). There were no significant changes using these same criteria with the 90MX extract. A majority of the genes (78%) were repressed by CE; Metallothionein 1F (MT1F) mRNA was increased fivefold while interferon-induced protein with tetratricopeptide repeats 5 (IFIT5) was reduced 10-fold relative to the DMSO-treated group.

Quantitative real-time PCR was used to confirm a subset of transcripts identified by the microarray experiments.

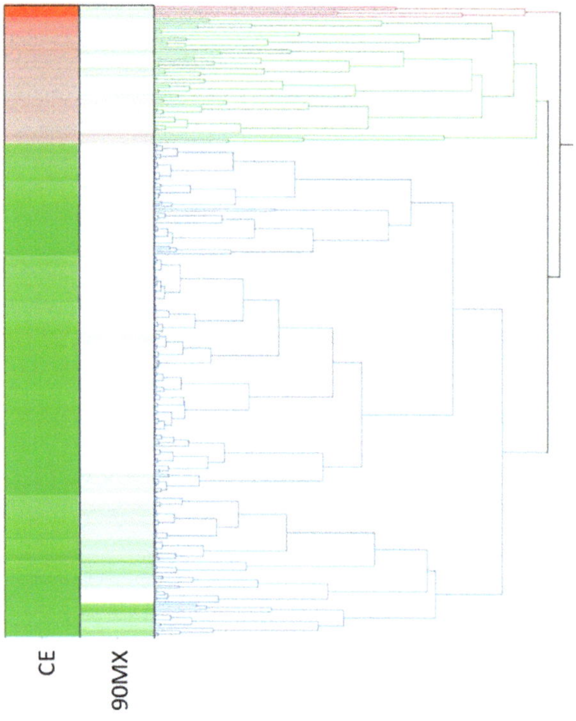

Figure 2. Comprehensive analysis of gene expression. Analysis of gene expression by high-density microarrays was performed by microarrays as described in Material and Methods. Average expression values (n = 3 arrays per group) were exported to JMP (SAS Institute, Cary NC) and hierarchical clustering performed. Data were expressed relative to the DMSO-treated group with green representing a decrease and red an increase relative to control (depicted as white).

Care was taken to choose genes that were both increased and decreased by CE treatment as well as those with known biological functions. THP-1 cells were treated as described above, with the exception that three doses of each extract was examined. As shown in Figure 3 (top panel), unlike the microarray experiment, the 90MX extract significantly regulated colony-stimulating factor 2 (CSF2) and cyclin L2 (CCNL2) mRNA accumulation. All genes studied, with the exception of solute carrier family 7A11 (SLC7A11), were significantly regulated by CE, albeit to a different extent and with varying potency (Fig. 3, bottom panel). However, in the ATP-binding cassette, the sub-family G, member 2 (ABCG2) mRNA was affected only at the highest dose, CSF2, 2′-5′-oligoadenylate synthetase 1 (OAS1), metallothionein 1F (MT1F), and CCNL2 mRNA were regulated at the 25 μg/mL dose.

GO and pathway analysis

The list of genes that were significantly regulated by the CE extract in THP-1 cells (twofold and $P < 0.05$, 236 genes) were classified according to their functional ontology terms (GO). Several GO biological processes were significantly enriched in these CE-regulated genes (http://pantherdb.org, see Table S2), including immune effector process, response to interferon, cell cycle checkpoint, cell cycle phase, and response to metal ion. The gene expression patterns were further examined to determine if they were consistent with certain diseases and functions (Ingenuity Pathway Analysis; Table 4 and Figures S1, S2). Genes regulated by CEs, such as ABCG2, CCNA2, CCNB1, and CDC25A were associated with cell cycle control and DNA repair processes. The majority of the genes in this network were decreased in expression relative to the DMSO-treated cells. Similarly, several CE-regulated genes were enriched in the inflammatory response network and most genes, with the exception of IL6, were repressed. Potential mechanisms by which CE regulates genes within these networks is shown in Table 5. Several transcription factors and signaling molecules are implicated, including HGF signaling, PPAR, LXR, or VDR activation and importantly inhibition of inflammatory signaling such as interferon, MAPK, or NFAT activity.

Discussion

Several berry fruits, including the American cranberry (*Vaccinium macrocarpon*), have recently received attention as a result of their effects in vitro and their associations with observational studies with lowered risk of some chronic diseases (Zafra-Stone et al. 2007; Blumberg et al. 2013). Cranberries, consumed in sauces, juices, dried fruit, or taken as a dietary supplement in powders or extract form, are a rich source of polyphenols that are associated with a variety of biological effects. In vitro studies have demonstrated antibacterial, antiviral, antimutagenic, anticarcinogenic, antitumorigenic, antiangiogenic, anti-inflammatory, and antioxidant properties (Yan et al. 2002; Bagchi et al. 2004; Ferguson et al. 2004; Seeram et al. 2004; Neto 2007; Zafra-Stone et al. 2007) (3,7,8). In vivo, animal models reveal that CEs: reduce proinflammatory interleukins (Kim et al. 2011); suppress Helicobacter pylori infection (Blumberg et al. 2013), and; improve pancreatic β-cell glucose responsiveness and β-cell mass (Zhu et al. 2011). The clinical effects of cranberry and their bioactives include: lowering LDL cholesterol and total cholesterol (Basu and Lyons 2012); improving markers of endothelial function (Bagchi et al. 2004; Dohadwala et al. 2011), lowering glycemic responses (Wilson et al. 2010), elevating plasma antioxidant capacity (McKay et al. 2015); modulation of gastric *Helicobacter pylori* infection (Shmuely et al. 2012); reducing biomarkers of metabolic syndrome (Wilson et al. 2010; Basu and Lyons 2012; Simão et al. 2013), and; protecting against urinary tract infections (UTIs) (Foxman et al. 2015).

Table 3. Genes significantly regulated by cranberry extracts (threefold, $P < 0.05$).

Probe set ID	Gene symbol	Gene title	90MX	CE
213629_x_at	MT1F	Metallothionein 1F	0.80	4.84
211906_s_at	SERPINB4	Serpin peptidase inhibitor, clade B (ovalbumin), member 4	0.70	4.47
210524_x_at	MT1F	Metallothionein 1F	0.81	4.10
212859_x_at	MT1E	Metallothionein 1E	0.75	3.87
220322_at	IL36G	Interleukin 36, gamma	0.72	3.56
203213_at	CDK1	Cyclin-dependent kinase 1	0.89	0.33
210764_s_at	CYR61	Cysteine-rich, angiogenic inducer, 61	0.87	0.33
203725_at	GADD45A	Growth arrest and DNA-damage-inducible, alpha	0.94	0.32
207386_at	CYP7B1	Cytochrome P450, family 7, subfamily B, polypeptide 1	1.05	0.32
211668_s_at	PLAU	Plasminogen activator, urokinase	1.04	0.32
218662_s_at	NCAPG	Non-SMC condensin I complex, subunit G	0.91	0.32
214453_s_at	IFI44	Interferon-induced protein 44	0.57	0.31
204747_at	IFIT3	Interferon-induced protein with tetratricopeptide repeats 3	0.63	0.31
203362_s_at	MAD2L1	MAD2 mitotic arrest deficient-like 1 (yeast)	0.94	0.31
219209_at	IFIH1	Interferon induced with helicase C domain 1	0.80	0.31
202127_at	PRPF4B	Pre-mRNA processing factor 4B	0.56	0.30
201291_s_at	TOP2A	Topoisomerase (DNA) II alpha 170 kDa	0.96	0.30
218883_s_at	CENPU	Centromere protein U	0.74	0.30
213226_at	CCNA2	Cyclin A2	0.80	0.29
202508_s_at	SNAP25	Synaptosomal-associated protein, 25 kDa	0.51	0.29
209969_s_at	STAT1	Signal transducer and activator of transcription 1, 91 kDa	0.80	0.29
210559_s_at	CDK1	Cyclin-dependent kinase 1	0.90	0.29
211597_s_at	HOPX	HOP homeobox	0.99	0.29
216442_x_at	FN1	Fibronectin 1	1.00	0.28
206513_at	AIM2	Absent in melanoma 2	0.85	0.28
203967_at	CDC6	Cell division cycle 6	0.77	0.28
204127_at	RFC3	Replication factor C (activator 1) 3, 38 kDa	0.81	0.28
204994_at	MX2	Myxovirus (influenza virus) resistance 2 (mouse)	0.63	0.28
210495_x_at	FN1	Fibronectin 1	0.98	0.28
212464_s_at	FN1	Fibronectin 1	0.95	0.27
203708_at	PDE4B	Phosphodiesterase 4B, cAMP-specific	0.78	0.27
211719_x_at	FN1	Fibronectin 1	0.98	0.27
202833_s_at	SERPINA1	Serpin peptidase inhibitor, clade A (alpha-1 antiproteinase, antitrypsin), member 1	1.03	0.27
205479_s_at	PLAU	Plasminogen activator, urokinase	1.02	0.27
201506_at	TGFBI	Transforming growth factor, beta-induced, 68 kDa	1.12	0.26
204823_at	NAV3	Neuron navigator 3	0.94	0.26
220104_at	ZC3HAV1	Zinc finger CCCH-type, antiviral 1	0.79	0.26
213293_s_at	TRIM22	Tripartite motif containing 22	0.41	0.26
222162_s_at	ADAMTS1	ADAM metallopeptidase with thrombospondin type 1 motif, 1	0.90	0.26
201340_s_at	ENC1	Ectodermal-neural cortex 1 (with BTB domain)	0.99	0.25
201341_at	ENC1	Ectodermal-neural cortex 1 (with BTB domain)	0.93	0.25
202628_s_at	SERPINE1	Serpin peptidase inhibitor, clade E (nexin, plasminogen activator inhibitor type 1), member 1	0.99	0.24
219148_at	PBK	PDZ-binding kinase	0.99	0.24
202086_at	MX1	Myxovirus (influenza virus) resistance 1, interferon-inducible protein p78 (mouse)	0.70	0.23
218039_at	NUSAP1	Nucleolar and spindle-associated protein 1	0.85	0.23
201890_at	RRM2	Ribonucleotide reductase M2	0.89	0.22
202589_at	TYMS	Thymidylate synthetase	0.85	0.21
219691_at	SAMD9	Sterile alpha motif domain containing 9	0.62	0.21
205552_s_at	OAS1	2′-5′-oligoadenylate synthetase 1, 40/46 kDa	0.54	0.20
202627_s_at	SERPINE1	Serpin peptidase inhibitor, clade E (nexin, plasminogen activator inhibitor type 1), member 1	1.01	0.20
214146_s_at	PPBP	Proplatelet basic protein (chemokine (C-X-C motif) ligand 7)	1.26	0.20
219684_at	RTP4	Receptor (chemosensory) transporter protein 4	0.72	0.20
219908_at	DKK2	Dickkopf WNT signaling pathway inhibitor 2	0.88	0.19
218585_s_at	DTL	Denticleless E3 ubiquitin protein ligase homolog (Drosophila)	0.95	0.19
203596_s_at	IFIT5	Interferon-induced protein with tetratricopeptide repeats 5	0.77	0.19

(*Continued*)

Table 3. Continued

Probe set ID	Gene symbol	Gene title	90MX	CE
213294_at	EIF2AK2	Eukaryotic translation initiation factor 2-alpha kinase 2	0.75	0.18
209773_s_at	RRM2	Ribonucleotide reductase M2	0.86	0.18
202869_at	OAS1	2′-5′-oligoadenylate synthetase 1, 40/46 kDa	0.54	0.16
205239_at	AREG	Amphiregulin	1.00	0.15
212977_at	ACKR3	Atypical chemokine receptor 3	1.06	0.15
203153_at	IFIT1	Interferon-induced protein with tetratricopeptide repeats 1	0.54	0.14
201289_at	CYR61	Cysteine-rich, angiogenic inducer, 61	0.83	0.13
218943_s_at	DDX58	DEAD (Asp-Glu-Ala-Asp) box polypeptide 58	0.69	0.11
203595_s_at	IFIT5	Interferon-induced protein with tetratricopeptide repeats 5	0.75	0.09

Cranberries are a particularly rich source of phenolic phytochemicals, including phenolic acids (benzoic, hydroxycinnamic, and ellagic acids) and flavonoids (anthocyanins, flavonols, and flavanols), and these bioactive molecules are believed to be associated with the health benefits described above. The major anthocyanins in cranberry are galactosides and arabinosides of cyanidin and peonidin (Neto 2007). Anthocyanin content varies widely among cranberry cultivars with averages between 25 and 65 mg per 100 g of ripe fruit at harvest. The primary flavonol in cranberries is quercetin, which exists in several glycosidic forms, and the total flavonol content of cranberry fruit typically in the range of 20–30 mg per 100 g of fresh fruit weight. In comparing the two CEs used in the present study (Martín et al. 2015), 90MX contained higher amount of organic acids while CE had higher quantities of highly bioactive compounds such as phenolic acids, flavonols, and flavanols (see Table 1). More specific, components with a high antioxidant capacity such as chlorogenic acid, epicatechin, and quercetin were found in

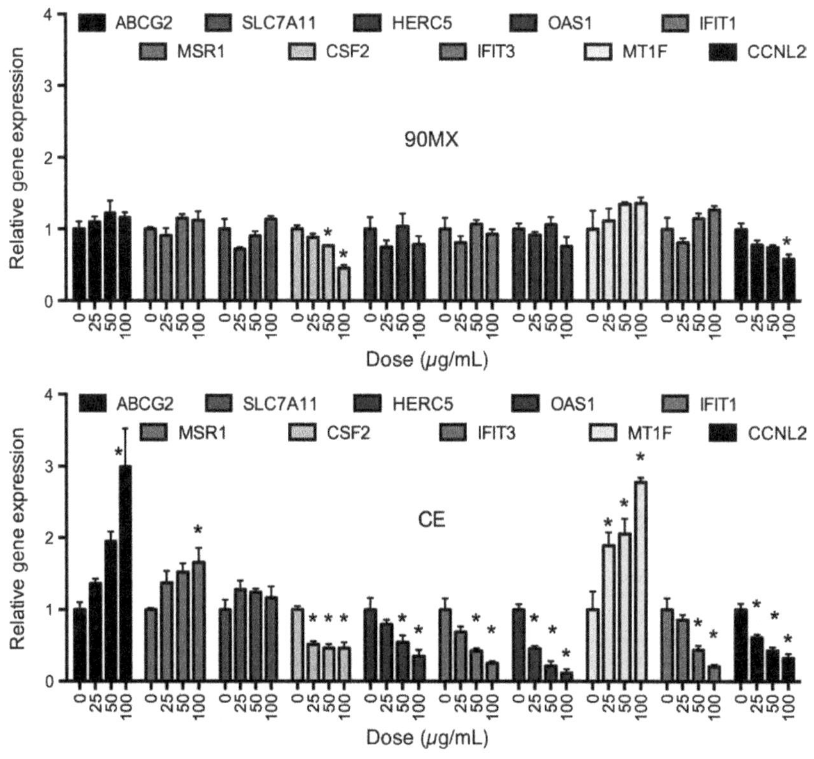

Figure 3. Expression of selected genes identified as responsive to cranberry extracts in THP-1 cells. Genes were selected from Table 2 to Figure 2 for validation by real-time PCR. Cells were treated and RNA extracted as described in Material and Methods. Gene expression following treatment with 90MX or CE (0, 25, 50, 100 μg/mL) is expressed relative to a housekeeping gene (18S) and normalized to vehicle control (DMSO). Asterisks denote significantly different than control ($P < 0.05$, $n = 3$, bars represent mean and SEM).

high concentrations in CE. The total PACs concentration was 18 times higher in CE than 90MX (51,000 vs. 2800 mg/100 g; [Martín et al. 2015]). In HepG2 cells, both CEs decreased ROSs and protected the cells from t-BOOH-induced cytotoxicity, albeit with CE being much more potent. Interestingly, stress-related signaling through the JNK pathway by t-BOOH was not averted by CE, indicating another mechanism such as redox regulation, might be primary in the protection from oxidative stress by CE in HepG2 cells.

The CEs significantly decreased expression of TNFα, CAT, and SOD1 mRNA (Fig. 1) relative to the vehicle control in LPS-stimulated THP-1 cells. In addition, the microarray studies showed mRNA for acute phase response genes (IL33, FOS, IL36G, IL1A, FN1, SERPINA1, SERPINE1) and interferon-signaling genes (IFIT3, IFIT1, OAS1, MX1, STAT1; Table 4) were decreased in these cells. These responses are consistent with several other studies showing an anti-oxidant and anti-inflammatory effect of cranberries and their bioactive molecules, in particular the PACs. In rats fed an atherogenic diet, C-reactive protein (CRP) and IL-1β were significantly lower in the cranberry powder groups compared to those in control rats (Kim et al. 2011). A CE (OptiBerry) significantly inhibited basal MCP-1 and inducible NF-κB transcription as well as the inflammatory biomarker IL-8 in a similar in vivo model (Zafra-Stone et al. 2007). Treatment of Caco-2 cells with these CEs prevented iron/ascorbate-mediated lipid peroxidation and counteracted LPS-mediated inflammation as evidenced by the decrease in proinflammatory cytokines (TNF-α and IL-6), cyclooxygenase-2 (COX-2) and prostaglandin E2 (PGE2, [Denis et al. 2015]). Networks of genes involved in the antimicrobial and inflammatory responses and infectious disease (Table 3) were identified as being coordinately affected by CE, adding support for the associations seen in observational studies. The moderate increase in IL-6 mRNA observed in the present studies, in the absence of increases in other proinflammatory markers such as COX-2 and IL-1α, may be the result of several factors. First, this suggests that CE is not causing generalized oxidative stress since other mRNAs would be coordinately affected. Second, this increase in IL6 mRNA may not be indicative of altered activity due to the small increase observed (2.5-fold), the fact that protein level of this factor was not examined and IL6-responsive genes (such as IL1) were not altered. Finally, it is obvious that CE, due to the complex mixture of bioactive molecules, has multiple mechanisms of action.

The mechanism of this anti-inflammatory effect has not been extensively studied, although PACs from cranberries and other sources have been proposed to act through oxygen free radical scavenging (Li et al. 2001) as well as metal chelation (Arola-Arnal and Bladé 2011), a contributor to ROS production. PACs affect the activity of signaling molecules associated with the inflammatory response, including the redox-sensitive transcription factor NF-κB (Liu et al. 2014), 5′-AMP activated protein kinase (AMPK)(Cui et al. 2012), p38 mitogen-activated protein

Table 4. Gene ontology analysis: top diseases and functions.

ID	Top diseases and functions	Molecules in network
1	Cell cycle, cellular assembly and organization, DNA replication, recombination, and repair	ABCG2, alcohol group acceptor phosphotransferase, ALT, ASAH1, AURKA, BUB1, BUB1B, CCNA2, CCNB1, CD163, Cdc2, CDC25A, CDK1, Cyclin B, ENO2, GADD45A, GINS1, HISTONE, Histone H1, Histone h3, HOPX, IL6, MCM4, MT1G, NASP, NCAPG, PRC1, PRPF4B, PTPase, RNA polymerase II, SFPQ, SMC4, SNX10, Sod, TTK
2	Cell cycle, embryonic development, organismal survival	AIM2, APC (complex), ATM/ATR, ATR, CDC6, CDC20, Cdk, Cyclin A, Cyclin D, Cyclin E, DTL, Dynein, E2f, FANCI, GMNN, HERC5, LUC7L3, MAD2L1, MCM10, MELK, NBN, NFkB (complex), NUSAP1, PCNA, PPP4R4, Rb, Rfc, RFC3, RFC4, RPA, RRM2, SKP2, TRIM22, TYMS, UNG
3	Antimicrobial response, inflammatory response, cell signaling	2′ 5′ oas, DDX58, DDX60, EIF2AK2, ERK, IFI16, IFI44, IFIH1, IFIT1, IFIT3, IFIT5, Ifn, IFN alpha/beta, IFN Beta, IFN type 1, Ifnar, IRF, ISG15, ISG20, ISGF3, JAK, MT1M, MX1, Oas, OAS1, OAS2, PARP12, RSAD2, STAT4, Stat1-Stat2, THEMIS2, USP18, XAF1, ZC3HAV1
4	Nervous system development and function, cancer, organismal injury and abnormalities	ACKR3, ACPP, ADAMTS1, ADCY, ADRB, Alpha catenin, AREG, BNIP3, CAP2, Cg, Creb, DUSP2, EMR2, FGF13, FSH, Gpcr, GPR56, GPR65, Hdac, HRH1, Lh, Mapk, Metalloprotease, MT1F, MT1X, NMDA Receptor, OXTR, Pdgfr, PLC, PVR, SLC7A11, SNAP25, STEAP1, TCF, Vegf
5	Infectious disease, cell morphology, hair and skin development, and function	AIF1, Akt, c-Src, Calcineurin A, Collagen(s), CYR61, Fascin, FCGR2B, FERMT1, Fgf, Fibrin, Fibrinogen, GDF15, Integrin, Integrin alpha 3 beta 1, Integrin alpha 4 beta 1, ITGA1, JINK1/2, KIAA0101, Laminin, Lfa-1, LRIG1, MAP2K1/2, MT1E, Notch, PBK, PMAIP1, PNISR, PNN, PPIG, SLC4A7, TLR2/TLR4, TRIB3, TRIM5, ZWINT

Table 5. Gene ontology analysis: top pathways.

Canonical pathways	*z*-score	Moleculesw
Cell cycle: G2/M DNA damage checkpoint regulation	1.134	GADD45A, TOP2A, ATR, AURKA, CDK1, SKP2, CCNB1
HGF signaling	1	MET, FOS, IL6, ELK3, PRKCB
PPAR signaling	1	IL33, FOS, IL36G, IL1A
LXR/RXR activation	0.447	IL33, IL36G, IL1A, SERPINA1, IL6
Activation of IRF by cytosolic pattern recognition receptors	−0.447	IFIH1, IL10, DDX58, IL6, STAT1, ISG15
PDGF signaling	−0.447	FOS, CAV1, EIF2AK2, STAT1, PRKCB
IL-6 signaling	−0.447	IL33, FOS, IL36G, IL1A, IL6
NF-κB signaling	−0.447	IL33, IL36G, IL1A, EIF2AK2, PRKCB
ERK/MAPK signaling	−0.447	FOS, STAT1, ELK3, DUSP2, PRKCB
Cholecystokinin/gastrin-mediated signaling	−0.816	IL33, FOS, IL36G, IL1A, MEF2C, PRKCB
Toll-like receptor signaling	−1	IL33, FOS, IL36G, IL1A, EIF2AK2
Growth hormone signaling	−1	FOS, IGFBP3, STAT1, PRKCB
JAK/stat signaling	−1	STAT4, FOS, IL6, STAT1
TREM1 signaling	−1	IL10, IL6, FCGR2B, CSF2
Tec kinase signaling	−1	STAT4, FOS, STAT1, PRKCB
Production of nitric oxide and reactive oxygen species in macrophages	−1	FOS, SERPINA1, STAT1, PRKCB
Colorectal cancer metastasis signaling	−1	FOS, IL6, STAT1, MMP19
Role of CHK proteins in cell cycle checkpoint control	−1.342	PCNA, RFC4, ATR, CDK1, CDC25A, RFC3, NBN
HMGB1 signaling	−1.342	FOS, IL1A, IL6, SERPINE1, CSF2, PLAT
p38 MAPK signaling	−1.342	IL33, IL36G, IL1A, MEF2C, STAT1
Aryl hydrocarbon receptor signaling	−1.342	CCNA2, FOS, IL1A, ATR, IL6
Acute phase response signaling	−1.414	IL33, FOS, IL36G, IL1A, FN1, SERPINA1, IL6, SERPINE1
VDR/RXR activation	−2	GADD45A, IGFBP3, CYP27B1, CSF2, PRKCB
UVA-induced MAPK signaling	−2	FOS, ZC3HAV1, PARP12, STAT1
Role of NFAT in regulation of the immune response	−2	FOS, MEF2C, FCGR2B, RCAN2
Interferon signaling	−2.236	IFIT3, IFIT1, OAS1, MX1, STAT1

kinase (MAPK, [Dinh et al. 2014]) and JNK (Guha et al. 2013; Liu et al. 2014). Data presented herein support the premise that CE decreases activity of NF-κB, p38 MAPK and NFAT in LPS-challenged macrophages. Quercetin, a polyphenol found in high concentration in CE (400 mg/100 g; [Martín et al. 2015]), induces metallothionein (MT) expression by activating the phosphorylation of JNK, p38 and PI3K/Akt as well as by enhancing Nrf2 DNA-binding activity in HepG2 cells (Weng et al. 2011). In CE-treated THP-1 cells, MT1E and 1F mRNA were among the most robustly induced transcripts, indicating that similar signaling pathways are affected in this cell line and that CEs may protect against metal-induced oxidative stress and toxicity.

Several in vitro studies suggest that cranberry bioactives are potential therapeutic agents for the treatment of cancer (Neto 2007; Zafra-Stone et al. 2007). For example, CEs and PACs decrease proliferation of the human breast (Ferguson et al. 2004; Sun and Liu 2006), glioblastoma multiforme (U87), colon (HT-29), prostate (DU145), and oral cancer cell lines (Seeram et al. 2004; Ferguson et al. 2006). Cell cycle arrest and apoptosis was induced by a cranberry PAC-rich extract in human esophageal adenocarcinoma (EAC) cells (Kresty et al. 2008) and prostate cells (MacLean et al. 2011). Although cell cycle and proliferation was not studied herein, several genes involved in checkpoint control such as PCNA, RFC4, ATR, CDK1, CDC25A, RFC3, and NBN (Tables 3, 5) were induced at the mRNA level by CE in THP-1 cells. Interestingly, cranberry ethanolic extract (CEE) prevents the DNA damage produced by benzo[a]pyrene (B[a]P) in an in vivo mouse peripheral blood micronucleus assay (Madrigal-Santillán et al. 2012). Our current study showed that several CE inducible genes are involved in G2/M DNA Damage checkpoint regulation, including GADD45A and CCNB1 (Tables 4, 5).

Taken together, these studies support the role of cranberry and its complex and rich phytochemical composition as an adjuvant for the treatment or prevention of chronic diseases with an inflammatory component. CEs decreased expression of several markers of inflammation and ROS signaling in the human monocyte cell line THP-1 that had been challenged with LPS. In addition, through the use of comprehensive gene expression analysis, the potential for cranberry or extracts for the prevention of metal-induced toxicity as well as cancer is supported. A limitation of the studies presented is that they are exclusively in vitro, using surrogate model systems for inflammation and oxidative stress. Although predictive of the potential of CE to affect human health, there must be consideration of availability of the bioactive constituents and the concentration achieved in vivo. In support of an in vivo response and hence bioavailability of active constituents, rats and mice-fed CEs exhibited reduced CRP, proinflammatory interleukins, and increase NO synthesis (Wang et al. 2012; Blumberg et al. 2013; Foxman et al. 2015). The range of doses of the cranberry phenolic powders was selected according to previous studies showing that concentrations in the μg/mL range with 30–40 μmol/L of cranberry phytochemicals have been found in plasma after cranberry juice intake (Martín et al. 2015). Although the identity of the specific cranberry-derived bioactive molecule or the molecular pathway involved has not been definitively identified, this study supports a wide range of in vitro, animal as well as nutritional invention studies showing this berry have unique and powerful health benefits.

Acknowledgments

This work was conducted under a contract between Ocean Spray and Indigo Biosciences Inc.

Conflict of Interest

JVH is an employee of Penn State University and has a financial stake with Indigo Biosciences Inc., which may constitute a conflict of interest.

References

Arola-Arnal, A., and C. Bladé. 2011. Proanthocyanidins modulate microRNA expression in human HepG2 cells. PLoS ONE 6:e25982.

Bagchi, D., C. K. Sen, M. Bagchi, and M. Atalay. 2004. Anti-angiogenic, antioxidant, and anti-carcinogenic properties of a novel anthocyanin-rich berry extract formula. Biochemistry (Mosc) 69: 75–80, 1 p preceding 75.

Basu, A., and T. J. Lyons. 2012. Strawberries, blueberries, and cranberries in the metabolic syndrome: clinical perspectives. J. Agric. Food Chem. 60:5687–5692.

Basu, A., N. M. Betts, J. Ortiz, B. Simmons, M. Wu, and T. J. Lyons. 2011. Low-energy cranberry juice decreases lipid oxidation and increases plasma antioxidant capacity in women with metabolic syndrome. Nutr. Res. 31:190–196.

Blumberg, J. B., T. A. Camesano, A. Cassidy, P. Kris-Etherton, A. Howell, C. Manach, et al. 2013. Cranberries and their bioactive constituents in human health. Adv. Nutr. 4:618–632.

Cassidy, A., É. J. O'Reilly, C. Kay, L. Sampson, M. Franz, J. P. Forman, et al. 2011. Habitual intake of flavonoid subclasses and incident hypertension in adults. Am. J. Clin. Nutr. 93:338–347.

Caton, P.W., M. R. Pothecary, D. M. Lees, N. Q. Khan, E. G. Wood, T. Shoji, et al. 2010. Regulation of vascular endothelial function by procyanidin-rich foods and beverages. J. Agric. Food Chem. 58:4008–4013.

Côté, J., S. Caillet, G. Doyon, J. F. Sylvain, and M. Lacroix. 2010. Bioactive compounds in cranberries and their biological properties. Crit. Rev. Food Sci. Nutr. 50:666–679.

Crozier, A., D. Del Rio, and M. N. Clifford. 2010. Bioavailability of dietary flavonoids and phenolic compounds. Mol. Aspects Med. 31:446–467.

Cui, X., X. Liu, H. Feng, et al. 2012. Grape seed proanthocyanidin extracts enhance endothelial nitric oxide synthase expression through 5′-AMP activated protein kinase/Surtuin 1-Krüpple like factor 2 pathway and modulate blood pressure in ouabain induced hypertensive rats. Biol. Pharm. Bull. 35:2192–2197.

Del Rio, D., A. Rodriguez-Mateos, J. P. E. Spencer, M. Tognolini, G. Borges, and A. Crozier. 2013. Dietary (poly)phenolics in human health: structures, bioavailability, and evidence of protective effects against chronic diseases. Antioxid. Redox Signal. 18:1818–1892.

Denis, M.-C., Y. Desjardins, A. Furtos, V. Marcil, S. Dudonné, A. Montoudis, et al. 2015. Prevention of oxidative stress, inflammation and mitochondrial dysfunction in the intestine by different cranberry phenolic fractions. Clin. Sci. (Lond.) 128:197–212.

Dinh, J., J. T. Angeloni, D. B. Pederson, X. Wang, M. Cao, and Y. Dong. 2014. Cranberry extract standardized for proanthocyanidins promotes the immune response of Caenorhabditis elegans to Vibrio cholerae through the p38 MAPK pathway and HSF-1. PLoS ONE 9:e103290.

Dohadwala, M. M., M. Holbrook, N. M. Hamburg, S. M. Shenouda, W. B. Chung, M. Titas, et al. 2011. Effects of cranberry juice consumption on vascular function in patients with coronary artery disease. Am. J. Clin. Nutr. 93:934–940.

Ferguson, P. J., E. Kurowska, D. J. Freeman, A. F. Chambers, and D. J. Koropatnick. 2004. A flavonoid fraction from cranberry extract inhibits proliferation of human tumor cell lines. J. Nutr. 134:1529–1535.

Ferguson, P. J., E. M. Kurowska, D. J. Freeman, A. F. Chambers, and J. Koropatnick. 2006. In vivo inhibition of growth of human tumor lines by flavonoid fractions from cranberry extract. Nutr. Cancer 56:86–94.

Foxman, B., A. E. W. Cronenwett, C. Spino, M. B. Berger, and D. M. Morgan. 2015. Cranberry juice capsules and urinary tract infection after surgery: results of a randomized trial. Am. J. Obstet. Gynecol. 213:194. e1–8.

Gu, L., M. A. Kelm, J. F. Hammerstone, G. Beecher, J. Holden, D. Haytowitz, et al. 2004. Concentrations of proanthocyanidins in common foods and estimations of normal consumption. J. Nutr. 134:613–617.

Guha, S., M. Cao, R. M. Kane, A. M. Savino, S. Zou, and Y. Dong. 2013. The longevity effect of cranberry extract in Caenorhabditis elegans is modulated by daf-16 and osr-1. Age (Dordr) 35:1559–1574.

Kim, M. J., J. Ohn, J. H. Kim, and H.-K. Kwak. 2011. Effects of freeze-dried cranberry powder on serum lipids and inflammatory markers in lipopolysaccharide treated rats fed an atherogenic diet. Nutr. Res. Pract. 5:404–411.

Kresty, L. A., A. B. Howell, and M. Baird. 2008. Cranberry proanthocyanidins induce apoptosis and inhibit acid-induced proliferation of human esophageal adenocarcinoma cells. J. Agric. Food Chem. 56:676–680.

Lee, Y., J. T. Thompson, and J. P. Vanden Heuvel. 2009. 9E,11E-conjugated linoleic acid increases expression of the endogenous antiinflammatory factor, interleukin-1 receptor antagonist, in RAW 264.7 cells. J. Nutr. 139: 1861–1866.

Li, W. G., X. Y. Zhang, Y. J. Wu, and X. Tian. 2001. Anti-inflammatory effect and mechanism of proanthocyanidins from grape seeds. Acta. Pharmacol. Sin. 22:1117–1120.

Liu, H., H. Liu, W. Wang, C. Khoo, J. Taylor, and L. Gu, 2011. Cranberry phytochemicals inhibit glycation of human hemoglobin and serum albumin by scavenging reactive carbonyls. Food Funct. 2:475–482.

Liu, C.-M., J.-Q. Ma, S.-S. Liu, G.-H. Zheng, Z.-J. Feng, and J.-M. Sun. 2014. Proanthocyanidins improves lead-induced cognitive impairments by blocking endoplasmic reticulum stress and nuclear factor-κB-mediated inflammatory pathways in rats. Food Chem. Toxicol. 72:295–302.

MacLean, M. A., B. E. Scott, B. A. Deziel, M. C. Nunnelley, A. M. Liberty, K. T. Gottschall-Pass, et al. 2011. North American cranberry (*Vaccinium macrocarpon*) stimulates apoptotic pathways in DU145 human prostate cancer cells in vitro. Nutr. Cancer 63:109–120.

Madrigal-Santillán, E., S. Fragoso-Antonio, C. Valadez-Vega, G. Solano-Solano, C. Z. Pérez, M. Sánchez-Gutiérrez, et al. 2012. Investigation on the protective effects of cranberry against the DNA damage induced by benzo[a] pyrene. Molecules 17:4435–4451.

Martín, M. A., S. Ramos, R. Mateos, J. P. Marais, L. Bravo-Clemente, C. Khoo, and L. Goya. 2015. Chemical characterization and chemo-protective activity of cranberry phenolic powders in a model cell culture. Response of the antioxidant defenses and regulation of signaling pathways. Food Res. Int. 71:68–82.

McKay, D. L., C.-Y. O. Chen, C. A. Zampariello, and J. B. Blumberg. 2015. Flavonoids and phenolic acids from cranberry juice are bioavailable and bioactive in healthy older adults. Food Chem. 168:233–240.

Neto, C. C. 2007. Cranberry and blueberry: evidence for protective effects against cancer and vascular diseases. Mol. Nutr. Food Res. 51:652–664.

Novotny, J. A., D. J. Baer, C. Khoo, S. K. Gebauer, and C. S. Charron. 2015. Cranberry juice consumption lowers markers of cardiometabolic risk, including blood pressure and circulating C-reactive protein, triglyceride, and glucose concentrations in adults. J. Nutr. 145:1185–1193.

Seeram, N. P., L. S. Adams, M. L. Hardy, and D. Heber. 2004. Total cranberry extract versus its phytochemical constituents: antiproliferative and synergistic effects against human tumor cell lines. J. Agric. Food Chem. 52:2512–2517.

Shmuely, H., I. Ofek, E. I. Weiss, Z. Rones, and Y. Houri-Haddad. 2012. Cranberry components for the therapy of infectious disease. Curr. Opin. Biotechnol. 23:148–152.

Simão, T. N. C., M. A. B. Lozovoy, A. N. C. Simão, S. R. Oliveira, D. Venturini, H. K. Morimoto, et al. 2013. Reduced-energy cranberry juice increases folic acid and adiponectin and reduces homocysteine and oxidative stress in patients with the metabolic syndrome. Br. J. Nutr. 110:1885–1894.

Stevenson, D. E., and R. D. Hurst. 2007. Polyphenolic phytochemicals–just antioxidants or much more? Cell. Mol. Life Sci. 64:2900–2916.

Sun, J., and Hai Liu. 2006. R. Cranberry phytochemical extracts induce cell cycle arrest and apoptosis in human MCF-7 breast cancer cells. Cancer Lett. 241:124–134.

Vinson, J. A., X. Su, L. Zubik, and P. Bose. 2001. Phenol antioxidant quantity and quality in foods: fruits. J. Agric. Food Chem. 49:5315–5321.

Wang, C.-H., C.-C. Fang, N.-C. Chen, S. S.-H. Liu, P.-H. Yu, T.-Y. Wu, et al. 2012. Cranberry-containing products for prevention of urinary tract infections in susceptible populations: a systematic review and meta-analysis of randomized controlled trials. Arch. Intern. Med. 172:988–996.

Watson, R. R., V. R. Preedy, and S. Zibadi. 2014. Polyphenols in human health and disease

Wedick, N. M., A. Pan, A. Cassidy, E. B. Rimm, L. Sampson, B. Rosner, et al. 2012. Dietary flavonoid intakes and risk of type 2 diabetes in US men and women. Am. J. Clin. Nutr. 95:925–933.

Weng, C.-J., M.-J. Chen, C.-T. Yeh, and G.-C. Yen. 2011. Hepatoprotection of quercetin against oxidative stress by induction of metallothionein expression through activating MAPK and PI3K pathways and enhancing Nrf2 DNA-binding activity. N. Biotechnol. 28:767–777.

Wilson, T., J. L. Luebke, E. F. Morcomb, E. J. Carrell, M. C. Leveranz, L. Kobs, et al. 2010. Glycemic responses to sweetened dried and raw cranberries in humans with type 2 diabetes. J. Food Sci. 75:H218–H223.

Wu, X., G. R. Beecher, J. M. Holden, D. B. Haytowitz, S. E. Gebhardt, and R. L. Prior. 2004. Lipophilic and hydrophilic antioxidant capacities of common foods in the United States. J. Agric. Food Chem. 52:4026–4037.

Yan, X., B. T. Murphy, G. B. Hammond, J. A. Vinson, and C. C. Neto. 2002. Antioxidant activities and antitumor screening of extracts from cranberry fruit (*Vaccinium macrocarpon*). J. Agric. Food Chem. 50:5844–5849.

Zafra-Stone, S., T. Yasmin, M. Bagchi, A. Chatterjee, J. A. Vinson, and D. Bagchi. 2007. Berry anthocyanins as novel antioxidants in human health and disease prevention. Mol. Nutr. Food Res. 51:675–683.

Zhang, J., P. M. Kris-Etherton, J. T. Thompson, and J. P. Vanden Heuvel. 2010. Effect of pistachio oil on gene expression of IFN-induced protein with tetratricopeptide repeats 2: a biomarker of inflammatory response. Mol. Nutr. Food Res. 54 (Suppl. 1): S83–S92.

Zhu, M., J. Hu, E. Perez, D. Phillips, W. Kim, R. Ghaedian, et al. 2011. Effects of long-term cranberry supplementation on endocrine pancreas in aging rats. J. Gerontol. A Biol. Sci. Med. Sci. 66:1139–1151.

3

Blanching influences the phenolics composition, antioxidant activity, and inhibitory effect of *Adansonia digitata* leaves extract on α- amylase, α- glucosidase, and aldose reductase

Emmanuel A. Irondi[1], Jacob K. Akintunde[1], Samson O. Agboola[2], Aline A. Boligon[3] & Margareth L. Athayde[3]

[1]Biochemistry Unit, Department of Biosciences and Biotechnology, Kwara State University, Malete, P.M.B. 1530, Ilorin, Nigeria
[2]Department of Veterinary Physiology, Biochemistry and Pharmacology, University of Ibadan, Ibadan, Nigeria
[3]Phytochemical Research Laboratory, Department of Industrial Pharmacy, Federal University of Santa Maria, Building 26, room 1115, Santa Maria, CEP 97105-900, Brazil

Keywords
Adansonia digitata leaves, blanching, carbohydrate-hydrolyzing enzymes, diabetic complications, phenolics, type 2 diabetes

Correspondence
Emmanuel A. Irondi, Biochemistry Unit, Department of Biosciences and Biotechnology, Kwara State University, Malete, P.M.B. 1530, Ilorin, Nigeria.
E-mail: irondi.emmanuel@yahoo.com

Funding Information
No funding Information provided.

Abstract

Adansonia digitata (*A. digitata*) leaves serve as food and has several medicinal uses in many parts of the world. This study evaluated the influence of blanching on the phenolics composition, antioxidant activity, and inhibitory effect of methanol extract of *A. digitata* leaves on the activities of some key enzymes (α-amylase, α-glucosidase, and aldose reductase) implicated in type 2 diabetes (T2D) in vitro. Reverse-phase HPLC analysis revealed that the leaves had appreciable levels of flavonoids and phenolic acids, including catechin, epicatechin, rutin, quercitrin, quercetin, kaempferol, and luteolin (flavonoids); gallic, chlorogenic, caffeic, and ellagic acids (phenolic acids). Blanching caused significant ($P < 0.05$) decrease in the flavonoids and phenolic acids contents; DPPH* (2,2 diphenyl-1-picrylhydrazyl radical) and ABTS^{*+} [2,2-azinobis (3-ethyl-benzothia zoline-6-sulfonic acid) radical cation] scavenging ability; reducing power; and Fe^{2+}-induced lipid peroxidation inhibitory capacity of the extract. Similarly, the inhibitory effect of the extract on the activities of α-amylase, α-glucosidase, and aldose reductase was significantly ($P < 0.05$) reduced due to blanching. Thus, *A. digitata* leaves extract could be effective for the management of T2D due to its flavonoids and phenolic acids content, antioxidant properties, and inhibitory potency on the activities of α-amylase, α-glucosidase, and aldose reductase. However, blanching militated against the levels of these functional attributes of the leaves and, therefore, may not be recommended for their optimal retention.

Introduction

Type 2 diabetes (T2D) is a heterogeneous disorder characterized by hyperglycemia resulting from insulin resistance and the inability of pancreatic β-cells to compensate for insulin resistance (DeFronzo 2004). The global prevalence of the disease is increasing alarmingly partly due to modern lifestyle and an increase in the consumption in high carbohydrate diets (Tappy and Le 2010), with its attendant postprandial hyperglycemia. Postprandial blood glucose level depends partly on the activities of carbohydrate-hydrolyzing enzymes, mainly, α-amylase and α-glucosidase, that breakdown dietary starch and sugars into glucose (Sim et al. 2010); thereby making more glucose available for absorption. Uncontrolled diabetic hyperglycemia precipitates other factors that accelerate the progression of diabetic complications (Oishi et al. 2006), including the major microvascular complications – nephropathy, neuropathy, and retinopathy. Hence, the inhibition of carbohydrate-hydrolyzing enzymes, with the resultant retardation of the digestion and absorption of dietary carbohydrate, is an important strategy for the prevention and management of T2D (Kwon et al. 2006; Oboh et al. 2010; Irondi et al. 2014). The inhibition of aldose reductase activity is also regarded as an important pharmacological strategy to prevent certain complications of diabetes (Saraswat et al. 2008).

Incidentally, acarbose and miglitol, the two leading oral hypoglycemic drugs that inhibit these enzymes have been reported to have some side effects such as diarrhea and other intestinal disturbances (Fujisawa et al. 2005), in addition to not being effective in maintaining euglycemia in diabetic patients. These limitations have necessitated more intensive research on plant products that could effectively reduce diabetic hyperglycemia and its associated complications possibly with less or no side effects (Ibrahim and Islam 2014). Interestingly, it has been suggested that about 90% of T2D cases could be possibly prevented by lifestyle modifications (Willett, 2002), including increased consumption polyphenolics-rich plant foods.

Adansonia digitata L. (African baobab) is a deciduous tree indigenous to Africa where it is popularly referred to as the "tree of life" due to its ability to sustain life as a result of its water-holding capacity, and its numerous ethnomedicinal and nutritional uses (Wickens and Lowe 2008). Various parts of the plant (including the leaves, pulp, fruits, seeds and bark) are sources of food, fiber and medicine for many people in Africa (Sibibe and Williams 2002; Chadare et al. 2009; De Caluwé et al. 2009). The various ethnomedicinal and food uses of *A. digitata* have attracted the interest of several pharmaceutical companies and researchers. Recently, the European Commission authorized the import of the fruit pulp as a novel food (Buchmann et al. 2010) and the Food and Drug Administration approved it as a food ingredient in the United States of America in 2009 (Addy 2009). In particular, the leaves of this plant which are eaten fresh or dried are the major source of food and folk medicine for many people in Africa (Ayele et al. 2013). For instance, the powdered leaves serve as a tonic and possess antihistamine and antitension properties. The leaves also possess antioxidant (Vertuani et al. 2002), anti-inflammatory, and antiviral activities (Vimalanathan and Hudson 2009). They also have several other medicinal uses such as treatment of diseases of the urinary tract, guinea worm, internal pains, dysentery, and ophthalmia (Sibibe and Williams 2002). Methanol and aqueous extracts of the leaves of the plant have been reported to contain glycosides, phytosterols, saponins, protein and amino acid, phenolic compounds and tannins, gums, mucilage, and flavanoids (Shri et al. 2004).

Blanching, as a vegetable processing method, involves the heating of the vegetables to a temperature sufficiently high to destroy the enzymes present in the tissue. It is a popular method of processing vegetables, including *A. digitata* leaves, that is intended to terminate the action of enzyme, shorten the drying and dehydration time, and set the color of the vegetables (Wen et al. 2010). However, how it impacts the phenolics composition, antioxidant activity, and inhibitory effect of *A. digitata* leaves extract on some enzymes associated with T2D has not been reported. This study was therefore designed to evaluate the influence of blanching on the phenolics composition, antioxidant activity, and inhibitory effect of *A. digitata* leaves extract on α-amylase, α-glucosidase, and aldose reductase in vitro.

Materials and Methods

Collection and preparation of samples

About 200 g of fresh leaves sample was randomly collected from *A. digitata* tree in a local farm settlement in Akingbile area of Moniya, Ibadan, Nigeria (Figure S1). The sample was authenticated at the Department of Botany, University of Ibadan, Nigeria. After sorting, the sample was divided into two portions; a portion was blanched, whereas the second portion was not. Blanching was carried out by immersing 50 g of whole Baobab leaves in 5 L of hot water (80°C) in a thermostatically regulated water bath (±0.5°C) for 10 min, using a wire mesh basket. After blanching, the basket was taken out and the water retained in the leaves was drained off using a plastic kitchen sieve.

Then the leaves were allowed to cool and dry under air-conditioner for 7 days. The raw leaves were also dried under the same condition. After drying, the samples were milled into fine particle size (0.5 mm), packed in air-tight plastic vials, and stored at −4°C until analysis.

Preparation of extract

Two gram of the sample was extracted by steeping in 100 mL of methanol overnight, after which it was filtered through Whatman No. 1 filter paper. The filtrate, subsequently referred to as extract, was stored at −4°C for further analysis.

Handling of experimental animal

Adult male Wister strain albino rats weighing 200–250 g were procured from the experimental animal breeding unit of Department of Veterinary Medicine, University of Ibadan, Nigeria. The rats were handled in accordance with our institution guide for the care and use of laboratory animals. The rats were kept in a cage to acclimatize for 7 days, during which they were maintained on a 12 h light/12 h dark cycle at 25°C, with free access to food and water.

Quantification of phenolic compounds by HPLC-DAD

Sample extracts at a concentration of 15 mg/mL were injected by means of Auto-sampler (Shimadzu, model

SIL-20A, Kyoto, Japan). Separations were carried out using Phenomenex C_{18} column (4.6 mm x 250 mm × 5 μm particle size). The mobile phase comprised solvent A [water: formic acid (98:2, v/v)] and solvent B (acetonitrile), at a flow rate of 0.6 mL/min and injection volume of 40 μL. Gradient program was started with 95% of A and 5% of B until 2 min and changed to obtain 25%, 40%, 50%, 70%, and 80% B at 10, 20, 30, 50, and 70 min, respectively, following the method described by Boligon et al. (2015), with slight modifications. The sample and mobile phase were filtered through 0.45 μm membrane filter (Millipore, USA) and then degassed by ultrasonic bath prior to use. Stock solutions of standards references were prepared in the HPLC mobile phase at a concentration range 0.025–0.300 mg/mL. Quantifications were carried out by integration of the peaks using the external standard method, at 254 nm for gallic acid and ellagic acid; 280 nm for catechin and epicatechin; 325 nm for caffeic acid and chlorogenic acid; and 366 for quercetin, quercitrin, kaempferol, luteolin, and rutin. The chromatography peaks were confirmed by comparing its retention time with those of reference standards and by DAD spectra (200–600 nm). Calibration curve for gallic acid: $Y = 13581x + 1195.7$ ($r = 0.9997$); catechin: $Y = 12609x + 1187.4$ ($r = 0.9996$); epicatechin: $Y = 12719x + 1356.9$ ($r = 0.9995$); caffeic acid: $Y = 12750x + 1352.9$ ($r = 0.9999$); chlorogenic acid: $Y = 11825x + 1383.6$ ($r = 0.9998$); ellagic acid: $Y = 13192x + 1176.5$ ($r = 0.9997$); quercitrin: $Y = 12641x + 1295.7$ ($r = 0.9999$); kaempferol: $Y = 11846x + 1283.9$ ($r = 0.9994$); rutin: $Y = 11792x + 1305.8$ ($r = 0.9995$); luteolin: $Y = 13894x + 1267.1$ ($r = 0.9998$); and quercetin: $Y = 12618x + 1196.3$ ($r = 0.9996$). All chromatography operations were carried out at ambient temperature and in triplicate.

LOD and LOQ of phenolic compounds

Limit of detection (LOD) and limit of quantification (LOQ) were calculated based on the standard deviation of the responses and the slope using three independent analytical curves, as defined by Khaliq et al. (2015). LOD and LOQ were calculated as 3.3 and 10 σ/S, respectively, where σ is the standard deviation of the response and S is the slope of the calibration curve.

Determination of ABTS*+ scavenging ability

The ABTS*+[2,2-azinobis (3-ethyl-benzothiazoline-6-sul fonic acid) radical cation] scavenging ability of the extracts was determined according to the method described by Sellappan and Akoh (2002). The ABTS*+ was generated by incubating equal volume of 7 mmol/L ABTS*+ aqueous solution with potassium persulfate (2.45 mmol/L) in the dark for 16 h at room temperature and adjusting the absorbance at 734 nm to 0.7 ± 0.02 with 95% ethanol. Then 0.2 mL appropriate dilution of the extract was added to 2.0 mL ABTS*+ solution and the absorbance were measured at 734 nm after 15 min. The ABTS*+ scavenging ability of the extracts was subsequently calculated and expressed in trolox equivalent (TE).

Determination of reducing power

The reducing power of the extracts was determined by assessing their ability to reduce $FeCl_3$ solution as described by Oyaizu (1986). An aliquot of 2.5 mL extract was mixed with 2.5 mL of 200 mmol/L sodium phosphate buffer (pH 6.6) and 2.5 mL of 1% potassium ferricyanide. The reaction mixture was incubated at 50°C for 20 min and then 2.5 mL of 10% trichloroacetic acid was added. This mixture was centrifuged at 650*g* for 10 min. Then 5 mL supernatant was mixed with an equal volume of water and 1 mL of 0.1% ferric chloride. The absorbance was measured at 700 nm. The reducing power of the extracts was subsequently calculated and expressed in gallic acid equivalent (GAE).

Determination of DPPH free radical scavenging ability

The DPPH* scavenging ability of the extracts was determined as described by Cervato et al. (2000). Briefly, different concentrations (0.10, 0.20, 0.30, and 0.40 mg/mL) of the extracts amounting to 1 mL were mixed with 3 mL of 60 μmol/L DPPH*; the mixture was left in the dark for 30 min before the absorbance was taken at 517 nm. A reference test (DPPH* solution without the extract) was included in the assay. The percentage DPPH* scavenging ability of the extract was calculated using the formula: % scavenging ability = $[(A517_{reference} - A517_{sample})/A517_{reference}] \times 100$; where $A517_{reference}$ is the absorbance of the reference test; and $A517_{sample}$ is the absorbance of the test containing the extract.

Inhibition of lipid peroxidation assay

The ability of the extracts to inhibit Fe^{2+}-induced lipid peroxidation in rat pancreas homogenate was assayed according to the modified method of Ohkawa et al. (1979). The rats were mildly anesthetized in ether, and their pancreas was rapidly excised and placed in ice. Then 10% (w/v) homogenate was prepared by homogenizing the pancreas in cold saline, and centrifuging for 10 min at 1400*g* to yield a low-speed supernatant (LSS) that was used for the assay. To a reaction mixture containing 100 μL of the LSS, 30 μL of 0.1 mol/L Tris-HCl buffer (pH 7.4) and different concentrations (0.10, 0.20, 0.30, and 0.40 mg/mL) of leaves extract, and 30 μL of freshly prepared 25 μmol/L ferric sulfate solution were added to initiate lipid peroxidation. The volume was made up to 300 μL with deionized water before incubation at 37°C for 1 h. The color reaction was initiated by adding 300 μL of 81 g/L sodium duodecyl sulfate to the reaction mixture containing the LSS, followed by the addition of 600 μL of acetic acid/HCl (pH 3.4) and 600 μL of 0.8% (v/v) TBA (Thiobarbituric acid). This mixture was incubated at 100°C for 1 h. The absorbance of thiobarbituric acid reactive species (TBARS) produced was measured at 532 nm in a UV-visible spectrophotometer. A reference test not containing the plant extract was carried out so as to obtain the absorbance of the maximum TBARS formed. The percentage inhibition of Fe^{2+}-induced lipid peroxidation by the extract was calculated using the formula: % Inhibition = $[(A532_{reference} - A532_{sample})/A532_{reference}] \times 100$; where $A532_{reference}$ is the absorbance of the reference test; and $A532_{sample}$ is the absorbance of the test containing the extract.

Alpha-amylase inhibition assay

Alpha-amylase inhibition assay was carried out following the procedure described by Kwon et al. (2008). Appropriate dilutions (0–200 μL) of the extracts amounting to 500 μL, and 500 μL of 0.02 mol/L sodium phosphate buffer (pH 6.9 with 0.006 mol/L sodium chloride) containing 0.5 mg/mL α-amylase solution (porcine pancreas α-amylase; Sigma, Cat. No. A3176, Chemical Co., St. Louis, MO, USA), were incubated at 37°C for 10 min. After preincubation, 500 μL of 1% starch solution in 0.02 mol/L sodium phosphate buffer was added. The reaction mixture was then incubated at 37°C for 15 min, and the reaction was terminated with 1.0 mL of DNSA color reagent (1% 3, 5-dinitrosalicylic acid and 12% sodium potassium tartrate in 0.4 mol/L NaOH). The reaction mixture was then incubated in a boiling water bath for 5 min, cooled to room temperature, and diluted with 10 mL distilled water. A reference test (without the plant extract) and a negative control test were carried out. The absorbance was measured at 540 nm. Percentage α-amylase inhibition was calculated using the formula: % Inhibition = $[(A540_{reference} - A540_{sample})/A540_{reference}] \times 100$; where $A540_{reference}$ is the absorbance of the reference test; and $A540_{sample}$ is the absorbance of the test containing the extract.

Alpha-glucosidase inhibition assay

The inhibitory effect of extracts against α-glucosidase activity was determined according to the method described by Kim et al. (2005), using α-glucosidase from *B. stearothermophillus* (Sigma, Cat. No. G 3651). Briefly, α-glucosidase (5 units) was preincubated with different dilutions (0–200 μL) of the extracts for 15 min. Next, 3 mmol/L para-nitrophenylglucopyranoside (PNPG) dissolved in 20 mmol/L phosphate buffer (pH 6.9) was added to start the reaction. The reaction mixture was further incubated at 37°C for 20 min, after which 2 mL of 0.1 mol/L Na_2CO_3 was added to stop the reaction. The absorbance of the yellow colored p-nitrophenol released from PNPG was measured at 400 nm. A reference test (without the plant extract) and a negative control test were carried out, and the percentage of α-glucosidase inhibition was calculated as follows: % Inhibition = $[(A400_{reference} - A400_{sample})/A400_{reference}] \times 100$; where $A400_{reference}$ is the absorbance of the reference test; and $A400_{sample}$ is the absorbance of the test containing the extract.

Aldose reductase inhibition assay

Partially purified rat lens aldose reductase was prepared following a procedure adapted from Hayman and Kinoshita (1965). Briefly, lenses were quickly removed from rats following anesthesia with ether, and homogenized in a glass homogenizer with a Teflon pestle in five volume of ice-cold distilled water. The homogenate was centrifuged at 10,000*g* at 0–4°C for 20 min. The supernatant was precipitated with saturated ammonium sulfate at 40%, 50%, and then at 75% salt saturation. The supernatant was retained after the first two precipitations. The pellet from the last step, possessing aldose reductase activity, was dispersed in 75% ammonium sulfate and subsequently used for the inhibition assay.

Inhibition of AR activity was assayed by estimating the consumption of NADPH at 340 nm as described by Da Settimo et al. (2005). The reaction mixture contained different dilutions (0–200 μL) of the extracts, 4.67 mmol/L D,L-glyceraldehyde as substrate, 0.11 mmol/L NADPH, 0.067 mol/L phosphate buffer (pH 6.2), and 0.05 mL of the enzyme preparation (rat lens homogenate) in a total volume of 1.5 mL. The enzyme reaction was initiated by addition of D,L-glyceraldehyde and was monitored for 4 min after an initial period of 1 min at 30°C. A reference test (without the plant extract) and a negative control test were carried out. A decrease in absorbance of sample test relative to the reference test at 340 nm is a function amount of NADPH consumed. Hence, % Inhibition = $[(A340_{reference} - A340_{sample})/A340_{reference}] \times 100$; where $A340_{reference}$ is the absorbance of the reference test; and $A340_{sample}$ is the absorbance of the test containing the extract.

Statistical analysis

Results of triplicate experiments were expressed as mean ± standard deviation (SD). *T*-test for independent samples was carried out on the result data at 95% confidence level using SPSS statistical software package, version 17, (SPSS Inc., Chicago). Half-maximal inhibitory concentration (IC_{50}) and half-maximal scavenging concentration (SC_{50}) were calculated from the % inhibition versus extract concentration nonlinear regression curve of each extract.

Results

Phenolics composition

The HPLC fingerprinting of the raw *A. digitata* leaves extract (Fig. 1) revealed the presence of gallic acid (Retention time, R_t = 10.19 min; peak 1), catechin (R_t = 16.07 min; peak 2), chlorogenic acid (R_t = 22.35 min; peak 3), caffeic acid (R_t = 26.97 min; peak 4), ellagic acid (R_t = 29.83 min; peak 5), epicatechin (R_t = 37.41 min; peak 6), rutin (R_t = 43.86 min; peak 7), quercitrin (R_t = 48.13 min; peak 8), quercetin (R_t = 52.01 min; peak 9), kaempferol (R_t = 57.69 min; peak 10), and luteolin (R_t = 64.15 min; peak 11). In contrast, the HPLC fingerprinting of the blanched leaves showed the presence of all the phenolic compounds found in the raw leaves except catechin and kaempferol that were not detected (Fig. 1).

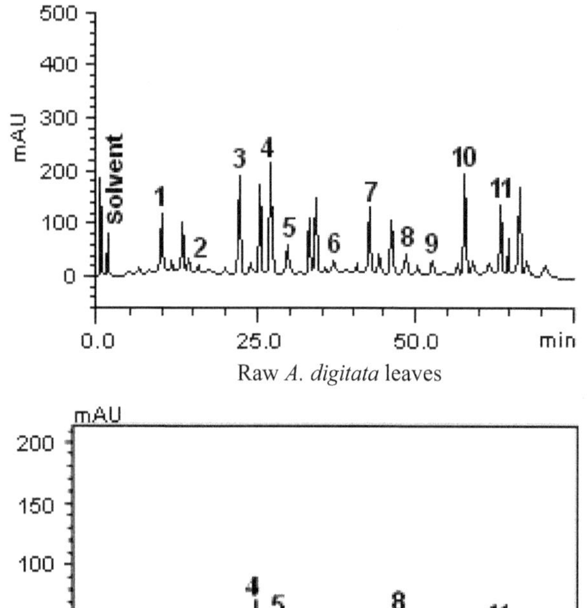

Raw *A. digitata* leaves

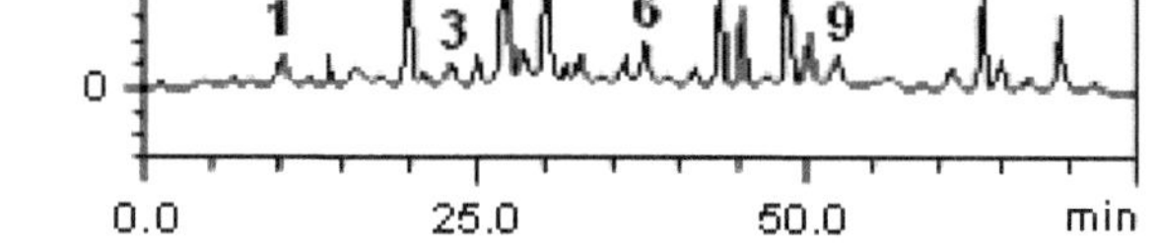

Blanched *A. digitata* leaves

Figure 1. Representative high-performance liquid chromatography profile of the extracts. UV detection was at 325 nm. Gallic acid (peak 1), catechin (peak 2), chlorogenic acid (peak 3), caffeic acid (peak 4), ellagic acid (peak 5), epicatechin (peak 6), rutin (peak 7), quercitrin (peak 8), quercetin (peak 9), kaempferol (peak 10), and luteolin (peak 11). Chromatographic conditions are described in the Material and Methods section.

Table 1 shows the phenolics composition of the raw and blanched leaves. Generally, the raw leaves had appreciable levels of the phenolics. The levels of the flavonoids were in the order of kaempferol > luteolin > quercetrin > quercetin > rutin > epicatechin > catechin; whereas the levels of the phenolic acids were in the order of chlorogenic acid > caffeic acid > gallic acid > ellagic acid. Blanching led to significant ($P < 0.05$) losses in the levels of both the flavonoids (except quercetin) and phenolic acids. Among the flavonoids, blanching resulted in 100% loss of catechin and kaempferol, as they were not detected in the blanched leaves. Interestingly, blanching led to 45.4% increase in the level of quercetin. Similarly, there were losses in the levels of the phenolic acids due to blanching; with chlorogenic acid (91.88% loss) and gallic acid (86.51% loss) being the most affected.

The antioxidant activity of the raw and blanched leaves was tested using four different assays, namely, $ABTS^{*+}$ and $DPPH^{*}$ scavenging assays, reducing power, and lipid peroxidation inhibition assays. The results, presented in Table 2, revealed that both the raw and blanched leaves extracts were able to scavenge $ABTS^{*+}$ and $DPPH^{*}$. The $ABTS^{*+}$ scavenging ability of the raw leaves extract (1.87 ± 0.09 mmol/L TE/g) was significantly ($P < 0.05$) higher than that of the blanched leaves extract (1.43 ± 0.06 mmol/L TE/g). The $DPPH^{*}$ SC_{50} of the raw leaves extract (0.23 ± 0.01 mg/mL) was significantly ($P < 0.05$) lower than that of the blanched leaves extract (0.30 ± 0.02 mg/mL), indicating that the raw leaves extract had stronger $DPPH^{*}$ scavenging ability than the blanched leaves extract. Similarly, the raw leaves extract had significantly ($P < 0.05$) higher reducing power than the blanched leaves extract. Extracts of both the raw and blanched leaves inhibited Fe^{2+}-induced lipid peroxidation in rat pancreas homogenate; however, the raw leaves (IC_{50}: 0.18 ± 0.01 mg/mL) had more inhibitory potency than the blanched leaves (IC_{50}: 0.27 ± 0.01 mg/mL).

The half-maximal inhibitory concentrations (IC_{50}) of the raw and blanched leaves extracts on α-amylase, α-glucosidase, and aldose reductase activities are presented in Table 3. The raw and blanched leaves were both able to inhibit the activities of these three carbohydrate-metabolizing enzymes that are implicated in T2D. However, the raw leaves extract was more potent in inhibiting the activities of these enzymes, as indicated by its lower IC_{50} values in comparison with those of the blanched leaves extract. Aldose reductase was the most inhibited, followed by α-glucosidase and α-amylase.

Table 1. Phenolics composition of raw and blanched *A. digitata* leaves.

Compounds (mg/g)	Raw	Blanched	LOD μg/mL	LOQ μg/mL	% Change
Gallic acid	4.15 ± 0.01^{a}	0.56 ± 0.02^{b}	0.024	0.079	−86.51
Catechin	0.75 ± 0.01	ND	0.013	0.042	−100.00
Chlorogenic acid	6.28 ± 0.03^{a}	0.51 ± 0.03^{b}	0.008	0.026	−91.88
Caffeic acid	6.31 ± 0.02^{a}	2.79 ± 0.01^{b}	0.019	0.061	−55.78
Ellagic acid	2.43 ± 0.01^{a}	2.34 ± 0.01^{a}	0.026	0.085	−3.70
Epicatechin	0.79 ± 0.04^{a}	0.55 ± 0.04^{b}	0.011	0.034	−30.38
Quercitrin	4.18 ± 0.01^{a}	2.13 ± 0.01^{b}	0.020	0.066	−49.04
Quercetin	1.63 ± 0.01^{b}	2.37 ± 0.02^{b}	0.027	0.089	45.40
Rutin	0.81 ± 0.03^{a}	0.53 ± 0.01^{b}	0.014	0.047	−34.57
Kaempferol	6.29 ± 0.02	ND	0.008	0.026	−100.00
Luteolin	4.54 ± 0.01^{a}	2.30 ± 0.02^{b}	0.017	0.056	−49.34

Results are expressed as mean ± standard deviations (SD) of three determinations. Values followed by different superscript letters in each row differ significantly at $P < 0.05$.
LOD, Limit of detection; LOQ, Limit of quantification.

Table 2. ABTS*+ scavenging ability, reducing power, DPPH SC_{50}, and Lipid peroxidation IC_{50} of raw and blanched *A. digitata* leaves extract.

Treatment	ABTS*+ scavenging ability (mM TE/g)	Reducing power (mg GAE/g)	DPPH SC_{50} (mg/mL)	Lipid peroxidation IC_{50} (mg/mL)
Raw	1.87 ± 0.09^{a}	20.02 ± 1.83^{a}	0.23 ± 0.01^{b}	0.18 ± 0.01^{b}
Blanched	1.43 ± 0.06^{b}	16.80 ± 1.02^{b}	0.30 ± 0.02^{a}	0.27 ± 0.01^{a}

Results are expressed as mean ± standard deviations (SD) of replicate determinations. Values followed by different superscript letters in each column differ significantly at $P < 0.05$.
ABTS*+, [2,2-azinobis (3-ethyl-benzothiazoline-6-sulfonic acid) radical cation]; GAE, gallic acid equivalent.

Table 3. IC_{50} of raw and blanched *A. digitata* leaves extracts on α-amylase, α-glucosidase, and aldose reductase activities.

Treatment	α-amylase IC_{50} (mg/mL)	α-glucosidase IC_{50} (mg/mL)	Aldose reductase IC_{50} (mg/mL)
Raw	1.18 ± 0.04^{b}	0.55 ± 0.01^{b}	0.43 ± 0.01^{b}
Blanched	1.79 ± 0.12^{a}	0.92 ± 0.01^{a}	0.87 ± 0.02^{a}

Results are expressed as mean ± standard deviations (SD) of replicate determinations. Values followed by different superscript letters in each column differ significantly at $P < 0.05$.

Discussion

Although blanching is intended to terminate the action of enzyme, shorten the drying and dehydration time, and set the color of vegetables (Wen et al. 2010), studies have shown that it influences the functional attributes of several plant products including the polyphenol content of *Coriandrum sativum* leaves and fruits (Kaiser et al. 2013); the total phenolics content and antioxidant activity of turnip greens (Martínez et al. 2013); the color, texture, polyphenols, and antioxidant capacity of Irish York cabbage (Jaiswal et al. 2012); and the inhibitory ability of *Amaranthus cruentus* extract on α-amylase and α-glucosidase activities (Oboh et al. 2013). Hence, the influence of blanching on the phenolics composition, antioxidant activity, and inhibitory effects of *A. digitata* leaves extract on the activities of α-amylase, α-glucosidase, and aldose reductase was evaluated in this study.

The phenolic compounds quantified in the leaves fall into two important classes of phenolics, namely, flavonoids and phenolic acids. The flavonoids include catechin, epicatechin, quercetrin, quercetin, rutin, kaempferol, and leuteolin; whereas the phenolic acids include gallic, chlorogenic, caffeic, and ellagic acids. Flavonoids are prominent as both electrons donors and terminators of chain reactions due to their hydroxyl groups, particularly at the 3′OH and 4′OH of their three-carbon chain (Kim et al. 2010; Cho et al. 2013). In contrast, phenolic acids contain a phenolic ring and an organic carboxylic acid function (Goufo et al. 2014), and the phenolic ring are capable of stabilizing and delocalizing unpaired electrons (Goufo and Trindade 2014). These distinguishing structural features confer antioxidant property on flavonoids and phenolic acids. Flavonoids and phenolic acids are also of pharmacological importance for the management and/or prevention of T2D (Ghasemzadeh and Ghasemzadeh 2011).

The raw leaves proved to be a rich source of these two classes of phenolics. Blanching resulted in significant ($P < 0.05$) losses in both the flavonoids (except quercetin) and phenolic acids content of the leaves; with ellagic acid (3.70% loss) as the least affected, and catechin and kaempferol (100% loss) as the most affected. Loss in the phenolics content of vegetables due to blanching has been reported by some previous studies (Sikora et al. 2008; Korus and Lisiewska 2011; Jaiswal et al. 2012), and this could be attributed to oxidation of the phenolics or their leaching into water during blanching (Roy et al. 2009). Phenolic compounds are known to occur in soluble forms and in combination with cell wall components in plants (Francisco et al. 2010). Thus, the high temperature of the blanching may have led to the disruption of the cell walls and the breakdown of the phenolics, thereby leading to their leaching into the blanching water. The differential losses in the levels of the individual flavonoids and phenolic acids after blanching may reflect variations in their individual solubility and thermo-stability in hot water. Francisco et al. (2010) have earlier demonstrated that the same method of cooking affects different types of flavonoids even within the same class differently. Thus, the absolute loss (100%) in catechin and kaempferol may suggest that these two flavonoids are highly water soluble and heat labile. Against the losses recorded for all other phenolics, the level of quercetin increased by 45.4% after blanching. This exclusive increase may be attributed to enhanced extractability (Wen et al. 2010), following the disruption of the cell wall of the leaves, as well as the hydrolysis of quercitrin.

The extracts scavenged DPPH* and ABTS*+, and reduced Fe^{3+} to Fe^{2+} (Table 2), and these represent their antioxidant activity. This finding corroborates previous reports that *A. digitata* leaves extract posses antioxidant activity (Vertuani et al. 2002; Ayele et al. 2013). Blanching attenuated the antioxidant activity of the leaves; this is also in agreement with several earlier studies that demonstrated that blanching reduces the antioxidant activity of vegetables (Korus and Lisiewska 2011; Jaiswal et al. 2012). This negative effect has been attributed to the loss in the phenolics and other water soluble antioxidants due to leaching and thermal degradation during blanching. However, Roy et al. (2009) noted that the influence of thermal processing on polyphenolics level and antioxidative activity is dependent on the type of product. In addition, Sikora et al. (2008) noted that the extent of polyphenolics degradation is very much dependent on processing time and the size of vegetables. Hence, Wen et al. (2010) reported that after blanching, the total phenolic content and antioxidant activity of five commonly consumed vegetables in Malaysia either decreased or increased depending on the type of vegetables.

Free radicals and reactive oxygen species (ROS) are notorious for the oxidative damage they cause to intra- and extracellular macromolecules, including damaging of the DNA, protein, lipids, and carbohydrates (Takemoto et al. 2009). Oxidative stress is induced when the free radicals and ROS (oxidants) burden of the cell overwhelms its antioxidant defense system, and it has been implicated in the pathogenesis and complications of diabetes (Giacco and Brownlee 2010). Lipid peroxidation, which is the oxidative damage of lipids (particularly, the polyunsaturated fatty acids that are very vulnerable to oxidative attack) by ROS and transition metal ions, also plays a major role in cell injury (Schafer et al. 2000), as it yields diverse cytotoxic products, mostly aldehydes such as malondialdehyde (MDA) (Shalaby and Shanab 2013). The toxic effects of these products are due to their ability to disrupt the function of membrane; inactivate membrane-bound receptors and enzymes, and compromise membrane permeability (Rahman 2003). As a chain reaction, lipid peroxidation in turn propagates the production of more free radicals that can induce oxidative damage to the body cells, including the β-cells of the pancreas (Shah and Fonseca 2011). This explains why tissue damages mediated by lipid peroxides have been observed in diabetes (Feillet-Coudray et al. 1999). However, these oxidative damages could be mitigated by a robust cellular antioxidant defense system. This therefore means that increasing the intake of *A. digitata* leaves rich in phenolics could prevent the onset of oxidative stress, and ameliorate its sequelae. Furthermore, as the leaves extract possesses reducing power, as seen in its reduction of Fe^{3+} to Fe^{2+}, it could reduce the oxidized intermediates of lipid peroxidation by acting as electron donor, thereby functioning as primary and secondary antioxidants (Chanda and Dave 2009). However, as in the radical scavenging results, blanching reduced the ability of the extract to inhibit Fe^{2+}-induced lipid peroxidation in rat's pancreas homogenate.

Plant foods rich in phenolics are important for the management and treatment of T2D. Studies have consistently shown that the inhibition of carbohydrate-hydrolyzing enzymes, including α-amylase, α-glucosidase, and aldose reductase, is one of the possible mechanisms through which plant-derived phenolics exhibit their antidiabetic activity (Adefegha and Oboh 2012; Irondi et al. 2014). Indeed, the hydrolytic activity of amylase and glucosidase on carbohydrates contributes to postprandial blood glucose level (Sim et al. 2010). Hence, by inhibiting α-amylase and α-glucosidase, with the concomitant decrease in the rate of glucose absorption, the phenolics in *A. digitata* leaves extract can reduce the rise in postprandial blood glucose. Interestingly, the inhibition of α-amylases and α-glucosidases activities has been reported as one of the most effective approaches to control hyperglycemia in T2D (Kim et al. 2005).

Activation of polyol pathway resulting from increased aldose reductase activity is one of the mechanisms underlying the development of secondary complications of T2D in diabetic patients. Aldose reductase is the rate-limiting enzyme in the polyol pathway that reduces excess D-glucose into D-sorbitol with concomitant conversion of NADPH into $NADP^+$ (Jesus and Sonia 2003). It is present in tissues such as retina, lens, nerve, and glomerulars cells (Ramasamy and Goldberg 2010), where glucose uptake is modulated by glucose transporters independent of insulin. Previous studies provided evidence for the involvement of this enzyme in diabetic complications including neuropathy, retinopathy, nephropathy, and cataract (Ramana 2011), and that its inhibition by plant extracts is a possible therapeutic strategy to ameliorating these complications (Karasu et al. 2012). In this study, *A. digitata* leaves extract inhibited aldose reductase, suggesting that it is capable of ameliorating the complications of T2D that are aldose reductase mediated. However, blanching reduced its inhibitory potency.

The inhibitory effect of the extracts on amylase, glucosidase, and aldose reductase could be attributed to the flavonoids and phenolic acids present in them. Previous studies have provided evidence for this; for instance, extracts of *Mangifera indica* and *Mucuna urens* seeds flours rich in these two classes of phenolics inhibited α-amylase, α-glucosidase, and aldose reductase in vitro (Irondi et al. 2014). The decrease in the inhibitory ability of the extract on the carbohydrate-hydrolyzing enzymes after blanching agrees with that reported by Oboh et al. (2013), who also observed a reduction in the inhibitory ability of *Amaranthus cruentus* extract on α-amylase and α-glucosidase activities after blanching. This observation could be a direct effect of the decrease in the phenolics levels, as they are responsible for the inhibition of these enzymes.

Conclusion

Adansonia digitata leaves proved to be a rich source of flavonoids and phenolic acids that are beneficial to health. These phenolics confered antioxidant activity and inhibitory effect against α-amylase, α-glucosidase, and aldose reductase on the leaves extract. Hence, the extract could be effective for the management of T2D. However, blanching reduced the levels of these functional attributes of the leaves, and may not be recommended for their optimal retention.

Conflict of Interest

We declare that we have no conflict of interest.

References

Addy, R. 2009. Baobab Fruit Approved as Food Ingredient in US. Available at: http://www.nutraingredients-usa.com/content/view/print/259574 (accessed: July 01, 2015)

Adefegha, S. A., and G. Oboh. 2012. *In vitro* inhibition activity of polyphenol-rich extracts from *Syzygium aromaticum* (L.) Merr. & Perry (Clove) buds against carbohydrate hydrolyzing enzymes linked to Type-2 diabetes and Fe^{2+}-induced lipid peroxidation in rat pancreas. Asian Pac. J. Trop. Biomed. 2:774–781.

Ayele, Y., J. Kim, E. Park, and Y. Kim, et al. 2013. A methanol Extract of *Adansonia digitata* L. Leaves Inhibits Pro-Inflammatory iNOS possibly via the Inhibition of NF-kB Activation. Biomol. Ther. 21: 146–152.

Boligon, A.A., M. Piana, T. F. Kubiça, and D. N. Mario, et al. 2015. HPLC analysis and antimicrobial, antimycobacterial and antiviral activities of *Tabernaemontana catharinensis* A. DC. J. Appl. Biomed. 13:7–18.

Buchmann, C., S. Prehsler, A. Hartl, and C. R. Vogl. 2010. The importance of baobab (*Adansonia digitata* L.) in rural West African subsistence—suggestion of a cautionary approach to international market export of baobab fruits. Ecol. Food Nutr. 49:145–172.

Cervato, G., M. Carabelli, S. Gervasio, A. Cittera, et al. 2000. Antioxidant properties of oregano (*Origanum vulgare*) leaf extracts. J. Food Biochem. 24:453–465.

Chadare, F. J., A. R. Linnemann, J. D. Hounhouigan, M. J. Nout, et al. 2009. Baobab food products: a review on their composition and nutritional value. Crit. Rev. Food Sci. Nutr. 49:254–274.

Chanda, S., and R. Dave. 2009. In vitro models for antioxidant activity evaluation and some medicinal plants possessing antioxidant properties: an overview. Afri. J. Microbiol. Res. 3:981–996.

Cho, J.-G., N.-Y. Song, T.-G. Nam, S. Shrestha, et al. 2013. Flavonoids from the grains of C1/R-S transgenic rice, the transgenic *Oryza sativa* spp. *japonica*, and their radical scavenging activities. J. Agric. Food Chem. 61:10354–10359.

Da Settimo, F., G. Primofiore, C. La Motta, S. Sartini, et al. 2005. Naphtho[1,2-d]isothiazole acetic acid derivatives as a novel class of selective aldose reductase inhibitors. J. Med. Chem. 48:6897–6907.

De Caluwé, E., K. Halamová, and P. Van Damme. 2009. Baobab (*Adansonia digitata* L.): a review of traditional uses, phytochemistry and pharmacology. Pp. 51–84 *in* H. Rodolfo, J. E. Simon and C.-T. Ho, eds. African natural plant products: new discoveries and challenges in chemistry and quality. Oxford Univ. Press, Washington D.C., USA.

DeFronzo, R. A. 2004. Pathogenesis of type 2 diabetes mellitus. Med. Clin. N Am. 88:787–835.

Feillet-Coudray, C., E. Rock, C. Coudray, K. Grzelkowska, et al. 1999. Lipid peroxidation and antioxidant status in experimental diabetes. Clin. Chem. Acta 284:31–43.

Francisco, M., P. Velasco, D. A. Moreno, C. García-Viguera, et al. 2010. Cooking methods of Brassica rapa affect the preservation of glucosinolates, phenolics and vitamin C. Food Res. Int. 43:1455–1463.

Fujisawa, T., H. Ikegami, K. Inoue, Y. Kawabata, et al. 2005. Effect of two α- glucosidase inhibitors, voglibose and acarbose, on postprandial hyperglycaemia correlates with subjective abdominal symptoms. Metabolism 54:387–390.

Ghasemzadeh, A., and N. Ghasemzadeh. 2011. Flavonoids and phenolic acids: role and biochemical activity in plants and human. J. Med. Plants Res. 5:6697–6703.

Giacco, F., and M. Brownlee. 2010. Oxidative stress and diabetic complications. Circ. Res. 107:1058–1070.

Goufo, P., and H. Trindade. 2014. Rice antioxidants: phenolic acids, flavonoids, anthocyanins, proanthocyanidins, tocopherols, tocotrienols, c-oryzanol, and phytic acid. Food Sci. Nutr. 2:75–104.

Goufo, P., J. Pereira, J. Moutinho-Pereira, C. M. Correia, et al. 2014. Rice (*Oryza sativa* L.) phenolic compounds under elevated carbon dioxide (CO_2) concentration. Environ. Exp. Bot. 99:28–37.

Hayman, S., and J. H. Kinoshita. 1965. Isolation and properties of lens aldose reductase. J. Biol. Chem. 240:877–882.

Ibrahim, M. A., and M. S. Islam. 2014. Anti-diabetic effects of the acetone fraction of *Senna singueana* stem bark in a type 2 diabetes rat model. J. Ethnopharmacol. 153:392–399.

Irondi, A. E., G. Oboh, A. A. Akindahunsi, A. A. Boligon, et al. 2014. Phenolic composition and inhibitory activity of Mango and Horse-eye bean seeds extracts against key enzymes linked to the pathology and complications of type 2 diabetes. Asian Pac. J. Trop. Biomed. 4:903–910.

Jaiswal, A. K., S. Gupta, and N. Abu-Ghannam. 2012. Kinetic evaluation of colour, texture, polyphenols and antioxidant capacity of Irish York cabbage after blanching treatment. Food Chem. 131:63–72.

Jesus, A. F., and M. Sonia. 2003. Aldose reductase inhibitors from natural. Nat. Prod. Rep. 20:243–251.

Kaiser, A., D. R. Kammerer, and R. Carle. 2013. Impact of blanching on polyphenol stability and antioxidant capacity of innovative coriander (*Coriandrum sativum* L.) pastes. Food Chem. 140:332–339.

Karasu, C., A. Cumaoğlu, A. R. Gurpinar, M. Kartal, et al. 2012. AR inhibitory activity and antioxidant capacity of pomegranate extracts. Interdiscip. Toxicol. 5:15–20.

Khaliq, A., S. M. Sabir, S. D. Ahmad, A. A. Boligon, et al. 2015. Antioxidant activities and phenolic composition of Olive (*Olea europaea*) leaves. J. Appl. Bot. Food Qual. 88:16–21.

Kim, Y. M., Y. K. Jeong, M. H. Wang, Y. H. Lee, et al. 2005. Inhibitory effect of pine extract on alpha-glucosidase activity and postprandial hyperglycaemia. Nutrition 21:756–761.

Kim, J. K., S. Y. Lee, S. M. Chu, S. H. Lim, et al. 2010. Variation and correlation analysis of flavonoids and carotenoids in Korean pigmented rice (*Oryza sativa* L.) cultivars. J. Agric. Food Chem. 58:12804–12809.

Korus, A., and Z. Lisiewska. 2011. Effect of preliminary processing and method of preservation on the content of selected antioxidative compounds in kale (*Brassica oleracea* L. var. *acephala*) leaves. Food Chem. 129:149–154.

Kwon, Y. I., H. D. Jang, and K. Shetty. 2006. Evaluation of *Rhodiola crenulata* and *Rhodiola rosea* for management of type II diabetes and hypertension. Asian Pac J Clin Nutr 15:425–432.

Kwon, Y. I., E. Apostolidis, and K. Shetty. 2008. Inhibitory potential of wine and tea against α-amylase and a-glucosidase for management of hyperglycemia linked to type 2 diabetes. J. Food Biochem. 32:15–31.

Martínez, S., N. Pérez, J. Carballo, and I. Franco. 2013. Effect of blanching methods and frozen storage on some quality parameters of turnip greens ("grelos"). LWT - Food Sci. Technol. 51:383–392.

Oboh, G., A. J. Akinyemi, A. O. Ademiluyi, and S. A. Adefegha. 2010. Inhibitory effects of aqueous extract of two varieties of ginger on some key enzymes linked to type-2 diabetes in vitro. J. Food Nutr. Res. 49:14–20.

Oboh, G., A. J. Akinyemi, A. O. Ademiluyi, and F. O. Bello. 2013. Inhibition of α-amylase and α-glucosidase activities by ethanolic extract of A*maranthus cruentus* leaf as affected by blanching. Afr. J. Pharm. Pharmaco. 7:1026–1032.

Ohkawa, H., N. Ohishi, and K. Yagi. 1979. Assay for lipid peroxides in animal tissues by thiobarbituric acid reaction. Anal. Biochem. 95:351–358.

Oishi, N., S. Morikubo, Y. Takamura, E. Kubo, et al. 2006. Correlation between adult diabetic cataracts and red blood cell aldose reductase levels. Invest. Ophthalmol. Vis. Sci. 47:2061–2064.

Oyaizu, M. 1986. Studies on products of browning reaction: antioxidative activity of products of browning reaction prepared from glucosamine. Jpn. J. Nutr. 44:307–315.

Rahman, I. 2003. Oxidative stress, chromatin remodeling and gene transcription in inflammation and chronic lung diseases. J. Biochem. Mol. Biol. 36:95–109.

Ramana, K. V. 2011. Aldose reductase: new insights for an old enzyme. Biomol. Concepts 2:103–114.

Ramasamy, R., and I. J. Goldberg. 2010. Aldose reductase and cardiovascular diseases, creating human-like diabetic complications in an experimental model. Circ. Res. 106:1449–1458.

Roy, M. K., L. R. Juneja, S. Isobe, and T. Tsushida. 2009. Steam processed broccoli (*Brassica oleracea*) has higher antioxidant activity in chemical and cellular assay systems. Food Chem. 114:263–269.

Saraswat, M., P. Muthenna, P. Suryanarayana, M. J. Petrash, et al. 2008. Dietary sources of aldose reductase inhibitors: prospects for alleviating diabetic complications. Asia Pac. J. Clin. Nutr. 17:558–565.

Schafer, F. Q., S. Y. Qian, and G. R. Buettner. 2000. Iron and free radical oxidations in cell membranes. Cell Mol. Biol. (Noisy-le-grand) 46: 657–662.

Sellappan, S., and C. C. Akoh. 2002. Flavonoids and antioxidant capacity of Georgia-grown vidalia onions. J. Agric. Food Chem. 50:5338–5342.

Shah, S. V., and V. A. Fonseca. 2011. Iron and diabetes revisited. Diabetes Care 34:1676–1677.

Shalaby, E. A., and S. M. M. Shanab. 2013. Antioxidant compounds, assays of determination and mode of action. Afr. J. Pharm. Pharmacol. 7:528–539.

Shri, V. T., D. Ramprasath, K. Karunambigai, D. Nagavalli, et al. 2004. Studies of pharmacognostical profiles of *Adansonia digitata* Linn. Ancient Sci. Life 24:60–64.

Sibibe, M., and J. T. Williams. 2002. Baobab – Adansonia digitata Fruits for the future. Int Centre Underutil Crops. University of Southampton, UK.

Sikora, E., E. Cieslik, T. Leszczynska, A. Filipiak-Florkiewicz, et al. 2008. The antioxidant activity of selected cruciferous vegetables subjected to aquathermal processing. Food Chem. 107:55–59.

Sim, L., C. Willemsma, S. Mohan, H. Y. Naim, et al. 2010. Structural basis for substrate selectivity in human maltase-glucoamylase and sucrase-isomaltase N-terminal domains. J. Biol. Chem. 285:17763–17770.

Takemoto, K., M. Tanaka, H. Iwata, R. Nishihara, et al. 2009. Low catalase activity in blood is associated with the diabetes caused by alloxan. Clin. Chim. Acta 407(1–2):43–46.

Tappy, L., and K. A. Le. 2010. Metabolic effects of fructose and the worldwide increase in obesity. Physiol. Rev. 90:23–46.

Vertuani, S., E. Braccioli, V. Buzzoni, and S. Manfredini. 2002. Antioxidant capacity of Adansonia digitata fruit pulp and leaves. Acta Phytotherapeutica 86:2.

Vimalanathan, S., and J. B. Hudson. 2009. Multiple inflammatory and antiviral activities in *Adansonia digitata* (Baobab) leaves, fruits and seeds. J. Med. Plants Res. 3:576–582.

Wen, T. N., K. N. Prasad, B. Yang, and A. Ismail. 2010. Bioactive substance contents and antioxidant capacity of raw and blanched vegetables. Innov. Food Sci. Emerg. Technol. 11:464–469.

Wickens, G. E., and P. Lowe. 2008. The Baobabs: pachycauls of Africa. Springer, Madagascar and Australia.

Willett, W. C. 2002. Balancing life-style and genomics research for disease prevention. Sci. 296:695–698.

4

Investigation of nutritional properties of three species of marine turban snails for human consumption

Roslizawati Ab Lah[1,2], Joshua Smith[1,3], Dale Savins[3], Ashley Dowell[3], Daniel Bucher[1] & Kirsten Benkendorff[1]

[1]Marine Ecology Research Centre, School of Environment, Science and Engineering, University of Southern Cross, Lismore 2480, New South Wales, Australia
[2]University Malaysia Terengganu, Kuala 21030, Terengganu, Malaysia
[3]Southern Cross Plant Science, University of Southern Cross, Lismore 2480, New South Wales, Australia

Keywords
Fatty acids, heavy metals, *n*−3/*n*−6 ratio, protein, trace elements, turban snails, Turbinidae

Correspondence
Kirsten Benkendorff, Marine Ecology Research Centre, School of Environment, Science and Engineering, University of Southern Cross, 2480 Lismore, New South Wales, Australia.
E-mail: kirsten.benkendorff@scu.edu.au

Funding Information
The research was funded by the postgraduate research funding from the School of Environment, Science and Engineering and Marine Ecology Research Centre, Southern Cross University The authors gratefully acknowledge the Ministry of Higher Education of Malaysia for the PhD scholarship for the first author.

Abstract

Turban snails (family Turbinidae) are gastropod molluscs that are harvested for human consumption yet little is known about the nutritional properties of these snails, particularly from Australian waters. This study compares the proximate composition (ash, moisture, protein, and lipid content), fatty acid profiles, mineral, and trace element content of three species of turbinid snails; *Turbo militaris, Lunella undulata,* and *Lunella torquata* from northern New South Wales, Australia. They were all found to have relatively high protein in their flesh (16.0% to 18.5% of the fresh weight). *L. torquata* had a significantly higher lipid content (8.5% w/w) than *L. undulata* (5.2% w/w), whereas *T. militaris* (5.6% w/w) was not significantly different to either. Analysis with gas chromatography showed there was no significant difference in monounsaturated fatty acid (MUFA) content, with an average of approximately 14% of the total fatty acids in all three species. However, saturated fatty acids (SFA) were significantly higher in *T. militaris* (41%), whereas polyunsaturated fatty acids (PUFA) were significantly higher in *L. undulata* (46%). The ratio of $n-3/n-6$ fatty acids ranged from 1.1 in *T. militaris* to 1.4 in *L. torquata,* which is good for human health and comparable to other high value gastropods. The results indicate that *T. militaris, L. undulata,* and *L. torquata* provide a good source of essential elements such as zinc, selenium, and iron. At the location studied, toxic metals and metalloids were below safe recommended standards for human consumption. Overall, this study confirms the suitability of turban snails as a nutritional food for human consumption.

Introduction

Many marine molluscs are harvested around the world for their meat. They are important resources that contribute considerable economic value to the world's fisheries (Leiva and Castilla 2002). In the year 2013, the commercial harvest of at least 9.8 million tons of molluscs was reported as part of the world fisheries catch (FAO, 2015a). The majority of the molluscan fishery is contributed by bivalves and cephalopods, with gastropods contributing less than 2% of the total harvest (FAO, 2015b), although some gastropods do have a relatively high economic value (Leiva and Castilla 2002). The demand for global fisheries product, including molluscs, increases every year as the human population grows (Naylor et al. 2000; Diana 2009) leading to exploitation of new stocks (Dey 2015). Consequently, there is a need for supplementing the current mollusc catch with new or underutilized species.

Molluscs have been recognized as a high-quality nutritious food source and many species are considered as culinary delicacies. A considerable amount of literature has been published on the nutritional composition of some molluscs. For example, several studies have reported relatively high protein levels found in mollusc flesh, including abalone *Haliotis diversicolor* (Chiou et al. 2001) and oysters *Crassostrea gigas* (Linehan et al. 1999; Dridi et al. 2007). The nutritional quality of mollusc flesh lies not only with the high quality of protein, but also in its relatively low lipid content and high proportion of polyunsaturated fatty acids (PUFAs) (Nichols et al. 1998; Mooney et al. 2002).

Molluscs are known to contain a wide variety of PUFAs, some of which are considered as essential fatty acids that humans cannot synthesize and must be obtained from food (Smoothey 2013). Among the PUFA's, long-chain omega-3 fatty acids, such as eicosapentaenoic (EPA), docosapentaenoic (DPA), and docosahexanoic (DHA), are thought to play beneficial roles in a healthful diet. The balanced intake of omega-3 ($n-3$) and omega-6 ($n-6$) fatty acid can help prevent cardiovascular disease (Mahaffey 2004; Mahaffey et al. 2008), coronary heart disease, arthritis (Simopoulos 1991), and other inflammation (Milinsk et al. 2003; Mahaffey 2004; Mahaffey et al. 2008). Since these $n-3$ and $n-6$ fatty acids cannot be synthesized by molluscs, they must be acquired from their food intake, such as phytoplankton or algae (Foster and Hodgson 1998). As a consequence, the fatty acid content is expected to vary within and between mollusc species depending on their specific diets and over time as the populations of algal species fluctuate. Physiological demand for certain fatty acids during the reproductive cycle could also contribute to temporal variation and differences between the sexes (Brazao et al. 2003).

The nutritional content and fatty acid compositions of molluscs has been intensively investigated in commercially important bivalve species, including oysters (Ostreidae) (Saito and Hashimoto 2010), scallops (Pectinidae) (Napolitano and Ackman 1992; Pazos et al. 1997a,b), pearl oyster (Pteriidae) (Saito 2004; Gokoglu et al. 2006), and mussels (Mytilidae) (Chan et al. 2004; Su et al. 2006). Nevertheless, there is less information available on the biochemical components of other molluscs. In particular, only a few studies have been published on fatty acid composition and nutritional quality of the flesh of gastropods, including members of the families Haliotidae (Dunstan et al. 1996; Chiou et al. 2001; Nelson et al. 2002; Su et al. 2006), Turbinidae (Freiji and Awadh 2010; Nooshin and Peyman 2011; Saito and Aono 2014), Babyloniidae (Periyasamy et al. 2011), and Muricidae (Woodcock and Benkendorff 2008; Vasconcelos et al. 2009).

Molluscs are also known to be among the best bioindicators for monitoring environmental pollution in coastal waters, due to their relative immobility and their ability to accumulate high concentrations of heavy metals from the surrounding environment (Metian et al. 2008; Jakimska et al. 2011). Increasing urbanization and industrialization could potentially increase the contamination of marine ecosystems through discharge of sewage, industrial runoff, and agricultural waste (Chouvelon et al. 2009; Pan and Wang 2012). The capacity to accumulate metals may vary between species and individuals depending on size or physiological condition (Cubadda et al. 2001; Duquesne et al. 2004; Mubiana et al. 2006; Bille et al. 2015). If the concentrations in molluscs exceed the permitted concentration, this may pose a health risk to humans.

A study on the turbinid gastropod *Cookia sulcata* highlighted the presence of essential dietary minerals such as zinc and other nutritional components (Mason et al. 2014). Several studies have been undertaken on the nutritional and elemental composition of other gastropods, such as the muricids *Chicoreus ramosus* (Xavier Ramesh and Ayyakkannu 1992), *Rapona venosa* (Celik et al. 2014) and the babyloniid *Babylonia spirata* (Periyasamy et al. 2011), as well as bivalves such as the oysters *Crassostrea rhizophorae* and *Ostra edulis* (Karakoltsidis and Zotos 1995; Martino and Cruz 2004), the venerid clams *Meretrix casta* and *Protothaca thaca* (Olmedo et al. 2013; Smoothey 2013), the mussel *Mytilus galloprovincialis* (Karakoltsidis and Zotos 1995; Olmedo et al. 2013) and the cockle, *Ostra edulis* (Karakoltsidis and Zotos 1995) and *Mytilus galloprovincialis*, *Cerastoderma edule* (Olmedo et al. 2013).

Turban snails are abundant in most coastal seas (Joll 1980; Smoothey 2013; Saito and Aono 2014). In Japan, Korea, and China, turban snails are highly valued as a food (Chen et al. 2004; Mason et al. 2014) and have been described as being "among the best gastropods for human consumption" by Yearsley et al. (1999). The turban snail fishery in Australia is currently a small-scale fishery with annual commercial landings of approximately 7 tons in New South Wales and approximately 6.5 tons in South Australia (PIRSA, 2010; Rodellar et al. 2010). However, the Turbinidae can also be subject to substantial recreational harvest (Cooling and Smith 2015). Three species in family of Turbinidae that commonly occur in temperate-to-subtropical waters of Australia are *Turbo militaris*, *Lunella torquata*, and *L. undulata*. They can be found in shallow rocky reef habitats along the eastern and southern coasts of Australia (Fig. 1). The distributions of all three species overlap in the subtropical waters of northern New South Wales (NSW). This provides an opportunity to directly compare the nutritional properties between these species without confounding effects from different locations. No previous studies have been undertaken to investigate the nutritional properties of these Australian Turbinidae species. Therefore, the aim of this study was

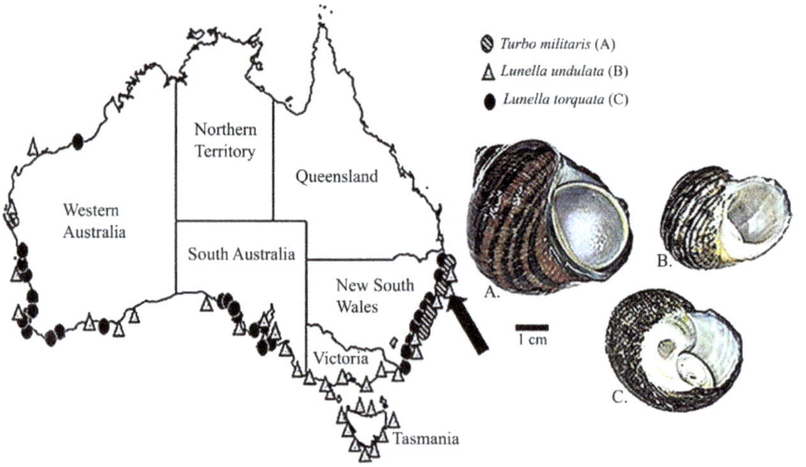

Figure 1. Map showing the distribution of the three turban snails: A) *Turbo militaris* Reeve, 1848; B) *Lunella undulata* Lightfoot, 1786; C) *Lunella (Ninella) torquata* Gmelin, 1791, in Australia with the arrow indicating the location of the sampling site (Woolgoolga NSW; -30.108300, 153.207003). Adapted from: (Bouchet 2015), Australian Faunal Directory (accessed Oct 2015).

to assess the nutritional content of *T. militaris, L. undulata,* and *L. torquata,* from NSW, Australia, specifically the proximate composition (i.e., protein, lipid, carbohydrate, moisture, and ash), fatty acid profiles and micronutrient and trace elemental concentrations.

Materials and Methods

Collection and preparation of specimens

The snails were all collected from Woolgoolga, Coffs Harbour, Australia (Fig. 1) under fisheries permit (permit number: P13/0002–1.0) in May 2014. To eliminate the effects of variations in trace elements associated with different localities and temporal variations in proximate composition due to the reproductive cycle and seasonal variations in food supply, three species were collected by hand from the same locality on the same low tides. In total, six specimens of *L. undulata*, four specimens of *T. militaris*, and four specimens of *L. torquata* were collected. All the specimens were transported to the laboratory in a 10 L bucket and processed within 4 h of collection. The shell was broken using a bench vice and the foot muscle and viscera removed. Foot tissue was used for all analyses, as this is the part of the animal used for human consumption. Each specimen was divided into four pieces weighing approximately 1 g each. All tissue weights were recorded for the proximate composition analysis using an analytical balance with precision of ± 0.0001 g (model ML 204/01; Mettler Toledo, Plainview, NY). One portion of each snail was used for moisture and ash analysis, another for lipid and fatty acid analysis, a third for protein analysis and the forth for elemental composition. Portions from each snail were analyzed separately to provide four to six replicate analyses per species.

Nutritional proximate analysis

All reagents and chemicals in this study were purchased from Sigma (St Louis, Mo). Moisture content was calculated based on the percentage weight loss after drying to a constant weight at 60°C for 24–48 h (Woodcock and Benkendorff 2008). To determine the ash content, the dry samples were weighed and transferred to a muffle furnace (model KSL 1700X; MTI Corporation, Richmond, CA) at 550°C for 4 h.

Lipids were extracted from a second piece of tissue from each specimen according to the methods of Woodcock and Benkendorff (2008) based on the original method by Bligh and Dyer (1959). Samples were immersed for 1.5 h in the solvent (1:2 chloroform methanol) (v/v) then filtered through Whatman #1 filter paper (Sigma-Aldrich; Munich, Germany) into a preweighed clean test tube (culture test tube with Teflon lined screw cap). Solvent replacements continued until no further color was extracted from the tissue. All the solvent fractions were then combined and the extracts were dried under a stream of high-purity nitrogen gas until no solvent remained, then reweighed.

Analysis of fatty acid composition

The lipid extracts were subject to fatty acid analysis by gas chromatography after derivatization into fatty acid methyl esters (FAMEs). To prepare the methyl esters, 1.5 mL of a 0.5 mol/L solution of sodium hydroxide in methanol was added to the lipid extracts (Kanthilatha et al. 2014). The samples were heated in a dry block at 100°C for 10 min. To complete the methylation of fatty acids, 2 mL of boron trifluoride in methanol was added and heated at 100°C for a further 30 min. The samples were then cooled to room temperature before 1 mL of hexane was added to extract the fatty acid methyl esters. The tube was shaken vigorously for at least 30 sec and 5 mL of saturated sodium chloride solution was added followed by shaking thoroughly for at least 5 sec. The polar and lipophilic solvent layers were allowed to separate and the upper hexane layer transferred to an autosampler vial for gas chromatography (GC) injection.

The composition of fatty acids was determined using standard FAMEs analysis by gas chromatography. The gas chromatograph used was an Agilent 6890 N, equipped with a FID (flame ionization detector). The Agilent 6890 split injector and FID were maintained at 230°C and 260°C, respectively. The capillary column used was BPX 70 (70% cyanopropyl polysilphenylene-siloxane, 50 m × 0.22 mm × 0.25 μm). The GC oven temperature was programmed with 100°C hold for 5 min and then increased at a rate of 5°C/ min until the final temperature 240°C was reached. The carrier gas was Helium. One microliter of the extract containing the fatty acids methyl esters was injected with a split ratio of 200:1, and a column flow of 1 mL/min. The retention time of each peak detected in the samples was compared to the FAMEs test mix (Sigma) and the area under the curve was calculated to determine the percent composition relative to all peaks.

Some supplementary analyses were undertaken using gas chromatography/mass spectrometry (GCMS) to confirm the identity of all fatty acid methyl esters and identify the unknown peaks that did not correspond to the FAMEs standards. The GCMS (Agilent 6890) was coupled with an Agilent 5973 mass selective detector. The mass spectra were recorded at 70 eV ionization voltage over the mass range 35–550 amu. The identification of unknown peaks was based on matching to a mass spectral library (WILEY 275 and NIST98).

Protein analysis

For protein determination, 1 g of foot tissue was digested in 10 mL of 1 mol/L sodium hydroxide (NaOH) until all tissue completely dissolved. After digestion 1 mL of sample was transferred to an Eppendorf tube and centrifuged in a rotary microfuge for 5 min at 96.15 g. Bovine serum albumin (BSA) was used as a standard protein solution (10 mg/mL) and a twofold dilution series was created (10.000–0.0195 mg/mL). The BSA standard protein solutions and all the digested snail protein samples were subjected to the Biuret Assay (Brooks et al. 1995). For a negative control, 1 mol/L NaOH was used. The absorbance of protein in the samples was measured at 550 nm on a spectrophotometer (model Victor X4; Perkin Elmer, Waltham, MA). The shift at 550 nm results from the reagents reacting with the peptide bonds of proteins, with absorbance intensity directly proportional to the concentration of protein (Okutucu et al. 2007). The concentration of all the unknown samples was determined using the linear regression equation from absorbance values generated by the BSA standard curve.

Analysis of mineral concentrations

For mineral analysis, 1 g samples of foot tissue were submitted to the Environmental Analysis Laboratory (EAL), Southern Cross University (NATA Accreditation Number 14,960). Samples of foot tissue were dissolved in a mixture of HNO_3 (25%) and HCL (75%) (1:3, v/v) and subjected to hot-block (Hot-Block; Environmental Express, Charleston, South Carolina) acid digestion procedure (APHA, 2012). Mineral concentrations were analyzed by inductively coupled plasma mass spectrometry (ICPMS) using a NexION 300 D series ICP spectrometer with an ESI SC-FAST Auto Sampler (Perkin Elmer, Waltham, MA).

Statistical analysis

The data are expressed as means ± standard error. For parametric univariate analyses, homogeneity of the data was explored with Levene's test. Log transformation was applied if the residuals of the data in the ANOVA model were not normally distributed (Kolmogorov–Smirnoff test). Data with homogeneous variances were analyzed using Analysis of Variance (ANOVA) and *post hoc* Tukey's LSD multiple comparisons to determine differences between species. ANOVA tests were performed using the software package SPSS for windows, version 20 (IBM Corp., Armonk, New York). Multivariate data and data that could not be transformed to meet the assumptions of ANOVA were tested using permutational analyses in PRIMER v 6 + PERMANOVA add-on (v.6, PRIMERe, Pty. Ltd., Plymouth, UK). Euclidean distance similarity matrices were created from the percentage composition data for fatty acids or after normalization to the same scale for the mineral and trace element concentration analysis. One-way PERMANOVAs were run using 9999 permutations of the data to determine overall differences between species. When there was a significant species effect, post hoc pairwise tests were used to determine which pairs of species differed. Principle component ordination (PCO) was also undertaken to visually display the differences between species in fatty acids and trace elements, with vector overlay using Pearson correlation >0.8 and >0.5, respectively. In all analyses, a significance of $\alpha = 0.05$ was used.

Results

Proximate analysis

The proximate compositions of the three turban snail species are reported on a fresh weight basis in Table 1. No significant difference ($P < 0.05$) in the ash content was observed between the three different species, with an average around 2% w/w. The moisture content of *L. torquata* (68.50%) was significantly lower than the other two species ($P < 0.05$, Table 1). The lipid content varied from <5 to >9% across all species (Table 1). A one-way ANOVA with post hoc tests revealed that *L. torquata* has a significantly higher percentage of lipids in the fresh weight compared to *L. undulata* ($P < 0.05$), but neither of these species were significantly different to *T. militaris* (Table 1). Conversely, analysis of protein found that *T. militaris* had significantly lower proportions than those of *L. torquata* ($P < 0.05$) and *L. undulata* ($P < 0.05$). Protein constituted between 16 and 20% w/w protein of the flesh (Table 1). The carbohydrate content was estimated indirectly as the remaining percent weight at around 3% w/w of the flesh and showed no significant differences between species (Table 1).

Fatty acids analysis

The fatty acid composition of the lipid extracts from the foot tissue of the three species is presented in Table 2. Fatty acid profiles show a high proportion (>45%) of polyunsaturated fatty acids (PUFA) and saturated fatty acids (SFA) (>39%), and only ~14% monounsaturated fatty acids (MUFA) (Fig. 2A). The mean ratio of saturated to unsaturated fatty acids is 0.63 for *L. undulata*, 0.65 for *L. torquata*, and 0.69 for *T. militaris*. Univariate PERMANOVA revealed no significant difference between species in the percentage of MUFA ($F = 2.26$, $P > 0.05$). However, there was a significant difference between species in the percentage of SFA ($F = 5.73$, $P < 0.05$) and PUFA ($F = 5.35$, $P < 0.05$). Pairwise analyses revealed a significantly higher proportion of SFA in *T. militaris* compared to *L. torquata* ($P < 0.05$) and *L. undulata* ($P < 0.05$), but there was no significant difference in SFAs between *L. undulata* and *L. torquata* ($P > 0.05$). Pairwise analyses in the percentage of PUFA showed a significantly higher proportion of PUFA in *L. undulata* compared to *T. militaris* ($P < 0.05$), but neither of these species was significantly different to *L. torquata* ($P > 0.05$).

In all species, the SFA were dominated by palmitic acid (C16), lignoceric acid (C24), and stearic acid (C18). The MUFA with the highest levels in all the three turban snails was oleic acid (C18:1(n−9)) (Table 2). Docosapentaenoic (C22:5(n−3)), arachidonic acid (C20:5(n−6)), docosadienoic (C22:2(n−6)), and eicosapentaenoic (20:5(n−3)) were identified as the primary PUFAs (Table 2).

The foot tissues of the three turban snails have a mean n−3: n−6 ratio of 1.36 for *L. torquata*, 1.15 for *L. undulata*, and 1.09 for *T. militaris* (Fig. 2B). Univariate PERMANOVA revealed a significant difference in the percent of n−3 ($F = 14.16$, $P < 0.05$) and n−6 ($F = 11.45$, $P < 0.05$) fatty acids between species. Pairwise analyses for the n−3 fatty acids revealed significantly lower levels in *T. militaris* compared to *L. undulata* ($P < 0.05$) and *L. torquata* ($P < 0.05$), whereas n−6 fatty acids were significant lower in *L. torquata* compared to *T. militaris* ($P < 0.05$) and *L. undulata* ($P < 0.05$) (Fig. 2B).

Multivariate analysis using PERMANOVA revealed that there was a significant difference in the overall fatty acid composition between the three species of turban snails ($F = 7.39$, $P < 0.05$). Pairwise tests revealed that the composition of fatty acids was different between each pair of species ($P < 0.05$). A Principal Component Ordination (PCO) was used to explore the differences in the fatty acid profiles of the three turban snails. Separation along the X axis distinguishes *L. torquata* which is characterized by higher docosapentaenoic (C22:5(n−3)) and palmitic acids (C16) and *L. undulata* which contains high stearic acid (C18) and a tendency toward high α linolenic (C18:3 (n−3)) and eicosenoic acid (C20:1(n−9)) (Fig. 3). Separated along the Y axis is driven by *T. militaris* which is characterized by higher docosadienoic (C22:2(n−6)), lignoceric (C24), and margaric acid (C17:0) (Fig. 3).

Table 1. Proximate analysis of the foot tissue from three different turban snails.

Species	Proximate contents (%)				
	Ash	Moisture	Lipid	Protein	Carbohydrate
L. torquata[1]	2.10 ± 0.14	68.50 ± 0.64^{a}	8.46 ± 0.52^{a}	18.03 ± 0.41^{a}	2.92 ± 0.50
L. undulata	1.97 ± 0.11	70.83 ± 0.95^{b}	5.20 ± 0.61^{b}	18.49 ± 0.47^{a}	3.51 ± 0.53
T. militaris[1]	2.14 ± 0.05	73.08 ± 1.15^{b}	5.57 ± 1.07^{ab}	16.19 ± 0.11^{b}	3.02 ± 0.52

Significant differences between species ($P < 0.05$) are indicated by different superscript letters in the same column.
[1]Means and ± SEs from 4 replicates (except *L. undulata* = 6 replicates).

Table 2. The fatty acid compositions of three turban snails (% of total fatty acids).

Fatty acid	Trivial name	*L. torquata* (*n* = 4)	*L. undulata* (*n* = 6)	*T. militaris* (*n* = 4)
C14:0	Myristic	0.55 ± 0.05	0.96 ± 0.05	0.13 ± 0.05
C15:0	Pentadecanoic	1.18 ± 0.12	1.08 ± 0.09	1.49 ± 0.10
C16:0	Palmitic	23.01 ± 0.41	21.62 ± 0.41	22.12 ± 0.37
C17:0	Margaric	2.39 ± 0.04	1.87 ± 0.09	2.99 ± 0.10
C18:0	Stearic	5.68 ± 0.14	6.59 ± 0.15	5.45 ± 0.08
C24.0	Lignoceric	7.14 ± 0.33	6.49 ± 0.35	7.65 ± 0.22
C16:1	Palmitoleic	3.24 ± 0.10	2.41 ± 0.14	3.00 ± 0.13
C18:1(*n*−9)	Oleic	8.21 ± 0.22	8.41 ± 0.17	7.89 ± 0.18
C20:1(*n*−9)	Eicosenoic	2.77 ± 0.07	3.56 ± 0.17	2.86 ± 0.12
C22:1(*n*−9)	Erucic	0.23 ± 0.03	0.45 ± 0.06	0.30 ± 0.04
C18:2(*n*−6)(LA)	Linoleic	1.60 ± 0.14	2.82 ± 0.09	2.92 ± 0.23
C18:3(*n*−3)(ALA)	a- Linoleic	0.87 ± 0.12	2.33 ± 0.09	1.87 ± 0.20
C20:2	11, 13- Eicosadienoic	0.06 ± 0.02	0.21 ± 0.03	0.13 ± 0.02
C20:3(*n*−3)(ETA)	Eicosatrienoic	0.16 ± 0.01	0.43 ± 0.05	0.27 ± 0.05
C20:4(*n*−6)(ARA)	Arachidonic	14.93 ± 0.44	16.01 ± 0.24	15.06 ± 0.25
C20:5(*n*−3)(EPA)	Eicosapentaenoic	5.29 ± 0.25	4.63 ± 0.30	3.70 ± 0.12
C22:2	5, 13- Docosadienoic	6.61 ± 0.35	5.83 ± 0.21	7.48 ± 0.24
C22:6(*n*−3)(DHA)	Docosahexaenoic	0.80 ± 0.23	0.53 ± 0.04	0.37 ± 0.02
C22:5(*n*−3)(DPA)	Docosapentaenoic	15.27 ± 0.52	13.79 ± 0.26	13.33 ± 0.10

Values are mean value ± SEs (% of total fatty acids)

Minerals

The mean concentrations of macronutrients and trace elements found in the foot tissue of the three Turbinidae species are summarized in Table 3. Sodium (Na), potassium (K), calcium (Ca), magnesium (Mg), phosphorus (P), sulfur (S), iron (Fe), copper (Cu), zinc (Zn), molybdenum (Mo), cobalt (Co), selenium (Se), manganese (Mn), aluminum (Al), arsenic (As), cadmium (Cd), chromium (Cr), nickel (Ni), cobalt (Co), lead (Pb), silver (Ag), and mercury (Hg) were assessed in edible foot tissue of the three species. The most abundant mineral was S with the lowest concentration of 8.37 mg/g of the fresh weight found in *T. militaris*. Na and K were also high in all three species, whereas Ca in *L. torquata* was found in higher concentrations than the other two species (Table 3). Among the other elements, *L. undulata* had the highest concentrations of Fe (41.10 ± 3.12 mg/Kg) and Zn (15.20 ± 0.99 mg/Kg).

PERMANOVA analysis on the normalized macroelemental composition revealed a significant difference between the three species ($F = 9.38$, $P < 0.05$). Pairwise tests confirmed that the composition of macroelements was different between all pairs of species ($P < 0.05$). The PCO plot illustrates the difference in macronutrient composition between the three species (Fig. 4A). There is greater variation between individuals of *L. torquata* and *T. militaris*, whereas *L. undulata* form a relatively tight cluster of points characterized by higher sulfur, potassium, and phosphorus. The X axis is largely driven by one outlier of T. militaris, which is characterized by higher sodium and magnesium (Fig. 4A).

For the microelements, PERMANOVA analysis found a significant difference between species ($F = 3.34$, $P < 0.05$). Pairwise analyses revealed significantly different microelement concentrations only between *L. undulata* and *T. militaris* ($P < 0.05$), whereas *L. torquata* was not different to either *T. militaris* ($P > 0.05$) or *L. undulata* ($P > 0.05$). PCO of the microelements (Fig. 4B) reveals a similar pattern as observed for the macroelements (Fig. 4B). *L. undulata* tends to have a relatively tight cluster of samples with relatively more zinc compared to the other species (Fig. 4B, Table 3), whereas *T. militaris* shows a tendency toward higher copper and relatively less Zn than *L. undulata*. Samples of *L. torquata* are interspersed across the full range of the other two species, consistent with no significant differences in the micronutrient composition.

PERMANOVA analysis identified a significant difference between three species ($F = 2.46$, $P < 0.05$) for trace heavy metals. However, pairwise comparison confirmed there was a significant difference only between *T. militaris* and *L. undulata* ($P < 0.05$), whereas *L. torquata* was not different to either *T. militaris* ($P > 0.05$) or *L. undulata* ($P > 0.05$). PCO was used to explore the differences in the heavy metal composition between the three species (Fig. 4 C). Tighter clustering in *L. undulata* with higher cadmium, appears to explain the difference between *L. undulata* and *T. militaris*, whereas *T. militaris* tends to

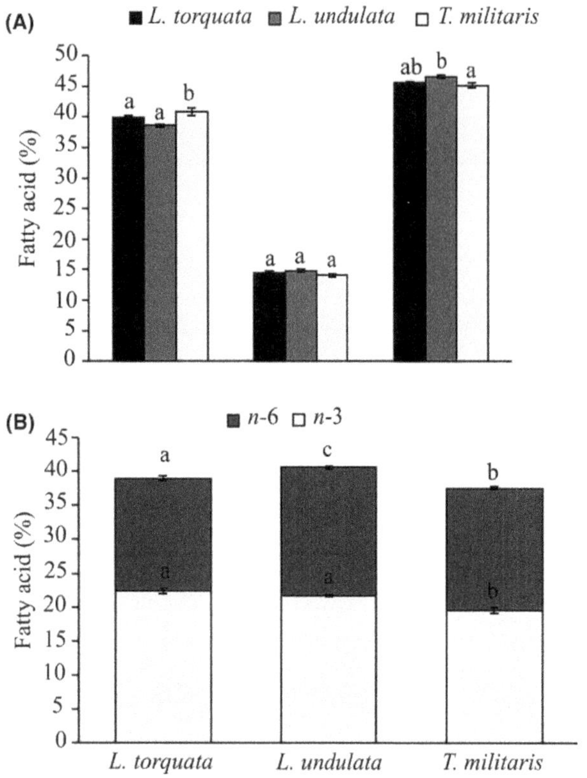

Figure 2. The composition of fatty acids for the three turbinid species with A) the proportion of saturated fatty acid; SFA, monounsaturated fatty acid; MUFA, and polyunsaturated fatty acid; PUFA and B) the proportion of n-3 and n-6 fatty acids. Results are presented as mean ± SE. Different superscripts above indicate significant difference between species, with separate univariate PERMANOVAs performed for each class of fatty acid ($P < 0.05$).

have higher nickel. The X axis is driven by one outlier of *L. torquata* which characterized by higher chromium, silver, and arsenic.

Discussion

Evaluation of the nutritional content of three Australian species in the Turbinidae family of gastropod molluscs indicates that these turban snails have good nutritional value, comparable to other shellfish from the other parts of the world. The main outcomes of this study are consistent with previous research on marine molluscs showing high protein (Linehan et al. 1999; Dridi et al. 2007; Periyasamy et al. 2011), as well as low lipid content, which is high in essential fatty acids (Nichols et al. 1998; Chan et al. 2004; Laxmilatha 2009) and a rich source of essential minerals such as zinc (Zn) and iron (Fe). Overall, this study supports the nutritional value of these Australian Turbinidae species and inclusion as part of a healthful human diet.

Protein plays a vital role in molluscs as it serves as an energy supply (Mao et al. 2006). The range of protein content in this study of 16% to 19% of the fresh weight is comparable to other herbivorous gastropods, for example, abalone (Haliotidae), which were reported to have 18.0 ± 0.7% (Chiou et al. 2001) and the turbinid *Cookia sulcata* which was found to contain 17.5 ± 1.5% of protein in the foot tissue (Mason et al. 2014). By comparison, studies on predatory gastropod whelks have generally found higher protein than that reported for herbivores, for example, the Muricidae *Chicoreus ramosus* 36% (Xavier Ramesh and Ayyakkannu 1992); *Hexaplex trunculus* 48% (Zarai et al. 2011); *Rapana venosa* 55.88 ± 2.04% (Celik et al. 2014) and as high as 80% in *Thais haemastoma* (Belisle and Stickle 1978). *Babylonia spirata*, which belongs to another family of predatory and scavenging whelks (Babyloniidae), was reported to exhibit a similar range of protein (53.86%), as found in Muricidae whelks (Periyasamy et al. 2011). Although the trophic niche appears to influence the protein content in gastropod molluscs, with higher contents in predators, the level of protein detected in Turbinidae in this study still suggests that these herbivorous snails are a very good potential source of protein. The protein content can vary depending on the organism, different body parts and seasonal variations (Smoothey 2013). In this study, only the foot tissue was sampled and all species were collected from the same place at the same time of year for standardized comparison. Future studies on the spatial and temporal changes of biochemical composition over the reproductive cycle are therefore recommended.

After proteins, lipids were the next most dominant organic component of the Turbinidae flesh. According to previous findings, the foot tissue of gastropods commonly has less than 10% w/w lipid content (Mclachlan and Lombard 1980; Chiou et al. 2001; Ramesh and Ravichandran 2008; Saito and Aono 2014). The lipid content often appears to be lower (0.5–5% w/w) in predatory gastropods (Belisle and Stickle 1978; Xavier Ramesh and Ayyakkannu 1992; Vasconcelos et al. 2009; Merdzhanova et al. 2014), in comparison to the herbivorous Turbinidae (5–9% w/w, Table 1). Similarly, herbivorous abalone *Haliotis tuberculata* were found to contain up to 6.46% lipid in their foot tissue (Hernandez et al. 2013). Lipid content in the viscera of gastropods appears to be higher than the foot tissue, ranging from 15 to 17% (Chiou et al. 2001). It has been suggested that the visceral tissue is the main storage of site for lipids in gastropods (Dunstan et al. 1996; Saito and Aono 2014). However, in this study we only focused on the foot tissue, since the viscera are not typically consumed by people in larger gastropods. Overall these findings confirm that the foot tissue of gastropods is suitable for inclusion in a high protein, low fat human diet.

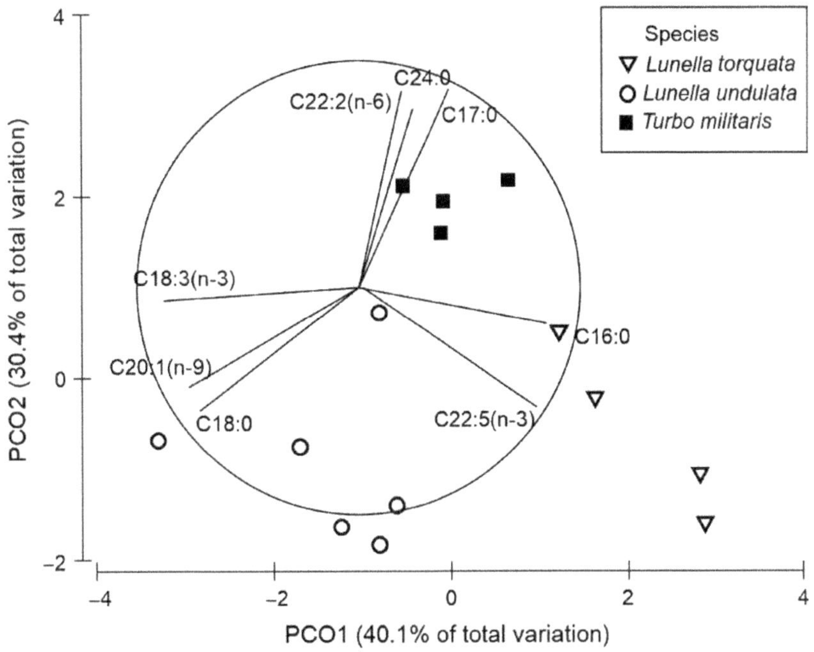

Figure 3. Principle component ordination (PCO) of the fatty acids profiles from the three turban snails based on a Euclidian distance similarity matrix of the percent composition data with vector overlay from Pearsons correlation >0.8.

Table 3. Trace elements compositions in three species of turban snails.

Elements	*L. torquata* (*n* = 4)	*L. undulata* (*n* = 6)	*T. militaris* (*n* = 4)
Macroelements (mg/g FW)			
Na	3.01 ± 0.12	2.70 ± 0.16	4.00 ± 0.34
K	3.05 ± 0.07	3.33 ± 0.06	2.73 ± 0.08
Ca	2.39 ± 1.11	0.44 ± 0.11	0.61 ± 0.28
Mg	0.69 ± 0.02	0.65 ± 0.03	0.77 ± 0.05
P	1.53 ± 0.09	1.64 ± 0.05	1.22 ± 0.03
S	11.22 ± 0.30	12.32 ± 0.31	8.37 ± 0.18
Microelements (mg/Kg FW)			
Fe	32.42 ± 6.93	41.10 ± 3.12	19.32 ± 1.04
Zn	14.01 ± 1.03	15.20 ± 0.99	12.21 ± 0.89
Cu	1.14 ± 0.12	0.55 ± 0.11	2.18 ± 0.29
Mo	0.15 ± 0.08	0.07 ± 0.004	0.10 ± 0.01
Co	0.03 ± 0.01	0.05 ± 0.01	0.02 ± 0.00
Se	0.177 ± 0.06	0.144 ± 0.02	0.177 ± 0.04
Toxic elements (mg/Kg FW)			
Mn	0.49 ± 0.08	0.45 ± 0.07	0.49 ± 0.14
Al	8.73 ± 4.80	11.12 ± 2.29	0
As	8.84 ± 3.69	5.03 ± 0.53	8.52 ± 1.44
Cd	0.06 ± 0.01	0.05 ± 0.004	0.04 ± 0.01
Cr	0.46 ± 0.33	0.10 ± 0.03	0.17 ± 0.01
Ni	0.05 ± 0.03	0.06 ± 0.02	0.14 ± 0.02
Pb	1.09 ± 0.19	1.04 ± 0.15	2.05 ± 0.62
Ag	0.15 ± 0.03	0.17 ± 0.05	0.04 ± 0.01
Hg	0.007 ± 0.004	0.004 ± 0.002	0.001 ± 0.001

All data presented based on fresh weight. Values are mean value and ± SE: n, number of samples.

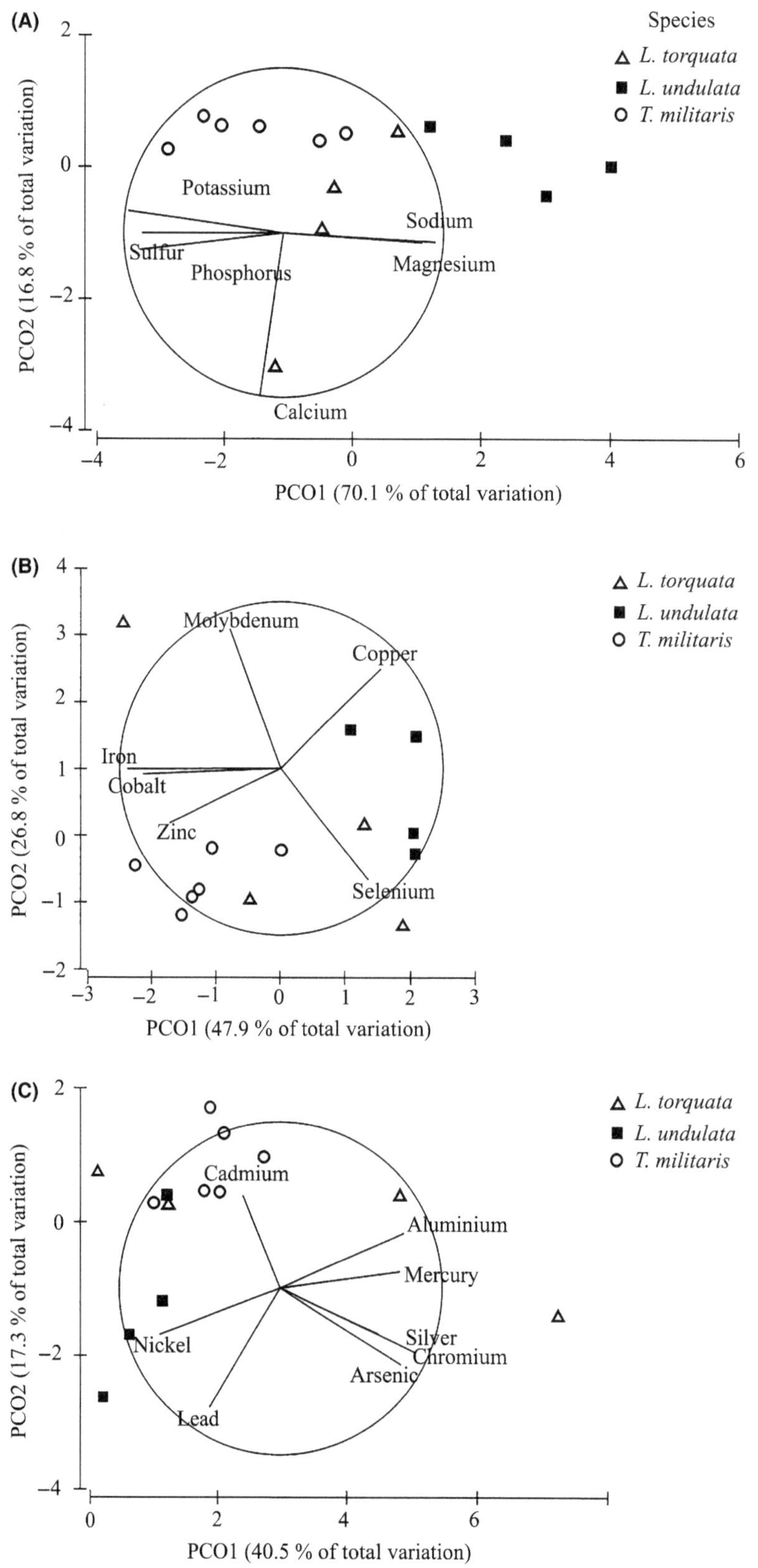

Figure 4. PCO plotted for (A) macro element, (B) microelement, and (C) toxic elements composition of the three turban snails based on a Euclidian distance similarity matrix of the percent composition data with vector overlay from Pearson's correlation >0.5.

This study presents the fatty acid compositions of the foot tissue of three edible Turbinidae *L. torquata*, *T. militaris*, and *L. undulata* from New South Wales, Australia. Palmitic acid (C16:0) is the dominant saturated fatty acid found in all three turban species. This finding is in agreement with previous studies on other molluscs, for example, *Haliotis fulgens*, the pulmonate land snail *Helix aspersa maxima* and the oyster *Crassostrea rhizophorae* (Nelson et al. 2002; Milinsk et al. 2003; Martino and Cruz 2004). According to Gabbott (1983), palmitic acid is the major end-product of fatty acid synthesis in animal tissue and is the precursor for *de novo* synthesis of long-chain saturated and unsaturated fatty acids. It is not surprising that Turbinidae have a high proportion of palmitic acid since they mainly feed on macroalgae, which have also been found to contain a high proportion of C16 saturated acid (Freiji and Awadh 2010; Saito and Aono 2014).

Other dominant fatty acids found in the Turbinidae (C18:1(n−9): oleic acid, C20:4(n−6): ARA, and C22:5(n−3): DPA) are very similar to those previously reported from other gastropods, including *Haliotis laevigata*, *Haliotis rubra*, and *Turbo cornutus* (Dunstan et al. 1996; Saito and Aono 2014). In contrast, previous studies on the lipid composition of bivalves (e.g., *Donax deltoides*, *Dosinia caerulea*, and *Perna canaliculus*) indicates that bivalves have relatively higher percentages of EPA and DHA, as opposed to ARA and DPA (Nichols et al. 1998; Mooney et al. 2002). Essential fatty acids such as EPA, DHA, and ARA, cannot be synthesized by molluscs and must be obtained from their food intake. Due to this, the quality and quantity of the food is likely to be the main source of variation in these PUFAs from molluscan tissue. Turban snails are generalist herbivores that feed on a variety of macroalgae (Foster and Hodgson 1998; Davis et al. 2005). Consequently, subtle differences in the macroalgal diet of the three species could explain the significant differences in fatty acid composition between these species collected from the same location.

Several studies comparing the fatty acid composition of marine algae have demonstrated differences between green, red, and brown algae. For example, the green macroalgae, *Caulerpa* sp. was found to be dominated by shorter chain trienoic acids including C16:3 and C18:3 (ALA), whereas the brown algae *Cladosiphon* sp. contained C18 and C20 PUFAs including C18:4(n−3), ARA, and EPA (Saito and Marty 2010). C16:3 was also found in the green alga *Enteromorpha*, but not in *Ulva* or several species of red and brown algae (Ragonese et al. 2014). A study on the dietary preferences of *Lunella undulatus* found that they will only consume low levels of *Caulerpa* when offered no choice and much prefer to feed on less chemically defended algae, such as *Ulva* and brown foliose algae (Davis et al. 2005). Furthermore, *L. torquata* feeding was significantly deterred by *Caulpera* extracts (Davis et al. 2005). This is consistent with absence of C16:3 in the turban snails. On the other hand, small amounts of DPA were detected in *Caulerpa* (Saito and Marty 2010), but not in a range of other algae (Ragonese et al. 2014). The turban snails have relatively, high proportions of DPA (>13%) compared to all algae (<1%), but lower proportions of DHA (<1%). DHA was primarily detected in brown algae (1–2%), but was absent in the green algae, including *Ulva* (Ragonese et al. 2014). A number of reports have confirmed the small DHA amount in other gastropod species such as *Littorina littorea* (Ackman and Hooper 1973), *Haliotis laevigata* and *Haliotis rubra* (Dunstan et al. 1996). A seasonal study on adult green abalone, *Haliotis fulgens* found that they have higher DPA in foot tissue when fed the chlorophyte *Ulva lobata* (8.3–12.2%), compared to those fed on the phaeophyte *Egregia menziesii* (5.7–11.8%) or the rhodophyte *Chondracanthus canaliculatus* (7.9–10.9%) (Nelson et al. 2002). These findings confirm that the macroalgae consumed by herbivorous gastropods can influence the overall fatty acid composition and may explain some of the differences between individuals and species. Other biotic and environmental factors such as reproductive status, salinity, temperature, and food availability can also influence the fatty acid compositions of marine organisms (Milinsk et al. 2003; Ozogul et al. 2005).

Among the fatty acids, long-chain PUFAs such as EPA, DHA, DPA, and ARA are found to have health, as well as nutritional benefits to humans, since they are important for reducing cholesterol levels and coronary heart disease, as well as helping to prevent arteriosclerosis and inflammation (Mahaffey 2004; Mahaffey et al. 2008). These PUFAs have been previously reported from a range of marine molluscs including *Ruditapes decussatus*, *Haliotis asinina*, *Unio terminalis*, *Patella depressa*, *Crassostrea gigas*, *Pinctada fucata martensii*, *Turbo cornutus*, and *Ifremeria nautilei* (Morais et al. 2003; Perez-Comacho et al. 2003; Saito 2004; Ersoy and Sereflisan 2010; Freiji and Awadh 2010; Saito and Hashimoto 2010, 2010; Bautista-Teruel et al. 2011). In this study, the levels of DHA in foot tissue of turban snails was relatively low, but high proportions of EPA, DPA, and the n−6 fatty acid ARA were detected. DHA was also found to be relatively low in abalone tissue (*Haliotis fulgens*) (Nelson et al. 2002). Another study confirmed that abalone (*Haliotis rubra* and *Haliotis laevigata*), have higher DPA, similar to the turbinids, which could due to the capability of the herbivorous gastropods to retrospectively convert DHA to DPA (Dunstan et al. 1996).

The ratio of n−3 to n−6 fatty acids is a good indicator for measuring the nutritional value of fatty foods. Based on the Department of Health (UK) guidelines, the maximum recommended ratio of n−3 to n−6 is 4 (Milinsk et al. 2003). In this study, the ratio of n−3 to n−6 in the three Turbinidae species was less than 1, which is a very healthful ratio, due to high quantities of ARA and DPA. This is consistent with a previous study on *L. undulata*, which reported a ratio of n−3 to n−6 = 0.9 (Mooney et al. 2002). By comparison, a study on *Turbo coronatus* from Bahrain reported that the ratio of n−3 to n−6 was almost 2 (Freiji and Awadh 2010), whereas Australian *Haliotis* spp. range from 1.2 to 1.7 (Mooney et al. 2002). There is much evidence that the early human ancestors consumed diets with n−3 to n−6 ratio 1:1 (Simopoulos 2002), but this ratio has changed considerably in recent centuries with a bias toward more n−6 (Martino and Cruz 2004). The imbalance of n−3 to n−6 ratio has been linked to a large number of diseases, such as cardiovascular disorders and cancer (Martino and Cruz 2004; Freiji and Awadh 2010). This study reveals that turban snails have potential to contribute to a healthful diet by providing a good source of long-chain PUFA, particularly DPA and ARA.

This study also investigated the ash content and inorganic elements from the Turbinidae flesh. The flesh was found to contain approximately 2% ash w/w. In a previous study on Haliotidae, the ash content of the abalone muscle was similar (1.8%) to Turbinidae, although a higher ash content was reported from the viscera tissue, with 2.8% w/w. Another study on the predatory gastropod *Dicathais orbita* revealed that the snails fed on different diets had different ash content (ranging from 3.5 to 8%) (Woodcock and Benkendorff 2008), thus suggesting that the percentage of ash could be influenced by the proportion of inorganic materials bioaccumulated at higher trophic levels. However, unlike the lipid composition, we found no significant difference in the total ash content of the three Turbinidae species (Table 1), despite the fact that they may have been feeding on different algae. Nevertheless, we did find interspecies differences in the mineral concentrations.

Molluscs have been considered as a good bioindicators for minerals and trace element availability in the surrounding environment (Cravo and Bebianno 2005). The most abundant macroelements in the turban snail's foot tissue were sulfur (S), potassium (K), and sodium (Na). These results are consistent with those of other studies on another turbinid *C. sulcata* as well as the land snail, *Helix pomatia* (Ozogul et al. 2005; Mason et al. 2014) with ranges of S, K, and Na of 5.5–6.0 mg/g, 0.8–3.0 mg/g, and 0.9–4.1 mg/g, respectively. However, sulfur was much higher in our study on east coast Australian turbinids (8–13 mg/g), when compared with *C. sulcata* from New Zealand (Mason et al. 2014). Sulfur is a common dominant inorganic mineral found in seawater and is one of the most essential elements present in animals, as it is incorporated into amino acids, proteins, enzymes, vitamins, and other biomolecules (Komarnisky et al. 2003; Waska et al. 2008). There is no maximum recommendation for sulfur intake in humans (Komarnisky et al. 2003). Turban snails also have relatively high concentrations of sodium (Na) (up to 4 mg/g) tissue, but a 100 g meal of any of these species remains well under the recommended upper level intake for humans, which is 2.3 g per day (National Health and Medical Research Council, 2006). The recommended daily intake (RDI) for potassium (K) is 3 g a day (National Health and Medical Research Council, 2006), which is corresponds to 1000 g of turban snails meat. Turban snails are not a very rich source of K but they appear to be a very good source of other microelements, which are considered essential minerals for human consumption. Iron (Fe) is among the major minerals found in all species and serves vital functions, such as carrying oxygen in hemoglobin of vertebrates (Erkan 2011). This oxygen carrying role is performed by copper (Cu) in hemocyanin in marine molluscs (Bryan et al. 1977; Stoeva et al. 1997), resulting in relatively high copper in the microelement composition. The turbinids in this study seem to have comparable Fe and Cu content to *Haliotis rubra* from southern Australian waters, which contain 7–31 mg/kg of Fe and 0.4–2.4 mg/kg of Cu (Skinner et al. 2004). All these gastropods fall under the upper limit of Fe and Cu uptake for humans, which is 45 mg/day for Fe and up to 10 mg/day for Cu (National Health and Medical Research Council, 2006) (WHO, 2003).

Zn is another important element with multiple biochemical functions in humans (Scherz and Kirchhoff 2006). For prevention of diseases, the recommended tolerable upper intake for Zn is 40 mg/day (National Health and Medical Research Council, 2006). The turban snails in this study contain up to 16 mg/kg of Zn in their tissue suggesting a 100 g meal of these snails could contribute up to 4% the daily required Zn intake. Previous studies have found a variable range in the Zn content of other molluscs, for example cockles 8.06 mg/kg and mussels 21.2 mg/kg (Guerin et al. 2011). In a previous study on abalone, Zn concentration was found to correlate with concentrations in algae and water; as the Zn increased in the algae, Zn also increased in water and abalone (Lin and Liao 1999). This further supports the idea that the level of microelements in an organism reflects the type of food that they feed on (Jakimska et al. 2011).

As a risk assessment, the Joint FAO/WHO Expert Committee on Food Additives (JECFA) have developed safe limit guidelines for chemicals, including heavy metals in human food, based on the recommendations by the

World Health Organization (Herrman and Younes 1999). These limits are represented as provisional tolerable weekly intakes (PTWI) (Table 4) to indicate the maximum safe levels an individual can consume each week per kilogram of body weight (Mamtani et al. 2011). Among the nonessential minerals, strikingly elevated arsenic (As) concentrations were found in the foot tissues of three species of turban snails, ranging from 5 to 9 mg/kg. Arsenic is relatively common in the marine environment and can often be concentrated in seafood (Moreda-Pineiro et al. 2012). However, Arsenic can exist in two forms: organic and inorganic (Ruttens et al. 2012; Mason et al. 2014), with the organic forms of relatively low toxicity, whereas inorganic forms present the greater hazard (Edmonds and Francesconi 1993). The Australian New Zealand food standard recommends the inorganic As concentration should be below a maximum of 1 mg/kg (FSANZ, 2004) (Table 4). In this study, we only measured total As levels and these ranged from 5 mg/kg in *L. undulata* to 8.8 mg/kg in *L. torquata*. In other gastropods, such as abalone, the inorganic As proportion constituted a maximum 1% of total As (Fabris et al. 2006) and a similar proportion was reported by Sloth et al. (2005) after analyzing a variety of seafood samples including fish, bivalves, and crustaceans. Assuming a similar ratio of less than 1% of the total arsenic is inorganic in Turbinidae flesh, the levels found in this study are not likely to constitute a risk to human health.

The highest level of aluminum (Al) concentrations were found in *L. undulata* (11.12 mg/kg) but this element was not detected at all in *T. militaris*. Mason et al. (2014) reported that Al concentrations in the *C. sulcata* ranged from 14.8 to 15.9 mg/kg. In contrast, two bivalve species, *Chamelea gallina* and *Donax trunculus* in Turkey had accumulated Al concentrations that were much higher (Özden et al. 2009). The PTWI for total Al is 2 mg/kg of body weight (Table 4), suggesting the Turbinids should not be consumed regularly in large quantities.

Lead (Pb) is a toxic element that exists in water mostly in particulate form and accumulates in marine organisms (Özden et al. 2009). In this study, Pb concentrations were higher in *T. militaris* (2.05 mg/kg) compared to the other species. This value only just exceeds the maximum range concentration for Australian and New Zealand food safety standard in molluscs of 2 mg/kg (Abbott et al. 2003) (Table 4). Colakoglu et al. (2011) reported that the highest Pb concentrations in the venerid clam from Turkey, *Chamelea gallina* was 3.24 mg/kg, which was higher than this study. As filter feeders, bivalves are more likely to ingest particulate lead than herbivorous gastropods. Average Pb concentration was 0.04 mg/kg in abalone (*H. tuberculata*) (Noel et al. 2011). It is recommended not to consume more than one kilogram of *T. militaris* in a day to maintain a daily lead intake below the recommended level. Gastropod meat rarely constitutes a major portion of people's diets, especially in more developed countries. So the occasional intake of metals above the recommended concentration does not necessarily equate to large intakes over time. In the case of lead the PWTI is 0.025 mg/kg of body weight (FSANZ (2011); Table 4), which is equivalent to 1.75 mg for a 70 kg adult. Serving of 100 g of turban snails could only contribute to 0.2 mg of Pb at the maximum detected level of total Pb of 2.05 mg/kg.

On the other hand, other toxic elements do not exceed the maximum amount as recommended (Table 4). However, similar to biochemical composition, mineral composition of marine foods can vary with seasonal and biological differences (species, size, age, sex, and sexual maturity), geographical area, food availability, and environmental conditions (temperature, contamination) (Cravo and Bebianno 2005; Scherz and Kirchhoff 2006; Kilic and Belivermis 2013; Bilandzic et al. 2014). Consequently, future studies should investigate the temporal and spatial variation in proximate and elemental composition of these Turbinidae from all major fisheries locations.

Table 4. The maximum permitted levels of toxic elements in seafood and their provisional tolerable weekly intake (PTWI) based on the Australian New Zealand standards.

Toxic element	Maximum Limit (mg/kg)	Reference	PTWI (mg/kg) body weight	Reference
Al	NA		2.0	(FSANZ, 2011)
As (inorganic)	1.0	(Abbott et al. 2003; FSANZ, 2004)	NA	(FSANZ, 2011)
Cd	2.0	(FSANZ, 2004)	0.03	(FSANZ, 2011)
Cr	NA		0.2	(FSANZ, 2013)
Pb	2.0	(Abbott et al. 2003)	0.025	(FSANZ, 2011)
Hg	0.5	(FSANZ, 2004)	0.004–0.005	(Rodellar et al. 2010; FSANZ, 2011)

NA= not applicable.

Conclusion

This study provides the first comprehensive assessment of the proximate and elemental composition of marine Turbinidae gastropods from NSW Australia. These findings suggest that in general, the three species of turbinids show minor differences in proximate content. However, all three species can be considered as a healthful food source, similar to other accepted molluscs such as abalone. Further research should be carried out to identify factors influencing variation in the proximate composition of the turbinid snails, including effects of the reproductive cycle, age/size, and site-specific environmental pollution. Further work could help promote consumer acceptance of Turbinidae as a new meat source and value-add the mollusc fishing industry in countries such as Australia, where relatively few species are consumed by the majority of the population.

Acknowledgments

The research was funded by the postgraduate research funding from the School of Environment, Science and Engineering and Marine Ecology Research Centre, Southern Cross University. The authors gratefully acknowledge the Ministry of Higher Education of Malaysia for the PhD scholarship for the first author. We also wish to thank Mrs. Roselyn Regino and Mrs. Bijayalakshmi Nongmaithem for commented on drafts of the paper.

Conflict of Interest

None declared.

References

Abbott, P., J. Baines, P. Fox, L. Graf, L. Kelly, G. Standley, et al. 2003. Review of the regulations for contaminants and natural toxicants. Food Control 14:383–389.

Ackman, R. G., and S. N. Hooper. 1973. Non-methylene-interrupted fatty acids in lipids of shallow-water marine invertebrates: A comparison of two molluscs (*Littorina littorea* and *Lunatia triseriata*) with the sand shrimp (*Crangon septemspinosus*). Comp. Biochem. Phys. 46B:153–165.

APHA. 2012. Standard methods for the examination of water and wastewater, 22nd ed.. American Public Health Association, Washington, D.C.

Bautista- Teruel, M., S. S. Koshio, and M. Ishikawa. 2011. Diet development and evaluation for juvenile abalone, *Haliotis asinina* Linne: Lipid and essential fatty acid levels. Aquaculture 312:172–179.

Belisle, B. W., and W. B. Stickle. 1978. Seasonal patterns in the biochemical constituents and body component indexes of the muricid gastropod, *Thais haemastoma*. Biol. Bull. 155:259–272.

Bilandzic, N., M. Sedak, M. Dokic, I. Varenina, B. S. Kolanovic, D. Bozic, et al. 2014. Determination of zinc concentrations in foods of animal origin, fish and shellfish from Croatia and assessment of their contribution to dietary intake. J. Food Composit Anal. 35:61–66.

Bille, L., G. Binato, V. Cappa, M. Toson, P. D. Pozza, G. Arcangeli, et al. 2015. Lead, mercury and cadmium levels in edible marine molluscs and echinoderms from the Veneto Region (north- western Adriatic Sea- Italy). Food Control 50:362–370.

Bligh, E. G., and W. J. Dyer. 1959. A rapid method of total lipid extraction and purification. Can. J. Biochem. Physiol. 37:911–917.

Bouchet, P. 2015. *Lunella undulata* (Lightfoot, 1786). In: MolluscaBase (2015). Accessed through: World Register of Marine Species. Available at www.marinespecies.org/aphia.php?p=taxdetails&id=579271 (accessed 15 December 2015).

Brazao, S., S. Morais, D. Boaventura, P. Re, L. Narciso, and S. J. Hawkins. 2003. Spatial and temporal variation of the fatty acid composition of *Patella* spp. (Gastropoda: Prosobranchia) soft bodies and gonads. Comp. Biochem. Physiol. Part B 136:425–441.

Brooks, S. P. J., B. J. Lampi, G. Sarwar, and H. G. Botting. 1995. A comparison of methods for determining total body protein. Anal. Biochem. 226:26–30.

Bryan, G. W., G. W. Potts, and G. R. Forster. 1977. Heavy metals in the gastropod mollusc Haliotis tuberculata (L.). J. Mar. Biol. Ass. U.K. 57:379–390.

Celik, M. Y., S. T. Culha, M. Culha, H. Yildiz, S. Acarli, I. Celik, et al. 2014. Comparative study on biochemical composition of some edible marine molluscs at Canakkale coasts. Turkey. Indian J. GeoMarine Sci. 43:601–606.

Chan, K. Y., Q. F. Gao, K. M. Yip, W. H. Wong, P. K. S. Shin, and S. G. Cheung. 2004. Lipid content and fatty acid composition in the green- lipped mussel *Perna viridis* (L.). J. Food Lipids 11:123–130.

Chen, M. H., Y. W. Chiu, A. Alf, K. Soong, and J. J. Li. 2004. Species and abundance of the edible turban snails *Turbo* spp. In intertidal areas of Hengchun Peninsula, southern Taiwan. Journal of National Parks 14:1–9.

Chiou, T., M. Lai, and C. Shiau. 2001. Seasonal variations of chemical constituents in the muscle and viscera of small abalone fed different diets. Fisheries Sci. 67:146–156.

Chouvelon, T., M. Warnau, C. Churlaud, and P. Bustamante. 2009. Hg concentrations and related risk assessment in coral reef crustaceans, molluscs and fish from New Caledonia. Environ. Pollut. 157:331–340.

Colakoglu, F. A., H. B. Ormanci, N. Berik, and I. E. Kunili. 2011. Proximate and elemental composition of *Chamelea gallina* from the Southern Coast of the Marmara Sea (Turkey). Biol. Trace Elem. Res. 143:983–991.

Cooling, K., and S. D. A. Smith. 2015. Population dynamics of *Turbo militaris* (Gastropoda: Turbinidae) on rocky shores in a subtropical marine park: implications for management. Molluscan Research. 35:173–181.

Cravo, A., and M. J. Bebianno. 2005. Bioaccumulation of metals in the soft tissue of *Patella aspera*: Application of metal/ shell weight indices. Estuar. Coast. Shelf Sci. 65:571–586.

Cubadda, F., M. E. Conti, and L. Campanella. 2001. Size-dependent concentrations of trace metals in four Mediterranean gastropods. Chemosphere 45:561–569.

Davis, A. R., K. Benkendorff, and R. D. Ward. 2005. Responses of common SE Australian herbivores to three suspected invasive *Caulerpa* spp. Mar. Biol. 146:859–868.

Dey, M. M. 2015. World and U.S. demand and supply relationships for seafood: Implications for aquaculture producers. Aquaculture Magazine. 41(2):44–45.

Diana, J. S. 2009. Aquaculture production and biodiversity conservation. J. Bioscience. 59:27–38.

Dridi, S., M. S. Romdhane, and M. Elcafsi. 2007. Seasonal variation in weight and biochemical composition of the Pacific oyster, *Crassostrea gigas* in relation to the gametogenic cycle and environmental conditions of the Bizert Lagoon. Tunisia. Aquaculture. 263:238–248.

Dunstan, G. A., H. J. Baillie, S. M. Barret, and J. K. Volkman. 1996. Effect of diet on the lipid composition of wild and cultured abalone. Aquaculture 40:115–127.

Duquesne, S., M. Liess, and D. J. Bird. 2004. Sub-lethal effects of metal exposure: physiological and behavioural responses of the estuarine bivalve *Macoma balthica*. Mar. Environ. Res. 58:245–250.

Edmonds, J. S., and K. A. Francesconi. 1993. Arsenic in seafoods: human health aspects and regulations. Mar. Pollut. Bull. 26:665–674.

Erkan, O. O. N. 2011. A preliminary study on amino acid and mineral profiles of important and estimable 21 seafood species. Brit. Food J. 113:457–469.

Ersoy, B., and H. Sereflisan. 2010. The proximate composition and fatty acid profiles of edibles parts of two freshwater mussels. Turk. J. Fish. Aquat. Sc. 10:71–74.

Fabris, G., N. J. Turoczy, and F. Stagnitti. 2006. Trace metal concentrations in edible tissue of snapper, flathead, lobster and abalone from coastal waters of Victoria. Australia. Ecotox. Environ. Safe. 63:286–292.

FAO, 2015a. Fishery Statistical Collections: Global Capture Production. Food and Agriculture Organization of the United Nations.

FAO, 2015b. Available at www.data.fao.org/dataset-data-filter?entryId=af556541-1c8e-4e98-8510-1b2cafba5935&tab=data&type=Dimension&uuidResource=6d56fdc7-9d21-410c-ae6d-ce8c57036ddb (accessed 18 May 2015).

Foster, G. G., and A. N. Hodgson. 1998. Consumption and apparent dry matter digestibility of six intertidal macroalgae by *Turbo sarmaticus* (Mollusca: Vetigastropoda: Turbinidae). Aquaculture 167:211–227.

Freiji, A. M., and M. N. Awadh. 2010. Fatty acid compositions of *Turbo coronatus* Gmelin 1791. Brit. Food J. 112:1049–1062.

FSANZ, 2004. Contaminants and natural toxicants. Food Standard Code, Food Safety Standard 1.4.1, 1.4.2. Food Standards, Australia, New Zealand.

FSANZ, 2011. The 23rd Australian total diet study. Food Standards, Australia, New Zealand

FSANZ, 2013. Australia New Zealand Food Standards Code- Standard 1.1.1 - Preliminary provisions-Application, interpretation and general prohibitions-F2013C00618. Food Standards, Australia, New Zealand.

Gabbott, P. A. 1983. Developmental and seasonal metabolic activities in marine molluscs. in P. W. Hochachka, ed. The Mollusca: Environmental Biochemistry and Physiology. Academic Press, United Kingdom.

Gokoglu, N., M. Gokoglu, and P. Yerlikaya. 2006. Seasonal variations in proximate and elemental composition of pearl oyster (*Pinctada radiata,* Leach, 1814). J. Sci. Food Agric. 86:2161–2165.

Guerin, T., R. Chekri, C. Vastel, V. Sirot, J. Volatier, J. Leblanc, et al. 2011. Determination of 20 trace elements in fish and other seafood from the French market. Food Chem. 127:934–942.

Hernandez, J., A. M. de la Parra, M. Lastra, and M. T. Viana. 2013. Effect of lipid composition of diets and environmental temperature on the performance and fatty acid composition of juvenile European abalone (*Haliotis tuberculata* L. 1758). Aquaculture 412–413:34–40.

Herrman, J. L., and M. Younes. 1999. Background to the ADI/TDI/PTWI. Regul. toxicol. pharm. 30:S109–S113.

Jakimska, A., P. Konieezka, K. Skora, and J. Namiesnik. 2011. Bioaccumulation of metals in tissues of marine animals, Part II: Metal concentrations in animal tissues. Pol. J. Environ. Stud. 20:1127–1146.

Joll, L. M. 1980. Reproductive biology of two species of Turbinidae (Mollusca:Gastropoda). Aust. J. Mar. Freshwater Res. 31:319–335.

Kanthilatha, N., W. Boyd, A. Dowell, A. Mann, N. Chang, H. Wohlmuth, et al. 2014. Identification of preserved fatty acids in archaeological floor sediments from prehistoric sites at Ban Non Wat and Nong Hua Raet in north east Thailand using gas chromatography. J. Archaeol. Sci. 46:353–362.

Karakoltsidis, P. A., and A. Zotos. 1995. Composition of the commercially important Mediterranean finfish, crustaceans and molluscs. J. Food Compost. Anal. 8:258–273.

Kilic, O., and M. Belivermis. 2013. Spatial and seasonal distribution of trace metal concentrations in mussel (*Mytilus galloprovincialis*) and sediment of Bosphorus and Golden Horn. Bull. Environ. Contam. Toxicol. 91:402–408.

Komarnisky, L. A., R. J. Christopherson, and T. K. Basu. 2003. Sulfur: its clinical and toxicologic aspects. Nutrition 19:54–61.

Laxmilatha, P. 2009. Proximate composition of the surf clam *Mactra violacea* (Gmelin 1791). Indian J. Fish. 56:147–150.

Leiva, G.E., and J. C. Castilla. 2002. A review of the world marine gastropod fishery: evolution of catches, management and the Chilean experience. Rev. Fish Biol. Fish. 11:283–300.

Lin, M., and C. Liao. 1999. ^{65}Zn (II) accumulation in the soft tissue and shell of abalone *Haliotis diversicolor* supertexta via the alga *Gracilaria tenuistipitata* var. *liui* and the ambient water. Aquaculture 178:89–101.

Linehan, L. G., T. P. O'Connor, and G. Burnell. 1999. Seasonal variation in the chemical composition and fatty acid profile of Pacific oysters (*Crassostrea gigas*). Food Chem. 64:211–214.

Mahaffey, K. R. 2004. Fish and shellfish as dietary sources of methylmercury and the omega-3 fatty acids, eicosahexaenoic acid and docosahexaenoic acid: risks and benefits. Environ. Res. 95:414–428.

Mahaffey, K. R., R. P. Clickner, and R. A. Jeffries. 2008. Methylmercury and omega-3 fatty acids: Co-occurrence of dietary sources with emphasis on fish and shellfish. Environ. Res. 107:20–29.

Mamtani, R., P. Stern, I. Dawood, and S. Cheema. 2011. Metals and disease: A global primary health care perspective. J. Toxicol. 1:1–11.

Mao, Y., Y. Zhou, H. Yang, and R. Wang. 2006. Seasonal variation in metabolism of cultured pacific oyster, *Crassostrea gigas*, in Sanggou Bay. China. Aquaculture. 253:322–333.

Martino, R. C., and G. M. Cruz. 2004. Proximate composition and fatty acid content of the mangrove oyster *Crassostrea rhizophorae* along the year seasons. Braz. Arch. Biol. Technol. 47:955–960.

Mason, S. L., J. Shi, A. E. Bekhit, and R. Gooneratne. 2014. Nutritional and toxicological studies of New Zealand *Cookia sulcata*. J. Food Composit. Anal. 36:79–84.

Mclachlan, A., and H. W. Lombard. 1980. Seasonal variations in energy and biochemical components of an edible gastropod, *Turbo sarmaticus* (Turbinidae). Aquaculture 19:117–125.

Merdzhanova, A., D. A. Dobreva, M. Stancheva, and L. Makedonski. 2014. Fat soluble vitamins and fatty acid composition of wild black sea mussel, rapana and shrimp. Ovidius University Annals of Chemistry. 25:15–23.

Metian, M., M. Warnau, R. P. Cosson, F. Oberhansli, and P. Bustamante. 2008. Bioaccumulation and detoxification processes of Hg in the king scallop *Pecten maximus*: Field and laboratory investigations. Aquat. Toxicol. 90:204–213.

Milinsk, M. C., R. G. Padre, C. Hayashi, N. E. Souza, and M. Matsushita. 2003. Influence of diets enriched with different vegetable oils on the fatty acid profiles of *Helix aspersa maxima*. Food Chem. 82:553–558.

Mooney, B. D., P. D. Nichols, and N. G. Elliot. 2002. Seafood the Good Food II: Oil profiles for further Australian seafoods and influencing factors. Hobart: CSIRO Division of Marine Research and Deakin, A.C.T.: Fisheries Research & Development Corporation (FRDC), Australia.

Morais, S., D. Boaventura, L. Narciso, P. Re, and S. J. Hawkins. 2003. Gonad development and fatty acid composition of *Patella depressa* Pennat (Gastropoda: Prosobranchia) populations with different patterns of spatial distribution, in expressed and sheltered sites. J. Exp. Mar. Biol. Ecol. 294:61–80.

Moreda-Pineiro, J., E. Alonso-Rodriguez, V. Romaris-Hortas, A. Moreda-Pineiro, P. Lopez-Mahia, S. Muniategui-Lorenzo, et al. 2012. Assessment of the bioavailability of toxic and non-toxic arsenic species in seafood samples. Food Chem. 130:552–560.

Mubiana, V. K., K. Vercauteren, and R. Blust. 2006. The influence of body size, condition index and tidal exposure on the variability in metal bioaccumulation in *Mytilus edulis*. Environ. Pollut. 144:272–279.

Napolitano, G. E., and R. G. Ackman. 1992. Anatomical distributions and temporal variations of lipid classes in sea scallops *Placopecten magellanicus* (Gmelin) from George Bank (Nova Scotia). Comp. Biochem. Physiol. 103B:645–650.

National Health and Medical Research Council. 2006. Nutrient reference values for Australia and New Zealand: Including recommended dietary intakes,National Health and Medical Research Council, Commonwealth of Australia.

Naylor, R. L., R. J. Goldburg, J. H. Primavera, N. Kautsky, M. C. M. Beveridge, J. Clay, et al. 2000. Effect of aquaculture on world fish supplies. Nature 405:1017–1024.

Nelson, M. M., D. L. Leighton, C. F. Phleger, and P. D. Nichols. 2002. Comparison of growth and lipid composition in the green abalone, *Haliotis fulgens*, provided specific macroalgal diets. Comp. Biochem. Physiol. Part B 131:695–712.

Nichols, P. D., P. Virtue, B. D. Mooney, N. G. Elliot, and G. K. Yearsley. 1998. Seafood the good food: the oil (fat) content and composition of Australian commercial fishes, shellfishes and crustaceans. Hobart: CSIRO Division of Marine Research and Deakin, A.C.T.:

Fisheries Research & Development Corporation (FRDC), Australia.
Noel, L., C. Testu, C. Chafey, P. Velge, and T. Guerin. 2011. Contamination levels for lead, cadmium and mercury in marine gastropods, echinoderms and tunicates. Food Control 22:433–437.
Nooshin, S., and E.-A. Peyman. 2011. Determination of fatty acid compositions as biomarkers in the diet of *Turbo coronatus* in Chabahar Bay. Journal of the Persian Gulf. 2:35–42.
Okutucu, B., A. Dincer, O. Habib, and F. Zihnioglu. 2007. Comparison of five methods for determination of total plasma protein concentration. J. Biochem. Biophys. Methods 70:709–711.
Olmedo, P., A. F. Hernandez, A. Pla, P. Femia, N. Navas-Acien, and F. Gil. 2013. Determination of essential elements (copper, manganese, selenium and zinc) in fish and shellfish samples. Risk and nutritional assessment and mercury- selenium balance. Food Chem. Toxicol. 62:299–307.
Özden, Ö., N. Erkan, and M. C. Deval. 2009. Trace mineral profiles of the bivalve species Chamelea gallina and Donax trunculus. Food Chem. 113:222–226.
Ozogul, Y., F. Ozogul, and A. I. Olgunoglu. 2005. Fatty acid profile and mineral content of the wild snail (*Helix pomatia*) from the region of the south of the Turkey. Eur. Food Res. Technol. 221:547–549.
Pan, K., and W-X. Wang. 2012. Trace element contamination in estuarine and coastal environments in China. Sci. Total Environ.. 421–422, 3–16.
Pazos, A. J., G. Roman, C. P. Acosta, M. Abad, and J. L. Sanchez. 1997a. Seasonal changes in condition and biochemical composition of the scallop *Pecten maximus* L. from suspended culture in the Ria de Arousa (Galicia, N.W. Spain) in relation to environmental conditions. J. Exper. Mar. Biol. Ecol. 211:169–193.
Pazos, A. J., G. Roman, C. P. Acosta, J. L. Sanchez, and M. Abad. 1997b. Lipid classes and fatty acid composition in the female gonad of *Pecten maximus* in relation to reproductive cycle and environmental variables. Comp. Biochem. Physiol. 117B:393–402.
Perez-Comacho, A., M. Delgado, M. J. Fernandez- Reiriz, and L. U. Labarta. 2003. Energy balance, gonad development and biochemical composition in the clam *Ruditapes decussatus*. Mar. Ecol. Prog. Ser. 258:133–145.
Periyasamy, N., M. Srinivasan, K. Devanathan, and S. Balakrishnan. 2011. Nutritional value of gastropod *Babylonia spirata* (Linnaeus, 1758) from Thazhanguda, Southeast coast of India. Asian Pac. J. Trop. Biomed. 12:249–252.
PIRSA, 2010. Ecological assessment of the South Australian scallop and turbo fisheries, prepared for the Australian Government Department of Environment and Heritage, Adelaide, South Australia.Available at www.environment.gov.au/system/files/pages/ecc294f7-30fc-4bf5-aa41-657b76d606de/files/sa-scallop-turbo-submission.pdf. (accessed 25 September 2013).
Ragonese, C., L. Tedone, M. Beccaria, G. Torre, F. Cichello, F. Cacciola, et al. 2014. Characterisation of lipid fraction of marine macroalgae by means of chromatography techniques coupled to mass spectrometry. Food Chem. 145:932–940.
Ramesh, R., and S. Ravichandran. 2008. Seasonal variation on the proximate composition of *Turbo brunneus*. Int. J. Zool. Res. 4:28–34.
Rodellar, S., M. Fontcuberta, J. F. Arques, J. Calderon, L. R. Barba, and L. Serra-Majem. 2010. Mercury and methylmercury intake estimation due to seafood products for the Catalonian population (Spain). Food Addit. Contam. 27:29–35.
Rowling, K., A. Hegarty, and M. Ives. 2010. Pp. 359–360 *in* Status of Fisheries Resources in NSW 2008/09., Turban Shells Industry & Investment NSW, Cronulla.
Ruttens, A., A. C. Blanpain, L. D. Temmerman, and N. Waegeneers. 2012. Arsenic speciation in food in Belgium Part 1: Fish, molluscs and crustaceans. J. Geochem. Explor. 121:55–61.
Saito, H. 2004. Lipid and FA composition of the pearl oyster *Pinctada fucata martensii*: influence of season and maturation. Lipids 39:997–1006.
Saito, H., and H. Aono. 2014. Characteristics of lipid and fatty acid of marine gastropod *Turbo cornutus*: High levels of arachidonic and n-3 docosapentaenoic acid. Food Chem. 145:135–144.
Saito, H., and J. Hashimoto. 2010. Characteristic of the fatty acid composition of the deep-sea vent gastropod, *Ifremeria nautilei*. Lipids 45:537–548.
Saito, H., and Y. Marty. 2010. High levels of icosapentaenoic acid in the lipids of oyster *Crassostrea gigas* ranging over both Japan and France. J. Oleo Sci. 59:281–292.
Saito, H., C. Xue, R. Yamashiro, S. Moromizato, and Y. Itabashi. 2010. High polyunsaturated fatty acid levels in the two subtropical macroalgae, *Cladosiphon okamuranus* Tokida and *Caulerpa lentillifera*. J. Phycol. 46:665–673.
Scherz, H., and E. Kirchhoff. 2006. Trace elements in foods: Zinc contents of raw foods- A comparison of data originating from different geographical regions of the world. J. Food Compost. Anal. 19:420–433.
Simopoulos, A. P. 1991. Omega-3 fatty acids in health and disease and in growth and development. American Society for Clinical Nutrition. 54:438–463.
Simopoulos, A. P. 2002. The importance of the ratio of omega-6/omega-3 essential fatty acids. Biomed. Pharmacother. 56:365–379.
Skinner, C., N. J. Turoczy, P. L. Jones, D. Barnett, and R. Hodges. 2004. Heavy metal concentrations in wild and cultures blacklip abalone (*Haliotis rubra* Leach) from southern Australian waters. Food Chem. 85:351–356.

Sloth, J. J., E. H. Larsen, and K. Julshamn. 2005. Survey of inorganic arsenic in marine animals and marine certified reference materials by anion exchange High-Performance Liquid Chromatography- Inductively Coupled Plasma Mass Spectrometry. J. Agric. Food Chem. 53:6011–6018.

Smoothey, A.F. 2013. Habitat- associations of turban snails on intertidal and subtidal rocky reefs. PLoS ONE 8:e0146911.

Srilatha, G., K. Chamundeeswari, K. Ramamoorthy, G. Sankar, and D. Varadharajan. 2013. Proximate, amino acid, fatty acid and minerals analysis of clam, Meretrix casta (Chemnitz) from Cuddalore and Parangipettai Coast, south east coast of India. J. Mar. Biol. Oceanogr 2. doi:10.4172/2324-8661.1000111.

Stoeva, S., P. Dolashka, K. Pervanova, N. Genov, and W. Voelter. 1997. Multidomain structure of the *Rapana thomasiana* (Gastropod) hemocyanin structural subunit RHSS1. Comp. Biochem. Physiol. 118B:927–934.

Su, X.-Q., K. Antonas, D. Li, and P. Nichols. 2006. Seasonal variations of total lipid and fatty acid contents in the muscle of two Australian farmed abalone species. J. Food Lipids 13:411–423.

Taylor, A. G., and S. Savage. 2006. Fatty acid composition of New Zealand green- lipped mussels, *Perna canaliculus*: Implications for harvesting for n-3 extracts. Aquaculture 261:430–439.

Vasconcelos, P., M. B. Gaspar, M. Castro, and M. L. Nunes. 2009. Influence of growth and reproductive cycle on the meat yield and proximate composition of *Hexaplex trunculus* (Gastropoda: Muricidae). J. Mar. Biol. Assoc.U.K. 89:1223–1231.

Waska, H., S. Kim, G. Kim, M. R. Kang, and G. B. Kim. 2008. Distribution patterns of chalcogens (S, Se, Te, and 210Po) in various tissues of a squid. Todarodes pacificus. Sci. Total Environ. 392:218–224.

WHO, 2003. Diet, nutrition and the prevention of chronic diseases: report of a joint WHO/FAO expert consultation, Technical Report Series 916, Geneva.

Woodcock, S. H., and K. Benkendorff. 2008. The impact of diet on the growth and proximate composition of juvenile whelks, *Dicathais orbita* (Gastropoda: Mollusca). Aquaculture 276:162–170.

Xavier Ramesh, X., and K. Ayyakkannu. 1992. Nutritive value of Chicoreus ramosus. A status report. Trop. Mar. Moll. Progm. 10:14.

Yearsley, G.K., R. D. Ward, and P. R. Last. 1999. Australian seafood handbook: an identification guide to domestic species. CSIRO Division of Marine Research, Hobart.

Zarai, Z., F. Frikha, R. Balti, N. Miled, Y. Gargouri, and H. Mejdoub. 2011. Nutrient composition of the marine snail (*Hexaplex trunculus*) from the Tunisian Mediterranean coasts. J. Sci. Food Agric. 91:1265–1270.

5

A nutritional supplement containing lactoferrin stimulates the immune system, extends lifespan, and reduces amyloid β peptide toxicity in *Caenorhabditis elegans*

Patricia Martorell[1], Silvia Llopis[1], Nuria Gonzalez[1], Daniel Ramón[1], Gabriel Serrano[2], Ana Torrens[2], Juan M. Serrano[2], Maria Navarro[2] & Salvador Genovés[1]

[1]Cell Biology Laboratory, Food Biotechnology Department, Biópolis SL, Paterna, Valencia 46980, Spain
[2]Research and Development Department, Sesderma Laboratories, Rafelbuñol, Valencia 46138, Spain

Keywords
Alzheimer's disease, *Caenorhabditis elegans*, immune system, lactoferrin, neuroprotection

Correspondence
Salvador Genovés, Cell Biology Laboratory, Food Biotechnology Department, Biópolis SL, Paterna, 46980 Valencia, Spain.
E-mail: salvador.genoves@biopolis.es

Funding Information
This work was funded by Sesderma S.L. The funders had no role in data collection and analysis or preparation of the manuscript.

Abstract

Lactoferrin is a highly multifunctional glycoprotein involved in many physiological functions, including regulation of iron absorption and immune responses. Moreover, there is increasing evidence for neuroprotective effects of lactoferrin. We used *Caenorhabditis elegans* as a model to test the protective effects, both on phenotype and transcriptome, of a nutraceutical product based on lactoferrin liposomes. In a dose-dependent manner, the lactoferrin-based product protected against acute oxidative stress and extended lifespan of *C. elegans* N2. Furthermore, Paralysis of the transgenic *C. elegans* strain CL4176, caused by Aβ1-42 aggregates, was clearly ameliorated by treatment. Transcriptome analysis in treated nematodes indicated immune system stimulation, together with enhancement of processes involved in the oxidative stress response. The lactoferrin-based product also improved the protein homeostasis processes, cellular adhesion processes, and neurogenesis in the nematode. In summary, the tested product exerts protection against aging and neurodegeneration, modulating processes involved in oxidative stress response, protein homeostasis, synaptic function, and xenobiotic metabolism. This lactoferrin-based product is also able to stimulate the immune system, as well as improving reproductive status and energy metabolism. These findings suggest that oral supplementation with this lactoferrin-based product could improve the immune system and antioxidant capacity. Further studies to understand the molecular mechanisms related with neuronal function would be of interest.

Introduction

Lactoferrin is an 80-kDa glycoprotein consisting of 703 amino acids and multiple sialic acid residues attached to N-linked glycan chains (Wolfson and Robbins 1971; Levay and Viljoen 1995). This protein is produced in the mucosal epithelial cells of various mammalian species including humans, cows, goats, horses, dogs, and rodents. Only low concentrations of lactoferrin are normally present in blood serum. In contrast, lactoferrin is abundant in exocrine fluids such as breast milk and colostrum, in mucosal secretions, and in secondary granules of neutrophils (Levay and Viljoen 1995; García-Montoya et al. 2012).

Because of its wide distribution in various tissues, lactoferrin is a highly multifunctional protein. Indeed, it is involved in many physiological functions, including regulation of iron absorption and immune responses. Lactoferrin also exhibits antioxidant properties and exerts both anticarcinogenic and anti-inflammatory activities (Connely 2001), and several enzymatic functions (Leffell and Spitznagel 1972). Moreover, lactoferrin exhibits strong antimicrobial activity against a broad spectrum of different viruses, microorganisms, and parasites (Yamauchi et al. 2006), although it seems to promote the growth of beneficial bacteria like *Bifidobacteria* and *Lactobacillus* (Sherman et al. 2004). In very low birth weight neonates, lactoferrin can prevent the development of necrotizing enterocolitis (Adamkin 2012). Moreover, it has been identified as an antioxidant protein with ability to increase antioxidant capacity and decrease reactive oxygen species (ROS) formation (Cohen et al. 1992; Maneva et al. 2003; Mulder et al. 2008; Safaeian and Zabolian 2014). Lactoferrin can cross the blood–brain barrier via receptor-mediated transcytosis (Kamemori et al. 2008) and has suppressive effects on psychological distress (Kamemori et al. 2004). These findings suggested a potential involvement of lactoferrin in neural functions of children. These include neuronal cell proliferation, differentiation, migration, and synaptic connections that are processes of critical importance in the development of cognitive functions (Wang 2012). Due to its multiple functions, lactoferrin has been used in clinical trials and industrial applications. One of the first applications of lactoferrin was in infant formula. Currently, it is added to immune system-enhancing nutraceuticals, cosmetics, pet-care supplements, drinks, fermented milks, chewing gums, and toothpaste (García-Montoya et al. 2012).

Alzheimer's disease (AD) is the most common form of dementia that results in the degeneration of neurons and synapses in the cerebral cortex and certain subcortical regions. It is characterized by the formation of amyloid plaques and neurofibrillary tangles in the brains of AD patients (Huang and Mucke 2012). The major components of amyloid plaques are β-amyloid (Aβ) peptide and the neurofibrillary tangles that mainly contain hyperphosphorylated tau protein. Aβ is a small peptide with 40–42 amino acids (Ab1–42), and is generated by step-wise cleavage of the larger β-amyloid precursor protein through the proteases named β-secretase and γ-secretase, respectively (Huang and Mucke 2012). The toxic nature of Ab1–42 makes it a marker of AD progression and a target of screening for new therapeutic treatments.

Transgenic *Caenorhabditis elegans* have been established as models for AD since 1995 (Link 1995). Nematode disease models have been used to study the mechanisms of AD toxicity (Link 2006) and to test the efficacies of drugs and nutritional supplements. A study using transgenic CL4176 worms, which express the human Ab1–42 in muscle tissues under a temperature-inducible system (Link 2006), reported that soybean isoflavone glycitein could protect worms from Ab-induced toxicity and this protection was credited to the antioxidative activity of glycitein (Gutiérrez-Zepeda et al. 2005). *Ginkgo biloba* extract EGb761 and ginkgolides were shown to suppress the Ab-induced pathological behaviors of several different Ab-transgenic *C. elegans*, not by reducing oxidative stress but rather by modulating Ab oligomeric species (Wu et al. 2006). Also a bioactive peptide obtained from a cocoa byproduct, showed antioxidant activity and functional properties against β-amyloid peptide toxicity related to AD (Martorell et al. 2013).

Iron is associated with neurodegenerative disorder etiopathology; an increase in brain iron concentration has been found in patients suffering AD. Moreover, iron is implicated in beta amyloid self-assembly and aggregation (Ayton et al. 2013). This has raised interest in metal chelation therapy. Previous studies provide evidence for the neuroprotective effect of lactoferrin conjugates in vivo and in vitro, acting as both iron-binding protein and inflammatory modulator (Kamalinia et al. 2013). In addition, there are reports of the accumulation of lactoferrin in the brain of Parkinson disease patients, and of coaccumulation of lactoferrin in senile plaques of a transgenic AD mouse model. Interestingly, the senile plaque formation precedes lactoferrin deposition, suggesting that could be an attempt by the brain to minimize the consequences of neurodegeneration (Wang et al. 2010; Rousseau et al. 2013). Moreover, oxidative stress-associated cell damage is one of the key factors in neurodegenerative disorders, including AD (Christen 2000), and lactoferrin has ability to decrease ROS formation (Safaeian and Zabolian 2014).

In this study, we used transgenic *C. elegans* CL4176 to evaluate the Ab toxicity-inhibitory effect of a lactoferrin-based product. We demonstrate that lactoferrin inhibits Ab toxicity and has antioxidant activity. We also performed a transcriptomic analysis in the nematode to determine the main metabolic targets of this product.

Material and Methods

Product

The commercial food supplement "Lactyferrin Classic Drinkable" (LfCD), a lactoferrin-based product (Sesderma S.L, Rafelbuñol, Valencia, Spain) has been used through this work. Lactoferrin was encapsulated in positively charged phosphatidylcholine liposomes (Lactyferrin Classic Drinkable Sesderma) at a concentration of 0.1%. The liposome preparation presented a unimodal size distribution with a diameter between 80 and 150 nm, a polidispersity index below 0.20, and a zeta potential of (30–150) mV. The size of the unillamelar nanoliposomes was between 80 and 150 nm in diameter (Delsa Nano C, particle analyzer, Beckman Coulter Inc., Brea, California, USA). The lactoferrin concentration was 0.1%, and the pH of the solution was 5–7. The nutritional composition is described in Table 1. The product contains 0.08 g of lactoferrin per 100 mL of product as functional ingredient (Table 1).

To perform the *C. elegans* assays, the product was added to the surface of nematode growth medium (NGM) plates containing *Escherichia coli* OP50 strain.

Table 1. Nutritional composition of the lactoferrin-based product LfCD.

Composition	(g/100 mL) of product
Proteins	2.1
Carbohydrates	0.60
Fat	2.80
Lactoferrin	0.08
Colostrum	0.02

Caenorhabditis elegans strains and maintenance

C. elegans wild-type strain N2 (Bristol) was obtained from the *Caenorhabditis* Genetics Centre (University of Minnesota, USA), and the transgenic strain CL4176 (smg-1ts [pAF29(myo-3/Ab1–42/let UTR)+pRF4(rol-6(su10069))]) was provided by Dr. Christopher D. Link. Paralysis was induced in the CL4176 strain by the expression of a muscle-specific Aβ_{1-42}, which depends on up-shifting temperature from 16 to 25°C (Link 1995).

Both *C. elegans* strains were routinely propagated on NGM plates with *E. coli* strain OP50 as a food source. *C. elegans* N2 strain was maintained at 20°C, whereas CL4176 strain was kept at 16°C.

Paralysis assays

Paralysis assays were carried out with *C. elegans* strain CL4176. Worms were synchronized by isolating eggs from gravid adults at 16°C in the NGM plates (control medium) and NGM supplemented with different amounts of LfCD (25, 50, 100, and 150 μL). *G. biloba* extract EGb 761®(1 μg/mL) (Tanakene, Ipsen Pharma, S.A., Sant Feliu de Llobregat, Spain) was used as an internal positive control. Nematode paralysis was assessed as described by Martorell et al. (2013). Experiments were carried out in duplicate.

Paralysis curves were statistically analyzed using the log rank survival test provided by GraphPad Prism 4 software package.

Oxidative stress assays

C. elegans strain N2 was egg-synchronized in the NGM plates (control medium) and NGM supplemented with the different doses of LfCD (50, 100, and 150 μL). Vitamin C (0.1 μg/mL, Sigma-Aldrich, St. Louis, MO) was used as an internal positive control. Experiments were performed according to a previously published protocol (Martorell et al. 2011). Assays were carried out in triplicate.

Statistical analysis of postoxidative stress worm viability was evaluated by means of one-way analysis of variance using Statgraphics plus (version 5.1) software (Manugistics, Rockville, MD).

Lifespan assays

Worms of the N2 strain were synchronized by isolating eggs from gravid adults and hatching them in NG agar plates (control media). When worms reached young adult stage, they were fed with LfCD product (25, 50 or 150 μL) for 24 h. A period of 24 h exposure was deemed long enough because this is approximately 1/3 of the *C. elegans*' life cycle. Afterward, worms were transferred to NGM control media. The animals were moved periodically to new NGM plates and were scored as dead if they failed to respond to a platinum wire (applied every 2 days). Two independent experiments were performed. Survival curves were compared using the log rank survival significance test, provided by GraphPad Prism 4 statistical software package.

Microarray analysis

Changes were studied in the gene expression of worms treated with LfCD. Age-synchronized embryos from wild-type strain N2 were obtained in NGM plates and NGM supplemented with 150 μL of the lactoferrin-based product. Worms were recovered at young adult stage with M9 buffer, washed three times and collected in eppendorf tubes for worm disruption by sonication. Total RNA was isolated with RNeasy Mini Kit (Qiagen, Hilden, Germany) and processed for hybridization using the GeneChip® *C. elegans* Genome Array of Affymetrix (UCIM, University of Valencia). Four biological replicates per condition were examined by bioinformatics.

Raw data obtained from Affymetrix arrays were background-corrected using RMA methodology (Irizarry et al. 2003). Signal intensity was standardized across arrays via quantile normalization algorithm. Differential gene expression was assessed between control and treated conditions using limma moderated *t*-statistics. To control the false discovery rate, *P*-values were corrected for multiple testing. Finally, gene set analysis was performed for each comparison using logistic regression models (Montaner and Dopazo 2010).

Results

Lactoferrin-based LfCD product has beneficial effects on body paralysis in CL4176

We examined whether the lactoferrin-based product LfCD reduced nematode body paralysis using the transgenic strain CL4176. We added different volumes to the agar media (25, 50, 100, and 150 μL) corresponding to different final doses of lactoferrin in 10 mL agar plates (2, 4, 8, and 12 μg/mL, respectively). A significant effect on the delay of nematode paralysis was observed at all doses assayed ($P < 0.0001$) (Fig. 1 and Table S1). The effect

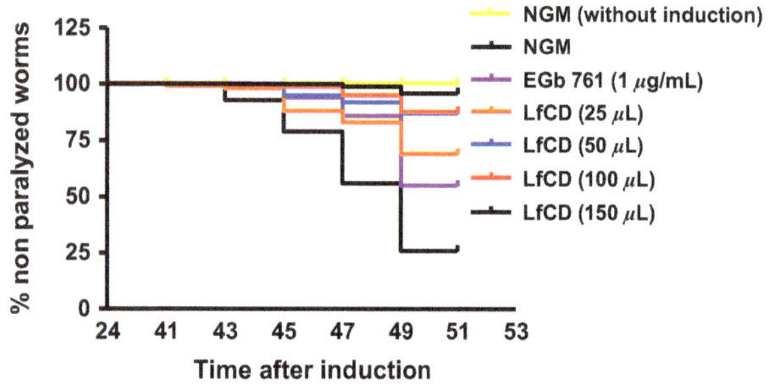

Figure 1. Measurement of body paralysis of *C. elegans* CL 4176 nematodes fed with LfCD product (25, 50, 100, and 150 μL) after temperature up-shift. *Gingko biloba* extract (1 μg/mL) was used as positive control. Worms without temperature-induction were included as negative control. Time refers to hours after Aβ_{42} induction by temperature up-shift. Data are the average of two independent experiments.

was dose-dependent. Specifically, delay of paralysis onset was obtained with doses ranging 50–150 μL ($P < 0.0001$), being 150 μL the most effective (onset paralysis: control: 41 h; treated: 47 h). Furthermore, the percentage of total paralysis at 49 h (end of experiment) was reduced with the LfCD treatment in a dose-dependent manner. This was especially remarkable at 150 μL, which almost completely inhibited paralysis rate (3.29% in treated nematodes vs. 73.6% in control NGM). These results show the strong protective activity of the lactoferrin-based product, even better than the positive control extract *G. biloba* (1 μg/mL) (Fig. 1 and Table S1).

Lactoferrin-based LfCD product shows antioxidant properties in *C. elegans*

To know whether the analyzed product has an in vivo antioxidant effect, we subjected worms N2 to oxidative stress with hydrogen peroxide after feeding with three doses of LfCD (50, 100, and 150 μL). All doses tested produced a significant effect on worm survival rates, increasing worm survival after stress compared with control conditions (medium NGM) (Fig. 2). Among the different doses assayed, 150 μL of the LfCD product provided the most significant protection (19.2 ± 2.6% increase of survival vs. control) ($P \leq 0.001$). The results indicate a marked antioxidant effect of the LfCD product, even greater than the positive control vitamin C (12.5 ± 1.9% increase in survival vs. control).

Lactoferrin-based LfCD product extends lifespan in *C. elegans*

In order to assess the effects of LfCD on the worm lifespan, this product was administered to nematodes in the adult stage for 24 h. Treatment with the product at two different doses (25 or 50 μL, corresponding to 2 and 4 μg/mL of lactoferrin, Fig. 3A and B, respectively) induced a significant increase in viability during the mature period of nematodes (from day 15 of life until death), whereas higher doses did not affect lifespan (data not shown). Specifically, the lactoferrin-based product at doses of 25 and 50 μL caused a significant increase in mean lifespan compared to control feeding (dose 25: 17 days ($P = 0.0025$); dose 50: 19 days ($P = 0.0006$); control: 15 days); which represents an increase of up to 26.6% (Fig. 3, Table S2). Moreover, the product at both doses, 25 and 50 μL, produced a final lifespan extension of 2 days (8.3% of extension). These results suggest that treatment with low doses of LfCD at early stages exerts beneficial effects on nematode lifespan.

Lactoferrin-based LfCD product induces upregulation of immune response, synaptic function, and antioxidative response in *C. elegans*

To determine which genes or pathways are affected by feeding *C. elegans* (N2) strain with the lactoferrin-based

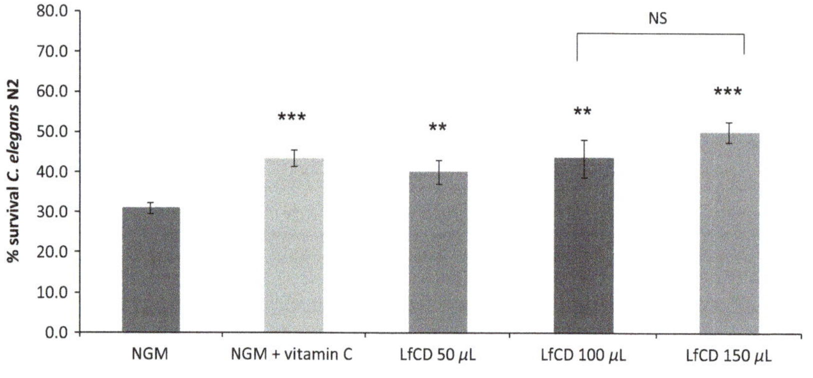

Figure 2. Survival of the *C. elegans* N2 nematodes treated with 2 mmol/L H_2O_2 on nematode growth medium plates in a worm population fed with different doses of the LfCD product. Vitamin C (10 μg/mL) was used as positive control. ***Significant at $P \leq 0.001$. **Significant at $P \leq 0.01$. NS: not significant. Data are the average of four independent experiments.

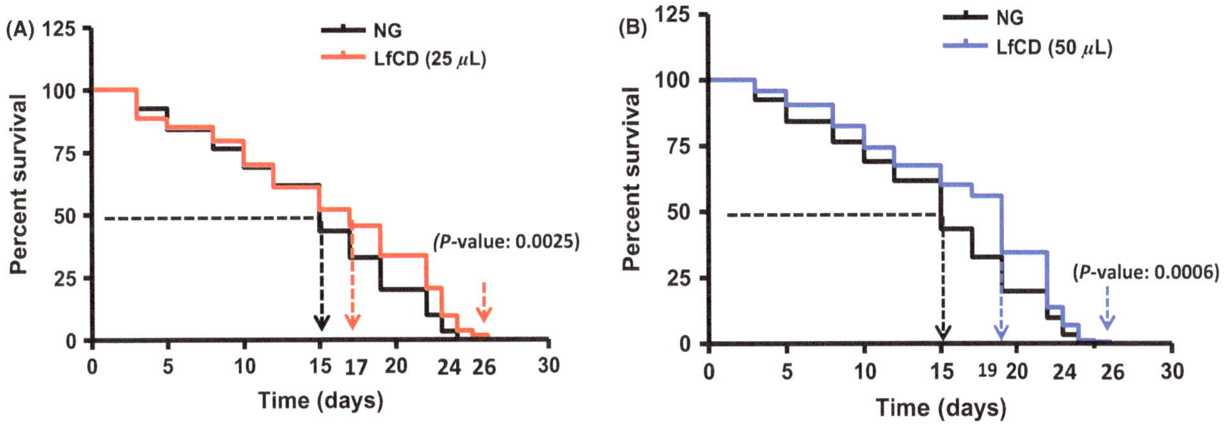

Figure 3. Survival curves of *C. elegans* wild-type strain N2 fed with nematode growth medium (NGM) medium (control) or with LfCD product during 24 h from adult stage with (A) 25 μL of LfCD; (B) 50 μL of LfCD. Two hundred worms per condition were used in two independent experiments. Mean lifespan, indicating the time in days where half of the worm population is still alive, is shown on the *X*-axis. *P*-values are shown in each curve comparison between control NGM and LfCD-treated nematodes. NS: no significant differences.

LfCD product, we analyzed gene expression using microarray experiments. Microarray data are available through the NCBI Gene Expression Omnibus data repository under accession GSE71482 (http://www.ncbi.nlm.nih.gov/geo/). Nematodes were fed with 150 μL of LfCD, which was the dose showing the most protective effect on body paralysis (Fig. 1), and it was found to have a strong antioxidant effect (Fig. 2) on nematodes after acute oxidative stress. Four biological replicates of *C. elegans* fed a 150 μL dose were compared with nematodes cultured in control conditions. RNA was isolated from nematodes and used for hybridization to Affymetrix *C. elegans* arrays.

First, we searched the data for significantly represented upregulated or downregulated gene sets, according to their fold-change ($P \leq 0.05$). We found a total of 540 upregulated genes and 244 downregulated genes in the nematodes fed with the lactoferrin product compared with nematodes under control feeding conditions. This showed the great impact that LfCD intake had on *C. elegans* gene expression. Focusing the analysis on these upregulated genes (the first 40 upregulated genes are listed in Table S3), we found genes related with the innate immune system of the nematode (recognition and defense against pathogens). Among these, we found saposins (spp-12, spp-23, spp-8), lysozymes (lys-1, lys-2, lys-8), and lectins (clec-66, clec-63, clec-62, clec-210, clec-143, clec-173, clec-83, clec-145, clec-3, clec-65, clec-266, clec-67, clec-49,clec-258, clec-74, clec-186, clec-174, and clec-222). Other defense-related genes were irg-3 and catalase (ctl-2). These results suggest that the LfCD product activates effector molecules in the immune system of the worm. Other genes are related with lipid metabolism (fatty acid β-oxidation, fatty acid elongation, fatty acid synthesis/degradation), xenobiotic metabolism and lysosomal degradation, neurotransmitter metabolism, glutathione metabolism, and glyoxylate cycle (Table S3).

With respect to metabolic pathways affected by the LfCD product, using the Kyoto Encyclopedia of Genes and Genomes (KEGG), we determined six pathways significantly upregulated ($P \leq 0.05$) in worms fed with the lactoferrin-based LfCD product (Table 2). These metabolic pathways were related with the activity of peroxisome (fatty acid β-oxidation organelle) and drug metabolism-cytochrome P450; which is in accordance with the overexpression of fatty acid β-oxidation genes and Cyp P450 genes (membrane proteins for endogen and exogen compounds metabolism). Upregulation of Wnt and TGF-beta signaling pathways was also observed under LfCD treatment. The first one is involved in cell proliferation, migration, polarity, differentiation, and axon growth. The TGF-beta pathway plays an important role in the *C. elegans* innate immune system, and defense against infections, also being involved in development, body size, and axonal guidance (Nicholas and Hodgkin 2004). These results would support the overexpression of different genes related with immune response in the presence of the analyzed product.

Another significantly upregulated pathway was the mammalian circadian rhythm. Finally, additional metabolic pathways were induced in response to the lactoferrin-based product ($0.05 \geq P \geq 1$). These were related with glutation metabolism, lipid metabolism, energy metabolism (oxidative phosphorilation, glioxilate metabolism), protein metabolism (ubiquitin-mediated proteolysis), retinol metabolism, and neuroactive ligand-receptor interaction.

Further data analysis focusing on biological processes showed a total of 31 significantly upregulated biological processes in treated worms ($P \leq 0.05$) (Table S4). The

Table 2. List of significantly ($P \leq 0.05$) upregulated kyoto encyclopedia of genes and genome (KEGG) pathways in nematodes fed with 150 μL of the lactoferrin-based LfCD product compared to control feeding conditions (in bold).

ID KEGGs	*P*-value	Name
04146	**0.0003**	**Peroxisome**
00982	**0.0009**	**Drug metabolism – cytochrome P450**
04710	**0.0014**	**Circadian rhythm – mammal**
00980	**0.002**	**Metabolism of xenobiotics by cytochrome P450**
04310	**0.048**	**Wnt signaling pathway**
04350	**0.048**	**TGF-beta signaling pathway**
00480	0.081	Glutathione metabolism
00071	0.081	Fatty acid metabolism
00190	0.127	Oxidative phosphorylation
04141	0.127	Protein processing in endoplasmic reticulum
00830	0.257	Retinol metabolism
00040	0.263	Pentose and glucuronate interconversions
04142	0.265	Lysosome
04120	0.265	Ubiquitin-mediated proteolysis
00514	0.284	Other types of O-glycan biosynthesis
00860	0.370	Porphyrin and chlorophyll metabolism
00630	0.386	Glyoxylate and dicarboxylate metabolism
00983	0.448	Drug metabolism – other enzymes
00500	0.584	Starch and sucrose metabolism
00053	0.825	Ascorbate and aldarate metabolism
04145	0.981	Phagosome
00520	0.985	Amino sugar and nucleotide sugar metabolism
00062	1	Fatty acid elongation in mitochondria
00600	1	Sphingolipid metabolism
04130	1	SNARE interactions in vesicular transport
00590	1	Arachidonic acid metabolism
01040	1	Biosynthesis of unsaturated fatty acids
04010	1	MAPK signaling pathway
04080	1	Neuroactive ligand-receptor interaction

Additional upregulated metabolic pathways ($0.05 \geq P \leq 1$) are shown.

nonredundant biological processes were grouped in seven processes (Table 3). The first set of genes was related with cell adhesion processes, which are involved in embryonic development, migration, cell differentiation and communication, and inflammation. These processes are mediated by adhesion molecules, like cadherins, which are membrane proteins involved in adhesion of growing axons. Likewise, our results also showed the overexpression of cdh-3 gene in LfCD-treated nematodes, a cadherin involved in epithelial cell morphogenesis (Pettitt et al. 1996). This increase in cellular adhesion could then be related with the upregulation of axon extension, which is essential for organelle and substances transport in neurons and nerve impulse conduction.

Table 3. List of significantly ($P \leq 0.05$) nonredundant upregulated biological processes in worms treated with 150 μL of the LfCD product.

ID gene ontology	Name	*P*-value
GO:0007155	Cell adhesion	0
GO:0018991	Oviposition	0.005
GO:0007411	Axon guidance	0.013
GO:0055114	Oxidation-reduction process	0.019
GO:0010172	Embryonic body morphogenesis	0.03
GO:0006366	Transcription from RNA polymerase II promoter	0.038
GO:0048675	Axon extension	0.049

Furthermore, reproductive behavior and oviposition, oxidation-reduction process, embryonic body morphogenesis and transcription were significantly upregulated after LfCD treatment in the nematode.

Discussion

In this study, we demonstrate that a lactoferrin-based product (LfCD) exhibits beneficial health properties. Lactoferrin rapidly degrades in the body due to enzymatic hydrolysis; therefore, an appropriate delivery system may improve its efficiency. In this product formulation, lactoferrin is encapsulated in phosphatidylcholine liposomes, designed for optimal delivery across the gastro-intestinal and blood–brain barriers. This encapsulation helps to protect it from the environment, increasing its bioavailability and bioactivity (Onishi 2011; Guan et al. 2012). In our study, we showed that the LfCD product provides an antioxidant activity and the capacity to protect *C. elegans* from acute oxidative stress. In addition to the observed increase in viability of the LfCD-treated worms, the transcriptomic analysis revealed upregulation of catalase (*ctl-2*) and glutathione peroxidase (*gpx-1*) genes in worms treated with LfCD. The *ctl-2* gene encodes an antioxidant enzyme with catalase and peroxidase activity, which protects cells from ROS, whereas *gpx-1* is a key enzyme in ROS neutralization. Furthermore, the glutathione metabolism pathway and redox process were upregulated. Glutathione scavenges free radicals and other ROS through enzymatic reactions, so it plays an important role in antioxidant defense (Wu et al. 2004). Oxidative stress occurs when ROS production exceeds the body's own natural antioxidant defense mechanisms, resulting in cellular damage. Moreover, oxidative stress is related with aging and pathogenesis, like Alzheimer's and Parkinson's disease (Christen 2000; Back et al. 2012). Therefore, our findings suggest that the lactoferrin-based product contributes to decreasing cellular oxidative stress. These results are in accordance with previous reports showing that lactoferrin has ROS-scavenging activity (Burrow et al. 2011; Ogasawara et al. 2014) and, therefore, displays antioxidant properties both in vitro and in vivo (Maneva et al. 2003; Safaeian and Zabolian 2014), including oral supplementation in clinical trials with healthy human males (Mulder et al. 2008).

In addition, our results showed an activation of the xenobiotics pathway, lysosome degradation, and genes related with these processes, such as cytochrome P450 and *gba-1* genes. Cytochrome P450 membrane-associated protein catalyzes the oxidative metabolism of a wide variety of exogenous and endogenous compounds including xenobiotics, drugs, environmental toxins, steroids, and fatty acids. Xenobiotics are molecules that are foreign to the body and must therefore be detoxified and eliminated. Abnormal microaggregates and pathological conformations of Aβ peptides might behave as xenobiotics. An increase in the xenobiotic metabolism pathway diminishes exposure to toxic compounds, and in the case of neuron cells, would decrease the accumulation of these compounds, thereby preventing Aβ deposition in AD (Dutheil et al. 2010). On the other hand, the *gba-1* gene encodes a glucosidase localized in the lysosome, involved in the destruction of toxic substances or in bacteria digestion. Deficiencies in this enzyme would contribute to the development of Parkinson's disease (Sidransky and López 2012). In fact, defective lysosomes play an important role in immune and neurological disorders and aging (Soukas et al. 2013).

In our study, the lactoferrin-based product showed the ability to extend the mean and final lifespan of nematodes with respect to control feeding conditions. This lifespan extension could be explained by the antioxidant activity of the product, which would improve the cellular redox status, decreasing ROS levels and hence favoring lifespan extension. Furthermore, the effect of lactoferrin on the immune system is known, and is thought to play a role in host defense, exhibiting antimicrobial activities, antiviral activities, and immunomodulation (Baveye et al. 1999; Chierici 2001; Zaczyńska et al. 2014). A recent study in humans provided evidence that oral supplementation with lactoferrin contributed to immune stimulation (Mulder et al. 2008). Our study shows that the lactoferrin-based product stimulates immune functions via induction of TGF-β and Wnt signaling pathways, and several genes encoding molecular effectors related with the innate immune response (Nicholas and Hodgkin 2004). This set of genes includes lysozymes (that mediate antibacterial defense through cleavage of bacterial cell walls), saposins (peptides with antibacterial activity that form ion-channels in the membranes of target cells), and lectins (proteins involved in pathogen detection). Concerning the signaling pathways, TGF-β pathway functions are related with protection against foreign microorganisms, axon pathfinding, body size/male tail development, and dauer formation (Patterson and Padgett 2000). Regarding the Wnt signaling pathway, it is formed by highly conserved secreted signaling molecules that regulate cell-to-cell interactions, cell proliferation, and differentiation during embryogenesis (Kim et al. 2013). It also has a role in central nervous system development (axis formation, neural growth, and development) in vertebrates (Rosso and Inestrosa 2013; Vargas et al. 2014). Both signaling pathways have previously been described as molecular targets of lactoferrin. Thus, lactoferrin was able to activate canonical TGF-β signaling in mice, contributing to protection against intestinal pathogens (Jang et al. 2014). Furthermore, lactoferrin stimulated cellular and intestinal development and immune system through the Wnt/β-catenin signaling pathway in an intestinal epithelial cell model (Jiang and Lönnerdal 2014). Furthermore, repression of Wnt signaling is associated with the progression of Alzheimer's pathology, whereas activation of Wnt signaling protects against Aβ toxicity and ameliorates cognitive impairment in AD patients (Wan et al. 2014; Riise et al. 2015).

In our study, the LfCD treatment displayed, in a dose-dependent manner, the ability to delay body paralysis in a *C. elegans* transgenic strain expressing the human Aβ(1–42) peptide in muscle. Although in this study, we did not confirm the potential activity of LfCD in preventing Aβ aggregation, additional experiments based on Aβ quantification in the presence/absence of the product would be decisive to understand additional mechanisms related with neurodegenerative disease. Moreover, our microarray analysis indicated an upregulation of several genes related with lipid metabolism at the neuronal level (Y48A6B.9 and *acs-7*). The Y48A6B.9 protein is an ortholog of human mitochondrial isoform of trans-2-enoyl-CoA reductase, involved in fatty acid elongation; *acs-7* gene encodes a human ortholog acyl-CoA synthetase family member 2, which intervenes in lipid synthesis and fatty acid degradation. The defects in these two genes cause alterations in the normal lipid homeostasis required for proper nervous system development, producing mental retardation and cognitive impairment in humans (Bhat et al. 2006; Çalışkan et al. 2011). Our results also showed an overexpression of *cat-4* gene (ortholog of the human GTP cyclohydrolase I), which participates in *C. elegans* neurotransmitter biosynthesis (serotonin and dopamine) involved in movement, mating behavior, and cell migration; animals bearing a cat-4 deletion reduces serotonin expression (Loer and Kenyon 1993) and causes dystonia in humans when mutated (Ichinose et al. 1994).

In addition, our study showed the activation of cell adhesion, neuroactive ligand-receptor interaction and neurogenesis and axon extension biological processes in the gene expression analysis. Cell adhesions are processes related with cell migration, cell differentiation, cell communication, and inflammation. In these processes, the adhesion molecules in the cell membrane, like cadherines, mediate adhesion in the growing axons. In our study, we observed the upregulation of the cadherine *cdh-3* gene, a Ca^{2+}-dependent adhesion molecule expressed in epithelial

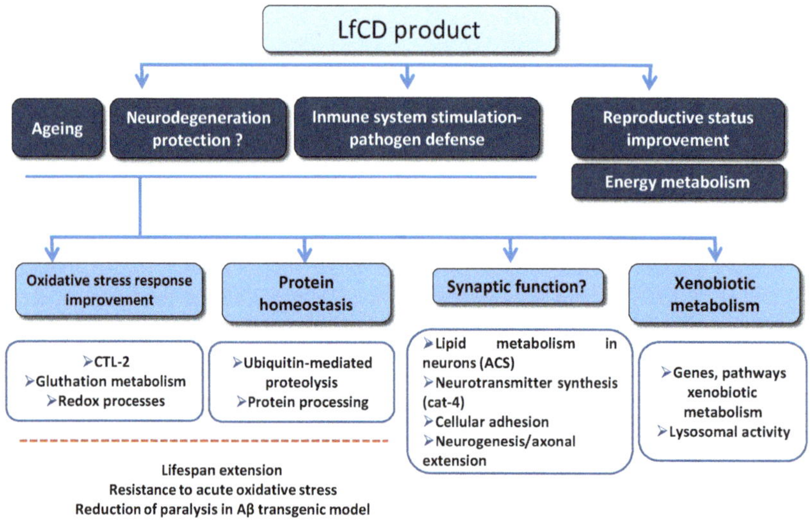

Figure 4. Model for the mechanism of action of LfCD product based on the different metabolic pathways targeted in *C. elegans*.

and neuroectodermal cells with a role in epithelial cell morphogenesis in *C. elegans* (Pettitt et al. 1996). This observed increase in cell adhesion could, hence, be related with the increase in axon guidance and neuroactive ligand-receptor interaction, suggesting that the lactoferrin-based product increased the expression of adhesion proteins in the growing axons. Taking into account that axons in neurons are essential for organelle transport and nerve impulse transmission, our hypothesis is that LfCD could improve the synaptic function in *C. elegans*. This would be in accordance with a recent work describing the protective effect of lactoferrin from degeneration in dopamine neurons of Parkinson's disease patients (Rousseau et al. 2013).

The LfCD-treated nematodes also showed an upregulation of the ubiquitin-mediated proteolysis process. This process takes places in the proteasome, degrading non-functional polyubiquitinated proteins to small peptides. Alterations in this pathway are implicated in the pathogenesis of many diseases, certain malignancies, and neurodegeneration (Glickman and Ciechanover 2002). A defect in protein homeostasis causes an accumulation of unfolded proteins or insoluble protein fibrils and aggregates, associated with AD (Alavez et al. 2011; Regitz et al. 2014). The observed overexpression of proteolysis suggests that lactoferrin would promote protein homeostasis in vivo, enhancing protein degradation. These results would support the potential attenuation of the toxicity produced by Aβ(1–42) peptide accumulation in transgenic nematodes, exerted by the LfCD product, and therefore in the delay of body paralysis. These data correlate well with previous studies, suggesting that lactoferrin shows neuroprotective effects against brain injury in rats (Van de Looij et al. 2014) and improves cognition in postnatal piglets through changes in the expression of some genes involved in neurodevelopment and cognition (Chen et al. 2014).

Finally, nematodes treated with the lactoferrin-based product experienced increased oviposition (Fig. S1) and energy metabolism. The ability of animals to regulate energy homeostasis is required for normal growth, development, and reproduction. Reproduction is a process with energy-intensive requirements, which depend on nutrient availability and metabolism. Several authors describe a connection between energy metabolism and reproductive behavior in *C. elegans* (Burks et al. 2000; Zhang et al. 2011; Martorell et al. 2012). These data may suggest that LfCD treatment upregulates the energy metabolism pathway, thereby having a positive effect on the reproductive status of *C. elegans*. Moreover, the reproductive pattern has been correlated with the activity of dopaminergic neurons (Nidheesh et al. 2016), which would support our hypothesis regarding the effect of the lactoferrin-based product on neuronal function.

In summary, this study demonstrates that a lactoferrin-based product displays antioxidant activity, extends lifespan and causes a delay in body paralysis in *C. elegans*. On the basis of our results and previously published data on lactoferrin's mode of action, we postulate that its mechanisms of action involve the activation of several metabolic pathways (Fig. 4). First, we propose that lactoferrin presents protection against aging and neurodegeneration by modulating processes involved in oxidative stress response, protein homeostasis, synaptic function, and xenobiotic metabolism. Second, we suggest lactoferrin would be able to stimulate the immune system and, finally, upregulate genes that improve reproductive status and energy metabolism.

Therefore, these findings indicate that oral supplementation with this lactoferrin-based product could improve immune system and antioxidant protection in humans. Further studies in *C. elegans* focused on neurotransmitter quantification, neurodegenerative protection or the ability to reduce Aβ aggregation would be of interest to confirm the role of LfCD on synaptic function. Finally, to confirm these results, clinical trials will be necessary.

Acknowledgments

This work was funded by Sesderma S.L. The funders had no role in data collection and analysis or preparation of the manuscript. We thank to C. Link for providing the *C. elegans* transgenic strain CL4176; and to the UCIM at University of Valencia for performing the DNA arrays.

Conflict of Interest

PM, SL, NG, DR, and SG are employees of Biopolis. GS, AT, JS, and MN are employees of Sesderma S.L. The authors declare no conflict of interest.

References

Adamkin, D. H. 2012. Mother's milk, feeding strategies, and lactoferrin to prevent necrotizing enterocolitis. JPEN J. Parenter. Enteral Nutr. 36:25S–29S.

Alavez, S., M. C. Vantipalli, D. J. Zucker, I. M. Klang, et al. 2011. Amyloid binding compounds maintain protein homeostasis during ageing and extend lifespan. Nature 472:226–229.

Ayton, S., P. Lei, and A. I. Bush. 2013. Metallostasis in Alzheimer's disease. Free Radic. Biol. Med. 62:76–89.

Back, P., B. P. Braeckman, and F. Matthijssens. 2012. ROS in aging *Caenorhabditis elegans*: damage or signaling? Oxid. Med. Cell. Longev. 2012:608478 doi:10.1155/2012/608478.

Baveye, S., E. Elass, J. Mazurier, and G. Spik. 1999. Lactoferrin: a multifunctional glycoprotein involved in the modulation of the inflammatory process. Clin. Chem. Lab. Med. 37:281–286.

Bhat, S. S., K. R. Schmidt, S. Ladd, K. C. Kim, et al. 2006. Disruption of *DMD* and deletion of *ACSL4* causing developmental delay, hypotonia, and multiple congenital anomalies. Cytogenet. Genome Res. 112:170–175.

Burks, D. J., J. Font de Mora, M. Schubert, D. J. Withers, et al. 2000. IRS-2 pathways integrate female reproduction and energy homeostasis. Nature 407:377–382.

Burrow, H., R. K. Kanwar, G. Mahidhara, and J. R. Kanwar. 2011. Effect of selenium-saturated bovine lactoferrin (Se-bLF) on antioxidant enzyme activities in human gut epithelial cells under oxidative stress. Anticancer Agents Med. Chem. 11:762–771.

Çalışkan, M., J. X. Chong, L. Uricchio, R. Anderson, et al. 2011. Exome sequencing reveals a novel mutation for autosomal recessive non-syndromic mental retardation in the TECR gene on chromosome 19p13. Hum. Mol. Genet. 20:1285–1289.

Chen, Y., Z. Zheng, X. Zhu, Y. Shi, D. Tian, et al. 2014. Lactoferrin promotes early neurodevelopment and cognition in postnatal piglets by upregulating the BDNF signaling pathway and polysialylation. Mol. Neurobiol. 52:256 [Epub ahead of print].

Chierici, R. 2001. Antimicrobial actions of lactoferrin. Adv. Nutr. Res. 10:247–269.

Christen, Y. 2000. Oxidative stress and Alzheimer disease. Am. J. Clin. Nutr. 71:621S–629S.

Cohen, M. S., J. Mao, G. T. Rasmussen, J. S. Serody, and B. E. Britigan. 1992. Interaction of lactoferrin and lipopolysaccharide (LPS): effects on the antioxidant property of lactoferrin and the ability of LPS to prime human neutrophils for enhanced superoxide formation. J. Infect. Dis. 166:1375–1378.

Connely, O. M. 2001. Antiinflammatory activities of lactoferrin. J. Am. Coll. Nutr. 438:389S–395S.

Dutheil, F., A. Jacob, S. Dauchy, P. Beaune, et al. 2010. ABC transporters and cytochromes P450 in the human central nervous system: influence on brain pharmacokinetics and contribution to neurodegenerative disorders. Expert Opin. Drug Metab. Toxicol. 6:1161–1174.

García-Montoya, I. A., T. S. Cendón, S. Arévalo-Gallegos, and Q. Rascón-Cruz. 2012. Lactoferrin a multiple bioactive protein: an overview. Biochim. Biophys. Acta 1820:226–236.

Glickman, M. H., and A. Ciechanover. 2002. The ubiquitin-proteasome proteolytic pathway: destruction for the sake of construction. Physiol. Rev. 82:373–428.

Guan, R., J. Ma, Y. Wu, F. Lu, et al. 2012. Development and characterization of lactoferrin nanoliposome: cellular uptake and stability. Nanoscale Res. Lett. 7:679.

Gutiérrez-Zepeda, A., R. Santell, Z. Wu, M. Brown, et al. 2005. Soy isoflavone glycitein protects against beta amyloid-induced toxicity and oxidative stress in transgenic *Caenorhabditis elegans*. BMC Neurosci. 6:54.

Huang, Y., and L. Mucke. 2012. Alzheimer mechanisms and therapeutic strategies. Cell 148:1204–1222.

Ichinose, H., T. Ohye, E. Takahashi, N. Seki, et al. 1994. Hereditary progressive dystonia with marked diurnal fluctuation caused by mutations in the GTP cyclohydrolase I gene. Nat. Genet. 8:236–242.

Irizarry, R. A., B. Hobbs, F. Collin, Y. D. Beazer-Barclay, et al. 2003. Exploration, normalization, and summaries of high density oligonucleotide array probe level data. Biostatistics 4:249–264.

Jang, Y. S., G. Y. Seo, J. M. Lee, H. Y. Seo, et al. 2014. Lactoferrin causes IgA and IgG2b isotype switching through betaglycan binding and activation of canonical TGF-β signaling. Mucosal Immunol.. doi:10.1038/mi.2014.121.

Jiang, R., and B. Lönnerdal. 2014. Transcriptomic profiling of intestinal epitelial cells in response to human, bovine and commercial bovine lactoferrins. Biometals 27:831–841.

Kamalinia, G., F. Khodagholi, F. Atyabi, M. Amini, F. Shaerzadeh, et al. 2013. Enhanced brain delivery of deferasirox-lactoferrin conjugates for iron chelation therapy in neurodegenerative disorders: in vitro and in vivo studies. Mol. Pharm. 10:4418–4431.

Kamemori, N., T. Takeuchi, K. Hayashida, and E. Harada. 2004. Suppressive effects of milk-derived lactoferrin on psychological stress in adult rats. Brain Res. 1029:34–40.

Kamemori, N., T. Takeuchi, A. Sugiyama, M. Miyabayashi, et al. 2008. Trans-endothelial and transepithelial transfer of lactoferrin into the brain through BBB and BCSFB in adult rats. J. Vet. Med. Sci. 70:313–315.

Kim, W., M. Kim, and E. H. Jho. 2013. Wnt/β-catenin signalling: from plasma membrane to nucleus. Biochem. J. 450:9–21.

Leffell, M. S., and J. K. Spitznagel. 1972. Association of lactoferrin with lysozyme in granules of human polymorphonuclear leukocytes. Infect. Immun. 6:761–765.

Levay, P. F., and M. Viljoen. 1995. Lactoferrin: a general review. Haematologica 80:252–267.

Link, C. D. 1995. Expression of human beta-amyloid peptide in transgenic *Caenorhabditis elegans*. Proc. Natl Acad. Sci. USA 92:9368–9372.

Link, C. D. 2006. *C. elegans* models of age-associated neurodegenerative diseases: lessons from transgenic worm models of Alzheimer's disease. Exp. Gerontol. 41:1007–1013.

Loer, C. M., and C. J. Kenyon. 1993. Serotonin-deficient mutants and male mating behavior in the nematode *Caenorhabditis elegans*. J. Neurosci. 13:5407–5417.

Maneva, A., B. Taleva, and L. Maneva. 2003. Lactoferrin-protector against oxidative stress and regulator of glycolysis in human erythrocytes. Z. Naturforsch. C. 58:256–262.

Martorell, P., J. V. Forment, R. de Llanos, F. Montón, et al. 2011. Use of *Saccharomyces cerevisiae* and *Caenorhabditis elegans* as model organisms to study the effect of cocoa polyphenols in the resistance to oxidative stress. J. Agric. Food Chem. 59:2077–2085.

Martorell, P., S. Llopis, N. González, F. Montón, et al. 2012. *Caenorhabditis elegans* as a model to study the effectiveness and metabolic targets of dietary supplements used for obesity treatment: the specific case of a conjugated linoleic acid mixture (Tonalin). J. Agric. Food Chem. 60:11071–11709.

Martorell, P., E. Bataller, S. Llopis, N. Gonzalez, et al. 2013. A cocoa peptide protects *Caenorhabditis elegans* from oxidative stress and β-amyloid peptide toxicity. PLoS One 8:e63283.

Montaner, D., and J. Dopazo. 2010. Multidimensional gene set analysis of genomic data. PLoS One 5:e10348.

Mulder, A. M., P. A. Connellan, C. J. Oliver, C. A. Morris, et al. 2008. Bovine lactoferrin supplementation supports immune and antioxidant status in healthy human males. Nutr. Res. 28:583–589.

Nicholas, H. R., and J. Hodgkin. 2004. Responses to infection and possible recognition strategies in the innate immune system of *Caenorhabditis elegans*. Mol. Immunol. 41:479–493.

Nidheesh, T., C. Salim, P. S. Rajini, and P. V. Suresh. 2016. Antioxidant and neuroprotective potential of chitooligomers in *Caenorhabditis elegans* exposed to Monocrotophos. Carbohydr. Polym. 135:138–144.

Ogasawara, Y., M. Imase, H. Oda, and H. Wakabayashi. 2014. Lactoferrin directly scavenges hydroxyl radicals and undergoes oxidative self-degradation: a possible role in protection against oxidative DNA damage. Int. J. Mol. Sci. 15:1003–1013.

Onishi, H. 2011. Lactoferrin delivery systems: approaches for its more effective use. Expert Opin. Drug Deliv. 8:1469–1479.

Patterson, G. I., and R. W. Padgett. 2000. TGF beta-related pathways. Roles in *Caenorhabditis elegans* development. Trends Genet. 16:27–33.

Pettitt, J., W. B. Wood, and R. H. Plasterk. 1996. Cdh-3, a gene encoding a member of the cadherin superfamily, functions in epithelial cell morphogenesis in *Caenorhabditis elegans*. Development 122:4149–4157.

Regitz, C., L. Dußling, and U. Wenzel. 2014. Amyloid-beta (Aβ(1-42))-induced paralysis in *Caenorhabditis elegans* is inhibited by the polyphenol quercetin through activation of protein degradation pathways. Mol. Nutr. Food Res. 58:1931–1940.

Riise, J., N. Plath, B. Pakkenberg, and A. Parachikova. 2015. Aberrant Wnt signaling pathway in medial temporal lobe structures of Alzheimer's disease. J. Neural. Transm. 122:1303 [Epub ahead of print].

Rosso, S. B., and N. C. Inestrosa. 2013. WNT signaling in neuronal maturation and synaptogenesis. Front. Cell. Neurosci. 7:103.

Rousseau, E., P. P. Michel, and E. C. Hirsch. 2013. The iron-binding protein lactoferrin protects vulnerable dopamine neurons from degeneration by preserving mitochondrial calcium homeostasis. Mol. Pharmacol. 84:888–898.

Safaeian, L., and H. Zabolian. 2014. Antioxidant effects of bovine lactoferrin on dexamethasone-induced hypertension in rat. ISRN Pharmacol.. doi:10.1155/2014/943523.

Sherman, M. P., S. H. Bennett, F. F. Hwang, and C. Yu. 2004. Neonatal small bowel epithelia: enhancing anti-bacterial defense with lactoferrin and *Lactobacillus* GG. Biometals 17:285–289.

Sidransky, E., and G. López. 2012. The link between the GBA gene and parkinsonism. Lancet Neurol. 11:986–998.

Soukas, A. A., C. E. Carr, and G. Ruvkun. 2013. Genetic regulation of *Caenorhabditis elegans* lysosome related organelle function. PLoS Genet. 9:e1003908.

Van de Looij, Y., V. Ginet, A. Chatagner, A. Toulotte, and E. Somm. 2014. Lactoferrin during lactation protects the immature hypoxic-ischemic rat brain. Ann. Clin. Transl. Neurol. 1:955–967.

Vargas, J. Y., M. Fuenzalida, and N. C. Inestrosa. 2014. In vivo activation of Wnt signaling pathway enhances cognitive function of adult mice and reverses cognitive deficits in an Alzheimer's disease model. J. Neurosci. 34:2191–2202.

Wan, W., S. Xia, B. Kalionis, L. Liu, et al. 2014. The role of Wnt signaling in the development of Alzheimer's disease: a potential therapeutic target? Biomed. Res. Int. 2014:301575.

Wang, B. 2012. Molecular mechanism underlying sialic acid as an essential nutrient for brain development and cognition. Adv. Nutr. 3:465S–472S.

Wang, L., H. Sato, S. Zhao, and I. Tooyama. 2010. Deposition of lactoferrin in fibrillar-type senile plaques in the brains of transgenic mouse models of Alzheimer's disease. Neurosci. Lett. 481:164–167.

Wolfson, D. R., and J. B. Robbins. 1971. Heterogeneity of human lactoferrin due to differences in sialic acid content. Pediatr. Res. 5:514–517.

Wu, G., Y. Z. Fang, S. Yang, and J. R. Lupton. 2004. Glutathione metabolism and its implications for health. J. Nutr. 134:489–492.

Wu, Y., Z. Wu, P. Butko, Y. Christen, et al. 2006. Amyloid-beta induced pathological behaviors are suppressed by *Ginkgo biloba* extract EGb761 and ginkgolides in transgenic *Caenorhabditis elegans*. J. Neurosci. 26:13102–13113.

Yamauchi, K., H. Wakabayashi, K. Shin, and M. Takase. 2006. Bovine lactoferrin: benefits and mechanism of action against infections. Biochem. Cell Biol. 84:291–296.

Zaczyńska, E., M. Kocięba, E. Śliwińska, and M. Zimecki. 2014. Bovine lactoferrin enhances proliferation of human peripheral blood lymphocytes and induces cytokine production in whole blood cultures. Adv. Clin. Exp. Med. 23:871–876.

Zhang, J., R. Bakheet, R. S. Parhar, C. H. Huang, et al. 2011. Regulation of fat storage and reproduction by Krüppel-like transcription factor KLF3 and fat-associated genes in *Caenorhabditis elegans*. J. Mol. Biol. 411:537–553.

6

Carotenoid profiling of the leaves of selected African eggplant accessions subjected to drought stress

Elias K. Mibei[1], Jane Ambuko[2], James J. Giovannoni[3], Arnold N. Onyango[1] & Willis O. Owino[1]

[1]Department of Food Science and Technology, Jomo Kenyatta University of Agriculture and Technology, Nairobi, Kenya
[2]Department of Plant Science and Crop Protection, University of Nairobi, Nairobi, Kenya
[3]Boyce Thompson Institute for Plant Research, Cornell University Campus, Ithaca, New York 14853

Keywords
African eggplants, Carotenoids, chlorophylls, drought stress, stress tolerance

Correspondence
Willis O. Owino, Department of Food Science and Technology, Jomo Kenyatta University of Agriculture and Technology, Nairobi 00200, Kenya.
E-mail: willis@agr.jkuat.ac.ke

Funding Information
The support for this research work was provided by U.S. Agency for International Development through the Partnerships for Enhanced Engagement in Research (PEER) program Sub-Grant Number: PGA-2000003426 to Dr. Willis Owino and Prof. James Giovannoni.

Abstract

African eggplants (*Solanum aethiopicum* and *S. macrocarpon*) are among the most economically important and valuable vegetable and fruit crops. They are a major source of biologically active nutritional substances and metabolites which are essential for plant growth, development, stress adaptation and defense. Among these metabolites are the carotenoids which act as accessory pigments for photosynthesis and precursor to plant hormones. Though African eggplants are known to be resistant to various abiotic stresses, the effect of these stresses on secondary metabolites has not been well defined. The objective of this study was to establish the effect of drought stress on carotenoid profiles of nineteen African eggplant accessions selected based on leaf and fruit morphological traits. Stress was achieved by limiting irrigation and maintaining the wilting state of the crops. Fresh leaves were sampled at different maturity stages; before stress, 2 weeks and 4 weeks after stress for carotenoid analysis. The fresh harvested leaf tissues were immediately frozen in liquid nitrogen and ground. Analysis was carried out using a Dionex HPLC machine coupled to Photo Array Detector and Chromeleon software package (Thermo Fisher Scientific Inc, Waltham, Massachusetts, USA). Major carotenoids viz;. Xanthophylls (neoxanthin, violaxanthin, zeaxanthin and lutein) and carotenes (β–carotene and α–carotene), phytofluene, lycopene, phytoene as well as chlorophylls (chlorophyll-b and Chlorophyll-a) were targeted. The carotenoids increased with maturity stage of the crop. Although the stressed crops reported significantly decreased amount of carotenes, chlorophylls, neoxanthin and violaxanthin, the concentration of zeaxanthin increased with stress whereas lutein had no significant change. Chlorophyll-a was significantly high in all the control accessions. Two accessions reported significantly higher contents of carotenoids as compared to the other accessions. The results of this study indicate that water stress has significant impact on the concentration of some carotenoids and photosynthetic pigments. This will definitely add value to the study of stress tolerance in crops.

Introduction

African eggplants (*Solanum aethiopicum* and *S. macrocarpon*) are among the nutritionally important and valuable crops in the Solanaceae family (Chadha and Mndiga 2007). They constitute important fruit and leaf vegetables in Africa (Shippers 2000) due to their dual value: leaves are used as cooked vegetables and the fruits are also edible. The leaves are appreciated for their slightly bitter taste and are eaten separately or in sauces. The fruit flesh on the other hand can be sweet or bitter in taste. The bitter cultivars have been used as medicine in many African countries (Chadha and Mndiga 2007). Besides, there is also increasing evidence that the intake of their leaves and fruits have favorable impact on the incidence of many chronic diseases including diabetes (Kwon et al. 2008). In addition, most indigenous vegetables have been reported to be rich in micronutrients and nutritional components (Mibei et al. 2011) and phytochemicals including alkaloids, flavonoids, tannins, saponins, steroids, phenols and antioxidants (Mibei and Ojijo 2011; Mibei et al. 2012). These are of health or nutraceutical significance therefore, authenticates their usefulness for medicinal purposes (Briskin 2000).

Despite the importance of many indigenous plants, stress has been reported as a major limiting factor leading to change in their growth and development thus disrupting metabolic homeostasis. This affects plants and requires an adjustment of metabolic pathways for acclimation (Suzuki et al. 2012). Metabolomics is an essential part of a systems biology approach to study plant defense, since different metabolic profiles are indicative of changes in metabolic pathways (Hankemeier 2007). Therefore, when plants are subjected to water stress, they change physically and chemically in numerous ways. In addition, they produce a huge number of metabolites to adapt to the stress conditions. Among these metabolites of interest are the carotenoids which are widely distributed in nature. They not only act as accessory pigments for photosynthesis and as precursors to plant hormones (Cazzonelli 2011), but also impart various benefits to human health (Johnson 2002; Rao and Rao 2007). They are potent antioxidants and free radical scavengers (Grassmann et al. 2002). This is believed to contribute to their ability to modulate the pathogenesis of coronary cancers (van Poppel and Goldbohm 1995) and coronary heart disease (Kritchevsky 1999). On the other hand, lycopene intake is associated with a decreased incidence of prostate cancer (Giovannucci 2002) and diabetes (Facchini et al. 2000).

Due to their importance in diet and health benefits, carotenoids have been extensively studied in different matrices to analyze their distribution and levels in plants. Based on this, the metabolic adjustments in response to the water stress conditions may be analyzed and this will highlight carotenoids that play important roles in metabolism and physiology of the plant. These carotenoids as well are important for human health as they have nutritional and medicinal properties.

Materials and Methods

Plant material

Seeds of seventy four African eggplant accession were obtained from the from local farmers, farmer groups and a variety of gene banks at local and regional centers and institutes which include, Kenya Agricultural Research Institute (KARI), Muguga Kenya and the Asian Vegetable Research Development Centre (AVRDC), Arusha, Tanzania.

Nineteen African eggplants accessions were selected (Table 1) based on their morphological traits. The traits were based on fruit size and weight, fruit shape, fruit length, flower color, leaf blade length and width. The selected accessions were grown alongside each other in the greenhouse at the Boyce Thomson Institute for Plant Research, Cornell University, USA during March - May, 2015 under carefully controlled and optimal growth conditions.

Table 1. List of selected African eggplants from the accessions provided by AVRDEC-ESA.

S/no	RVI code	Genus	Species	Name
1	RVI00343	*Solanum*	*macrocarpon*	CN012
2	RVI00199	*Solanum*	*sp*	EX-DAR
3	RVI00201	*Solanum*	*aethiopicum*	GKK-AE-158
4	RVI00332	*Solanum*	*aethiopicum*	RNL187-194
5	RVI00271	*Solanum*	*aethiopicum*	Line 87
6	RVI00445	*Solanum*	*sp*	S0004
7	RVI00333	*Solanum*	*aethiopicum*	SANGAWILI
8	RVI00259	*Solanum*	*aethiopicum*	Line 55
9	RVI00265	*Solanum*	*aethiopicum*	Line 21
10	RVI00273	*Solanum*	*aethiopicum*	Line 89
11	RVI00511	*Solanum*	*aethiopicum*	SENGEREMA 1
12	RVI00432	*Solanum*	*sp*	N4
13	RVI00246	*Solanum*	*aethiopicum*	Line 112
14	RVI00328	*Solanum*	*aethiopicum*	LOCAL MALI
15	RVI00327	*Solanum*	*aethiopicum*	AUBERGINE BLANCHE
16	RVI00342	*Solanum*	*aethiopicum*	OFARIWA'A
17	RVI00330	*Solanum*	*aethiopicum*	Local Gaya
18	GBK 050591	*Solanum*	*aethiopicum*	Kenya
19	RVI00438	*Solanum*	*aethiopicum*	MM1308

RVI-Accession registration code used in AVRDEC, sp - species.

Treatments

The African eggplant seeds were germinated in the greenhouse in trays and the seedlings transplanted after 4 weeks of germination. Normal irrigation was maintained before and 5 days after transplanting of the seedlings to keep the soil moisture at over 90% field capacity. The seedlings (one per pot) were grown in 15 cm-diameter pots containing growth media using randomized complete block design with three replications. The experiment had two treatments; water stress and control experiments. Water stress treatments were initiated after 5 days of transplanting. This was achieved by stopping irrigation for a few days and soil moisture monitored every day using Delmhorst model KS-D1 Digital Soil Moisture Tester (Delmhorst Instrument Co., Towaco, NJ). The wilting state of the crops was maintained and losses in soil moisture below 60% represented transpiration and evaporation. Therefore irrigation was done after every 2 days with equal amount of water (approximately 1 L) to compensate for this. For the control treatment, continued watering with sufficient amount of water (normal irrigation) was maintained throughout.

Chemicals

Tetrahydrofuran, petroleum ether, ethyl acetate, methanol and methyltert-butyl ether were purchased from Fischer Scientific (Fair Lawn, NJ). All reagents were analytical or HPLC grade. All mobile phases and samples were filtered before use.

Sample collection

Fresh leaves were sampled early in the morning at different growth and development stages (before stress, 2 weeks and 4 weeks after stress) for carotenoid analysis. The materials were harvested from equivalent fully expanded leaves from each plant at each stage. The harvested leaf tissues were immediately plunged (snap-frozen) in liquid nitrogen to quench further metabolism. Afterwards, they were ground in liquid nitrogen and stored in 15 mL falcon tubes at −80°C. The frozen leaf tissues were later used for carotenoid analysis by HPLC.

Carotenoid extraction

Carotenoids were extracted from the frozen leaf tissues using a modified protocol from Alba et al. (2005). About 200 mg of each tissue was weighed into 2 mL Eppendorf tubes and 2 beads added. Fifty microliters (50 μL) of 3 mg/mL magnesium carbonate suspension was added to each tube and 300 μL of tetrahydrofuran (THF) added to each tube. The mixture was homogenized in FastPrep machine (FastPrep-24, MP Biomedicals, Santa Ana, California, USA) (45 sec, speed = 5.0) and incubated at 4°C (in ice) for 20 min in dark. 300 μL of methanol was also added and homogenized then incubated at 4°C for 10 min. The homogenate was then transferred to Spin-X filter, centrifuged for 1 min at 1487 × g (4°C). 150 μL of THF and 150 μL of methanol were added to original extraction tube and vortexed. 1 mL pipettor (cut tip) was used to transfer all THF/methanol/debris to spin-X filter and centrifuged again. The filtered extract was then transferred to new 2 mL tube and 450 μL of THF added to debris pellet in spin-X filter and incubated on ice for 15 min (dark); centrifuged for 5 min at maximum speed. The filtered extracts were combined and 375 μL petroleum ether and 150 μL of 25% NaCl were added to each combined extract and vortexed vigorously. It was then centrifuged at maximum speed at 4°C for 3 min to separate phases and the upper phase transferred to new 2 mL tube. The interphase/lower phase was re-extracted with 500 μL petroleum ether and the upper phases removed and combined with like samples. The petroleum ether extract was then rotor evaporated for 20 min at 45°C (to near dryness). When HPLC was not conducted immediately, the dried extracts were stored under nitrogen (N_2) at −80°C (dark). 500 μL ethyl acetate was added and incubated at room temperature for 15 min to resuspend carotenoids; vortexed well and carotenoid suspension filtered through 0.45 μm nylon syringe filter (Cameo 3N syringe filter, GE Water and Process Technologies Trevose, Pennsylvania, USA).

HPLC analysis (YMC C_{30} column)

Carotenoid analysis was carried out using a Dionex HPLC machine (P680 HPLC pump, ASI-100 Automated Sample Injector; PDA-100 Photo Array Detector) and Chromeleon (v6.40 software package). Carotenoids were separated with a polar to non-polar gradient (0–5 min 100% methanol:0.1% ammonium acetate; 6–25 min ramp to 4% methanol:0.1% ammonium acetate and 96% methyl t-butyl ether; 26–30 min ramp to 100% methanol:0.1% ammonium acetate; 31–35 min 100% methanol:0.1% ammonium acetate) through a guard cartridge (YMC Carotenoid S-5, 4.0 mm × 20 mm DC guard; Waters), C30 column (YMC Carotenoid S-5, 4.6 mm × 250 mm; Waters) assembly. Five channels were used for data acquisition: channel 1 (286 nm); channel 2 (348 nm); channel 3 (434 nm); channel 4 (450 nm) and channel 5 (471 nm).

Identification and quantification of carotenoids

Peak identification was performed as described in Alba et al. (2005). The carotenoids were identified by comparing their retention time and spectra with respective authentic standards analyzed under identical analytical conditions. Peak areas of each of the standards were used to draw the standard curve and quantify the carotenoids.

Data analysis

The data were subjected to the statistical analysis of the variance (ANOVA) to evaluate significant differences between the different developmental stages and treatments of African eggplants. The analysis was performed using GenStat discovery 14th Edition (Payne et al. 2011) at 5% level of significance. Mean separation was done by Fisher's protected least significant difference (LSD) test using GenStat at $P = 0.05$.

Results

The difference in plant morphology under stress is illustrated in Figure 1.

Carotenoids profile of African eggplant leaves

The HPLC fingerprinting of the African eggplant leaf extracts revealed the presence of the carotenoids such as neoxanthin, violaxanthin, zeaxanthin, α-carotene, β-carotene, lutein and other unknowns. The chlorophylls (chlorophyll a and chlorophyll b) were also identified (Table 2). Phytoene, phytofluene and lycopene were not detected.

The total carotenoids of the leaves of the selected African eggplants subjected to drought stress and controls are reported in Figure 2. The concentration increased with the growth stages of the African eggplants with 4 weeks sampled leaves recording significantly higher amount ($P < 0.05$). The highest of the estimated carotenoids in mature leaves was reported in RV100327 (1049.4 ± 43.7 μg/g FW), RV100343 (1020.9 ± 26.9 μg/g FW), RV100438 (969.7 ± 30.3 μg/g FW) and RV100511 (996.2 ± 32.3 μg/g FW) stressed accessions whereas for the control RV100343 (1182.3 ± 33.6 μg/g FW), RV100332 (1027.2 ± 43.9 μg/g FW) and RV100438 (998.9 ± 37.6 μg/g FW) accessions had considerable high concentration of the total carotenoids. Unlike the other accessions, the concentration of the total carotenoids for GBK50591, RV100271, RV100265, RV100511, RV100327, RV100330 and RV100199 significantly increased ($P < 0.05$) in stressed crops as compared to the controls. Contrary to the trend for the other accessions, RV100201, RV100432, and RV100342 reported significantly higher ($P < 0.05$) carotenoids at 2 weeks then the content reduced as the plant grows at 4 weeks.

During the growth of the plant, increase in the carotenoids occurred in almost all the accessions. This was evident in the leaves sampled after 4 weeks (Fig. 2) reporting higher contents as compared to other stages. The chlorophyll contents of the leaves were also significantly higher ($P < 0.05$) as compared to the carotenoids. Zeaxanthin and α-carotene on the other hand reported low concentrations in both the stressed and control plants.

The individual carotenoid and chlorophyll concentrations of each African eggplant accession are shown in Figure 3. The concentration of the different carotenoids varied within between the different accessions.

The identified compounds were grouped into chlorophylls (chlorophyll a and chlorophyll b) (Fig. 4), carotenes (alpha carotene and beta carotene) (Fig. 5) and xanthophylls (lutein, zeaxanthin, violaxanthin and neoxanthin) (Fig. 6).

Chlorophylls

The chlorophyll contents decreased with stress (Fig. 4) since a significantly higher ($P < 0.05$) concentration of chlorophylls was reported in the controls as compared to the drought stressed crops. Chlorophylls also increased with plant growth and development with mature leaves (4 weeks) reporting higher concentration.

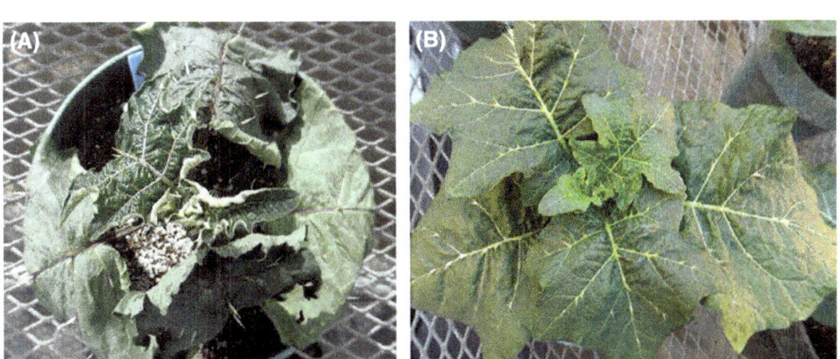

Figure 1. The picture of African eggplant (RV100332) accession (A) Water stressed (B) Control treatments.

Table 2. Carotenoids separated on a reverse-phase C30 HPLC system and spectral characteristics used in identification from photodiode array detection.

Carotenoid	Spectral characteristics (nm λ_{max})	Retention time (min)
Neoxanthin	466	6.99
Violaxanthin	433	7.68
Chlorophyll b	465, 471	10.6
Phytoene 1	284–286	~10.8
Lutein	442, 450	~11
Chlorophyll a	430	12.73
Zeaxanthin	430	13.33
Phytoene 2	284–286	~13.5
Phytofluene 1	343/348	~14.3
Phytofluene 2	343	~15.1
Others (unknown)	441, 443	15.96, 16.44
α-Carotene	407	17.03
β-carotene	450	~17.1, 17.6
Cis-Lycopene	471	~22.2
Trans-Lycopene	471	~24

Carotenes

The concentration of carotenes; β-carotene and α-carotene are reported in Figure 5. Similar to the chlorophylls, a significant increase in the concentration was also seen as the crop grows. Likewise the trend was also the same as stressed crops had significantly lower concentration of carotene as compared to the controls. In addition, the β-carotene was significantly higher ($P < 0.05$) as compared to α-carotene.

Xanthophylls

The concentration of xanthophylls lutein, zeaxanthin, violaxanthin and neoxanthin is reported in Figure 6. Contrary to the other xanthophylls, zeaxanthin reported increased concentration with the stress as compared to the control. Lutein had no significant difference between the stress and the control whereas violaxanthin and neoxanthin had significantly higher content in the control as compared to the stress.

Discussion

In this study, a comparative analysis of the carotenoid and chlorophyll composition of leaves of 19 African eggplant accessions at different stages of maturity under adequate water availability or water stress conditions was done. Maturity in the leaves reflected enhanced

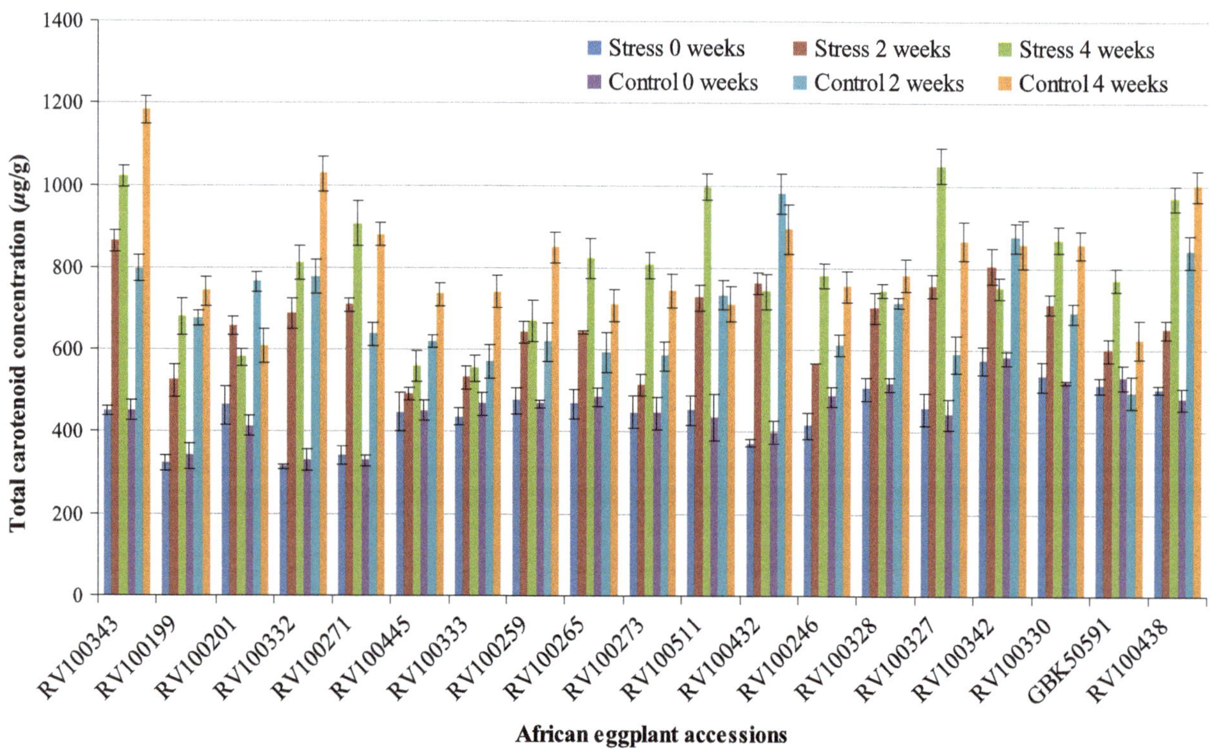

Figure 2. The total carotenoid concentration in the leaves of African eggplant subjected to stress and control at different growth and development stages; 0 weeks, 2 weeks and 4 weeks. Total carotenoid contents were calculated by taking the sum of each compound in all African eggplants. The results are presented as μg/g ± SD fresh weight.

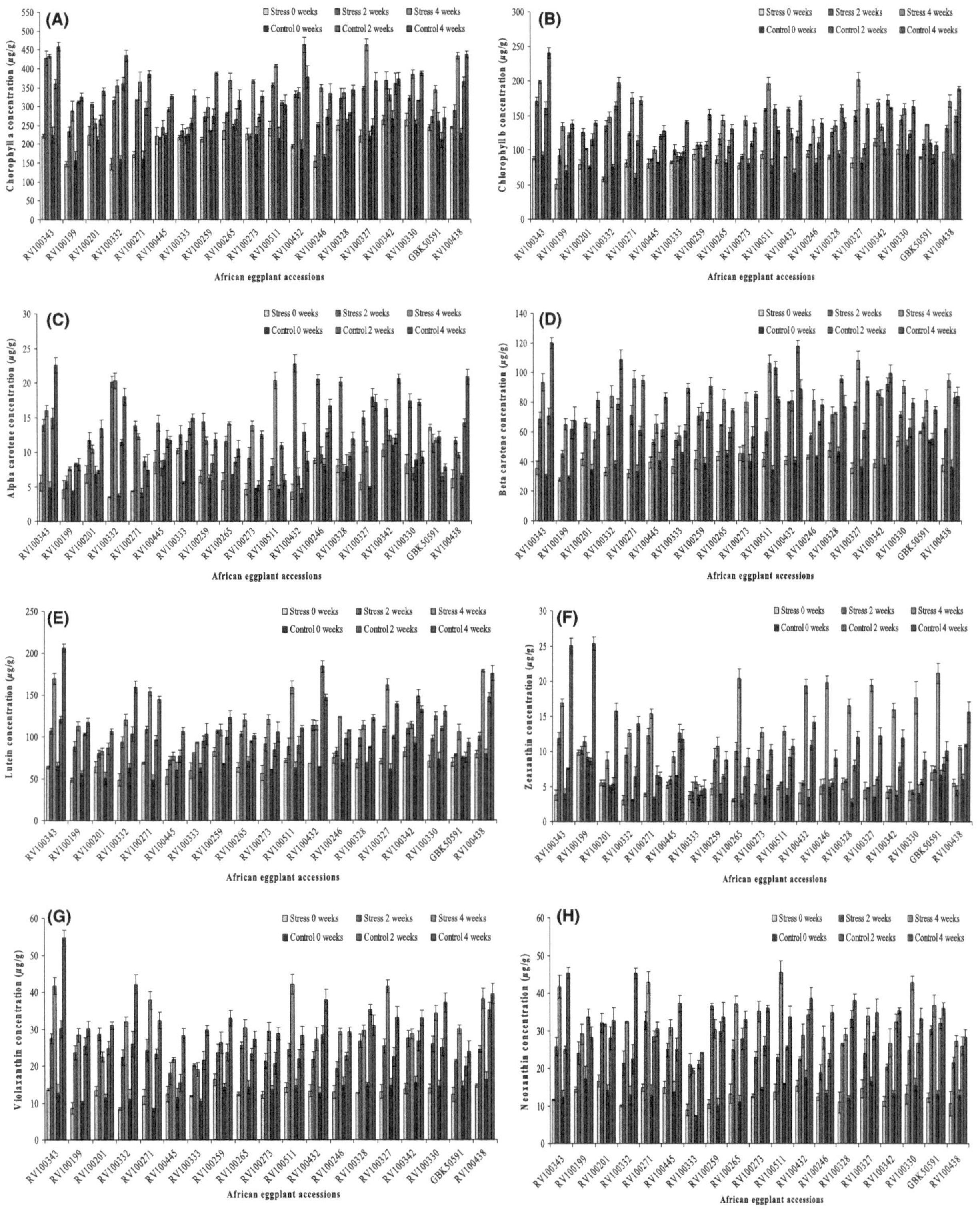

Figure 3. The carotenoid and chlorophyll concentration of different accessions expressed as µg/g ± SD fresh weight (n = 3) at different growth and development stages (0 weeks, 2 weeks and 4 weeks) for stress and control treatments. (A) Chlorophyll a, (B) chlorophyll b, (C) alpha carotene, (D) beta carotene, (E) lutein, (F) zeaxanthin, (G) violaxanthin and (H) neoxanthin.

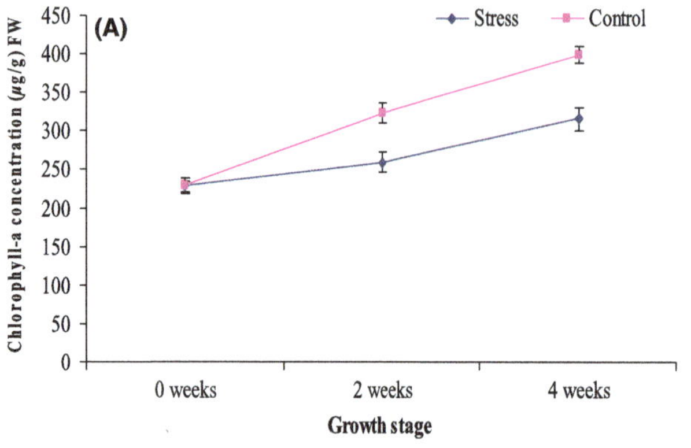

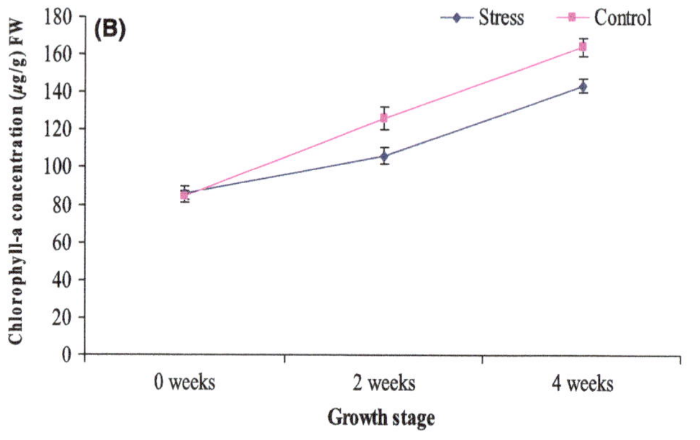

Figure 4. Average concentration of chlorophylls (A) chlorophyll a and (B) chlorophyll b of the stressed and control treatments of African eggplant accessions during different growth and development stages. Three independent leaf tissues were measured and expressed as mean ± SD (µg/g) fresh weight. The leaves were sampled before stress (0 weeks), 2 and 4 weeks after stress.

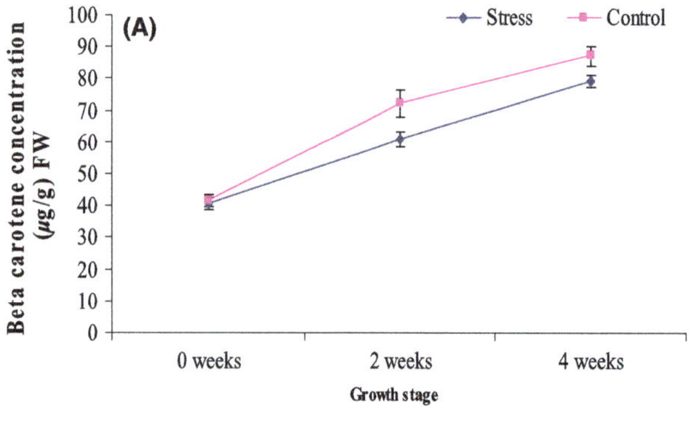

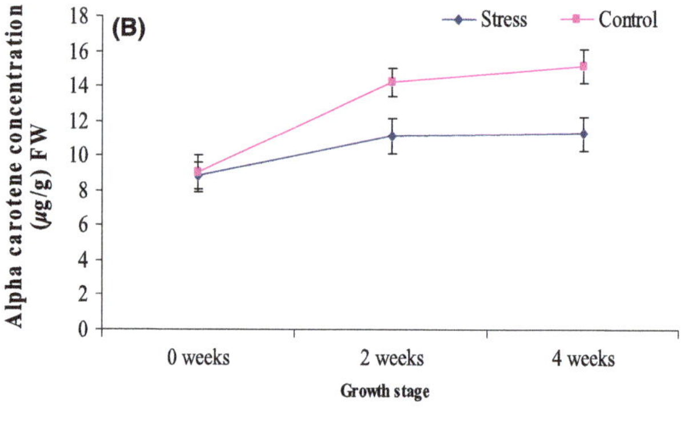

Figure 5. Average concentration of carotenes (A) β-carotene and (B) α-carotene of the stressed and control treatments of African eggplant accessions during different growth and development stages. Three independent leaf tissues were measured and expressed as mean ± SD (µg/g) fresh weight. The leaves were sampled before stress (0 weeks), 2 weeks and 4 weeks after stress.

carotenoid metabolic activities occurring during plant growth and development. This is reported by results showing changing concentrations with progressive plant growth and development as well as differences between in the stressed and control crops. There were significant differences in carotenoid concentration among the accessions used in the study. The concentration of all the carotenoids increased with growth and development of the plant. The most significant increase in the pigment concentration was recorded with 4 weeks after transplanting. This clearly indicates that the plant pigments accumulate as the plant grows. Some carotenoids were markedly characteristic of some accessions such as RV100343 and RV100342 which reported significantly higher contents ($P < 0.05$) of carotenoids as compared to the other accessions. These two accessions had a characteristic morphology of small leaf size as compared to the others.

Water stress, among other changes, has been reported to have the ability to reduce the tissue concentrations of chlorophylls and carotenoids (Kiani et al. 2008), primarily with the production of reactive oxygen species in the thylakoids (Reddy et al. 2004). The data from the study showed that the photosynthetic pigments such as the chlorophylls significantly reduced with stress. In general, the results obtained from this study agree with those reported in the literature and the values fall within the wide ranges of data found in the literature.

The variations in the levels of the major carotenoids lutein, β-carotene and neoxanthin, were similar to those observed for the chlorophylls, with decreases observed under water stress. The major carotenoids, violaxanthin and β-carotene increased progressively in control, whereas the proportion of lutein did not significantly change during the stress treatment. This is an indication that lutein is not significantly affected by water stress and this is an

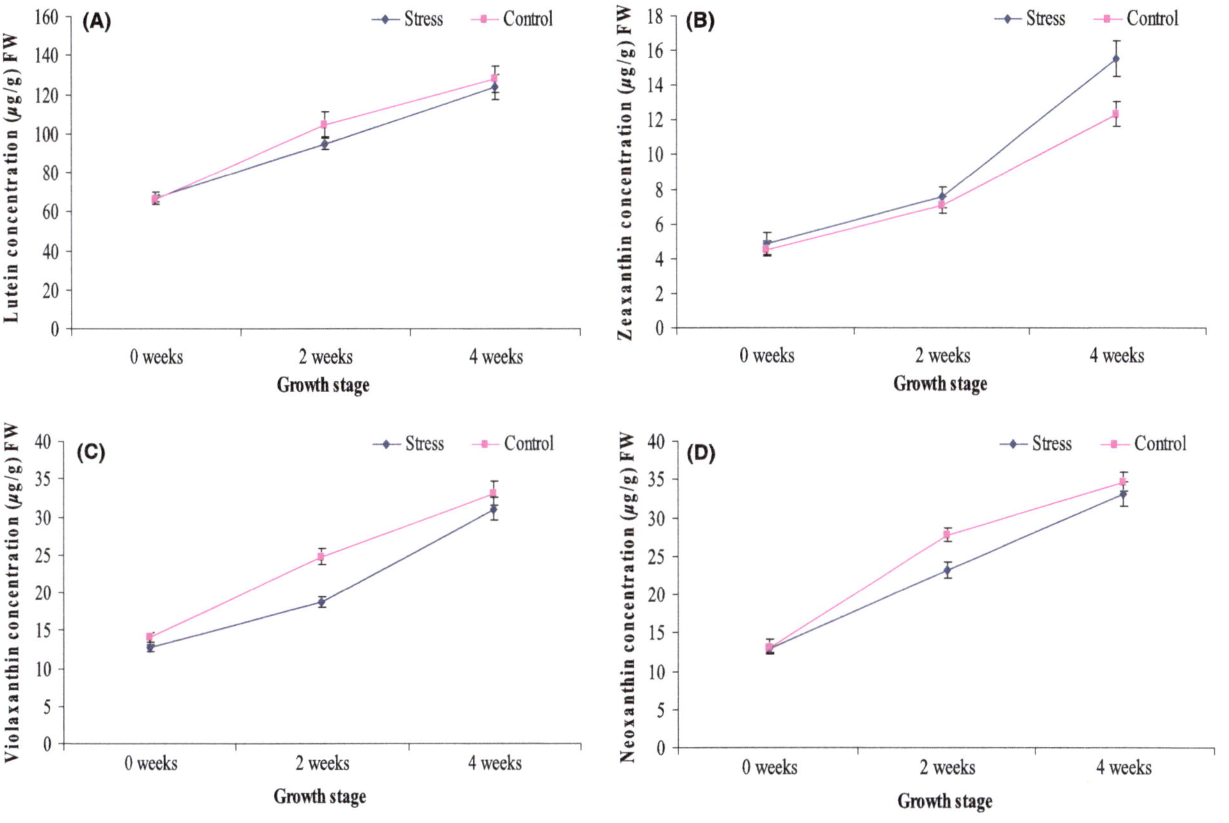

Figure 6. Average concentration of xanthophylls (A) lutein (B) zeaxanthin (C) violaxanthin and (D) neoxanthin of the stressed and control treatments of African eggplant accessions during different growth and development stages. Three independent leaf tissues were measured and expressed as mean ± SD (µg/g) fresh weight. The leaves were sampled before stress (0 weeks), 2 and 4 weeks after stress.

important avenue in the study of plan tolerance to stress. Variations similar to those of chlorophyll have also been observed for lutein, b-carotene and neoxanthin in rosemary plants (Munné-Bosch and Alegre 2000).

The proportions of zeaxanthin, neoxanthin, and violaxanthin were largely altered by the water stress treatment. During the stress treatment zeaxanthin increased whereas violaxanthin and neoxanthin decreased. On the contrary, RV100201, RV100432 and RV100342 accessions reported significantly higher carotenoids at 2 weeks and the contents reduced as the plant grows at 4 weeks. The fact that mature leaves suffered more stress than young leaves in these accessions suggests that developmental stages of these leaves might contribute to the differential prevention of oxidative damage in mature plants.

The decrease in chlorophyll content under drought is a commonly observed phenomenon (Heba and Samia 2014). This confirms the statement by Farooq et al. (2009) that both chlorophyll a and b are prone to soil drying. A reduction in chlorophyll content has also been reported in drought stressed cotton (Massacci et al. 2008) and Catharanthus roseus (Jaleel et al. 2009). In addition, the findings concur with that of the study by Kumar et al. (2011) who reported that chlorophyll content decreases under drought stress. This is because drought stress has been reported to cause closing of stoma, limitation of gas exchange and reduction of leaf area (Jaleel et al. 2009; Kumudini 2010); consequently decreasing photosynthetic pigments and activity. Similarly, this might be attributed to reduced synthesis of the main chlorophyll pigment complexes encoded by the cab gene family (Nikolaeva et al. 2010), or to destruction of the pigment protein complexes which protect the photosynthetic apparatus, or to oxidative damage of chloroplast lipids and proteins, therefore formation of chlorophyll a, b and other carotenoids decreases. Therefore, both stomatal and non-stomatal limitations (metabolic impairment) are generally accepted to be the main determinant of reduced photosynthetic pigments under drought stress (Farooq et al. 2009).

A concerted action of both enzymatic (ascorbate peroxidase, superoxide dismutase, peroxidase, ascorbate peroxidase, catalase, polyphenol oxidase and glutathione reductase) and non-enzymatic antioxidant (ascorbate, reduced glutathione, α-tocopherol and carotenoids) systems alleviates oxidative damage generated by drought stress in the plant tissue (Prochazkova et al. 2001). Nevertheless, carotenes form a key part of the plant antioxidant defense system, but they are very susceptible to oxidative destruction. In severe stress, β-carotene may be rapidly destroyed and therefore are no longer available to protect against oxidative damage (Young and Britton 1990). This explains the significant reduction in the concentrations of the stressed crops from the study.

The concentration of carotenoids and chlorophylls provide information about the level of stress experienced by the plant as well as its ability to endure these stresses (Strzalka et al. 2003). Therefore, due to the significant decrease in carotenoids during drought stress, it is evident that drought may lead to reduction in plant productivity. This is mainly by inhibiting growth and photosynthesis, and is one major limiting factor in agriculture worldwide leading to huge reductions in crop yield (Chaves and Oliveira 2004).

Conclusion

This study focused on the quantification of carotenoids of the leaves of African eggplants commonly consumed as leafy and fruit vegetables. The results gave comparative profiles of carotenoids at different growth and developmental stages and under drought stress. Perhaps the carotenoid levels increase with plant maturity, therefore in any case, mature leaves can provide high amounts of carotenoids that are important to human health. As well water stress affects the levels of carotenoids especially the chlorophylls which are the primary photosynthetic pigments. With this it is evident that plants subjected to drought stress have reduced levels of plant pigments such as chlorophylls and carotenes and increased xanthophylls. This adversely affects the functioning of the plant as it hinders the process of photosynthesis. Some of the observed carotenoid compositional changes could directly be related to known phenomenon associated with plant development, stress and photosynthetic activity. These changes may not only affect the nutritional value of the leaves abut also the health and medicinal value of the crops. The study therefore, presents data that attests to the importance of African eggplants in providing the much-needed dietary neutraceutical potential since they have substantial amounts of the important carotenoids. There is need to characterize other secondary metabolites of medicinal value such as the flavonoids, anthocyanins so as to state the effects of stress on these. This will help define the effect of stress on different plant metabolites and might also help in study of stress tolerance in plants.

Acknowledgments

The authors thank Dr. Tsvetelina Stoilova of Seed repository, AVRDC- World Vegetable Center in Arusha, Tanzania for the provision of the African eggplant seeds. We also thank the Staff of Boyce Thomson Institute for Plant Research (BTI), Cornell University, USA for being wonderful hosts and technical assistance. We specifically thank Ryan McQuinn, Itay Gonda, Betsy Ampofo, Grace Wacheke, and Meena M. Haribal of BTI for the technical assistance and Bryan K. Bell for efficient and excellent care of the eggplants in the greenhouse.

Conflict of Interest

None declared.

References

Alba, R., P. Payton, Z. J. Fei, R. McQuinn, P. Debbie, G. B. Martin, et al. 2005. Transcriptome and selected metabolite analyses reveal multiple points of ethylene control during tomato fruit development. Plant Cell 17:2954–2965.

Briskin, D. P. 2000. Medicinal plants and phytomedicines. Linking plant biochemistry and physiology to human health. Plant Physiol. 124:507–514.

Cazzonelli, C. I. 2011. Carotenoids in nature: insights from plants and beyond. Funct. Plant Biol. 38:833–847.

Chadha, M. L., H. H. Mndiga. 2007. African Eggplant - From Underutilized to a Commercially Profitable Venture. In: Proceedings of the 1st International Conference on Indigenous Vegetables and Legumes—Prospectus for Fighting Poverty, Hunger and Malnutrition. Eds. M.I. Chadha, G. Kuo, C. L. L. Gowda, Acta Horticulturalae. International Society for Horticultural Sciences (ISHS): Korbeek-Lo, Belgium, 2007; pp. 521–523.

Chaves, M. M., and M. M. Oliveira. 2004. Mechanisms underlying plant resilience to water deficits: prospects for water-saving agriculture. J. Exp. Bot. 55:2365–2384.

Facchini, F. S., M. H. Humphreys, C. A. DoNascimento, F. Abbasi, and G. M. Reaven. 2000. Relation between insulin resistance and plasma concentrations of lipid hydroperoxides, carotenoids, and tocopherols. Am. J. Clin. Nutr. 72:776–779.

Farooq, M., A. Wahid, N. Kobayashi, D. Fujita, and S. M. A. Basra, 2009. Plant drought stress: effects, mechanisms and management. Agronomy for Sustainable Development. Springer Verlag, Germany. 29(1), pp. 185–212.

Giovannucci, E. 2002. Lycopene and prostate cancer risk. Methodological considerations in the epidemiologic literature. Pure Appl. Chem. 74:1427–1434.

Grassmann, J., S. Hippeli, and E. F. Elstre. 2002. Plant's defence mechanism and its benefits for animals and medicine: role of phenolics and terpenoids in avoiding oxygen stress. Plant Physiol. Biochem. 40:471–478.

Hankemeier, T. 2007.Medical system biology. *In* Abstracts Book. The 11th International Congress, Phytopharm. Leiden, The Netherlands; 20.

Heba, I. M., and A. A. Samia. 2014. Influence of Garlic Extract On Enzymatic and Non Enzymatic Antioxidants in Soybean Plants (Glycine Max) Grown under Drought Stress. Life Sci. J. 11:47–58.

Jaleel, C. A., P. A. Manivannan, A. Wahid, M. Farooq, H. J. Al-Juburi, R. A. Somasundaram, et al. 2009. Drought stress in plants: a review on morphological characteristics and pigments composition. Int. J. Agric. and Biol. 11:100–105.

Johnson, E. J. 2002. The role of carotenoids in human health. Nutr. Clin. Care 5:56–65.

Kiani, S. P., P. Maury, A. Sarrafi, and P. Grieu. 2008. QTL analysis of chlorophyll fluorescence parameters in sunflower (Helianthus annuus L.) under well-watered and water-stressed conditions. Plant Sci. 175:565–573.

Kritchevsky, S. B. 1999. Beta carotene, carotenoids and the prevention of coronary heart disease. J. Nutr. 129:5–8.

Kumar, R. R., K. Karajol, and G. R. Naik. 2011. Effect of polyethylene-glycol-induced water stress on physiological and biochemical responses in Pigeonpea (Cajanus cajan L. Millsp.). Recent Res. Sci.Technol. 3:148–152.

Kumudini, S. 2010. Soybean Growth and Development. Pp. 48–73 *in* B. Singh, ed. The Soybean: botany, Production and Uses. CAB International, Oxfordshire, UK.

Kwon, Y. I., E. Apostolidis, and K. Shetty. 2008. In vitro studies of eggplant (Solanum melongena) phenolics as inhibitors of key enzymes relevant for type 2 diabetes and hypertension. Bioresour. Technol. 99:2981–2988.

Massacci, A., S. M. Nabiev, L. Pietrosanti, S. K. Nematov, T. N. Chernikova, K. Thor, et al. 2008. Response of the photosynthetic apparatus of cotton (Gossypium hirsutum) to the onset of drought stress under field conditions studied by gas-exchange analysis and chlorophyll fluorescence imaging. Plant Physiol. Biochem. 46:189–195.

Mibei, E. K., and N. K. O. Ojijo. 2011. Effects of processing on chemical composition of four African leafy vegetables. Electronic J. Environ., Agric. Food Chem. 10:3121–3131.

Mibei, E. K., N. K. O. Ojijo, S. M. Karanja, and J. K. Kinyua. 2011. Compositional attributes of the leaves of some indigenous African leafy vegetables commonly consumed in Kenya. Annals. Food Sci. Technol. 12:146–154.

Mibei, E. K., N. K. O. Ojijo, S. M. Karanja, and J. K. Kinyua. 2012. Phytochemical and antioxidant analysis of methanolic extracts of four African indigenous leafy vegetables. Annals. Food Sci. Technol. 13:37–42.

Munné-Bosch, S., and L. Alegre. 2000. Changes in carotenoids, tocopherols and diterpenes during drought and recovery, and the biological significance of chlorophyll loss in Rosmarinus officinalis plants. Planta 210:925–931.

Nikolaeva, M. K., S. N. Maevskaya, A. G. Shugaev, and N. G. Bukhov. 2010. Effect of drought on chlorophyll content and antioxidant enzyme activities in leaves of three wheat cultivars varying in productivity. Russ. J. Plant Physiol. 57:87–95.

Payne, R. W., D. A. Murray, S. A. Harding, D. B. Baird, and D. M. Soutar. 2011. An introduction to GenStat for Windows, 14th ed.. VSN International, Hemel Hempstead, UK.

van Poppel, G., and R. A. Goldbohm. 1995. Epidemiological evidence for b-carotene and cancer prevention. Am. J. Clin. Nutr. 62:1493–1503.

Prochazkova, D., R. K. Sairam, G. C. Srivastava, and D. V. Singh. 2001. Oxidative stress and antioxidant activity as the basis of senescence in maize leaves. Plant Sci. 161:765–771.

Rao, A. V., and L. G. Rao. 2007. Carotenoids and human health. Pharmacological research 55:207–216.

Reddy, A. R., K. V. Chaitanya, and M. Vivekanandan. 2004. Drought induced responses of photosynthesis and antioxidant metabolism in higher plants. J. Plant Physiol. 161:1189–1202.

Shippers, R. R. 2000. African indigenous vegetables: an overview of cultivated species. Natural resource institute, Chatham, UK. 214.

Strzalka, K., A. Kostecka-Gugala, and D. Latowski. 2003. Carotenoids and environmental stress in plants: significance of carotenoid-mediated modulation of membrane physical properties. Russ. J. Plant Physiol. 50:168–172.

Suzuki, N., S. Koussevitzky, R. Mittler, and G. Miller. 2012. ROS and redox signalling in the response of plants to abiotic stress. Plant, Cell Environ. 35:259–270.

Young, A., and G. Britton. 1990. Carotenoids and stress. Pp. 87–112 *in* R. G. Alscher and J. R. Cummings, eds. Stress responses in plants: adaptation and acclimation mechanisms. Wiley-Liss, NY.

7

The relationship between agricultural biodiversity, dietary diversity, household food security, and stunting of children in rural Kenya

Florence K. M'Kaibi[1,*], Nelia P. Steyn[2], Sophie A. Ochola[3] & Lissane Du Plessis[4]

[1]Stellenbosch University, Cape Town, South Africa
[2]Division of Human Nutrition, Department of Human Biology, University of Cape Town, Anzio Road, Cape Town, South Africa
[3]Department of Foods, Nutrition and Dietetics, Kenyatta University, Nairobi, Kenya
[4]Division of Human Nutrition, Stellenbosch University, Cape Town, South Africa

Keywords
Agricultural biodiversity, dietary diversity, household food security & stunting

Correspondence
Florence K. M'Kaibi, Kenya Technical Trainers College, P.O. Box 44600-00100, Nairobi, Kenya.
E-mail: fkkaibi@gmail.com

***Current address**
Kenya Technical Trainers College, Nairobi, Kenya

Funding Information
This work was funded by National Commission for Science, Technology and Innovation-Kenya, (Grant/Award Number: 'Kenya/South Africa Research grant'.

Abstract

The study was to determine the role of Dietary diversity (DD), household food security (HFS), and agricultural biodiversity (AB) on stunted growth in children. Two cross-sectional studies were undertaken 6 months apart. Interviews were done with mothers/caregivers and anthropometric measurements of children 24–59 months old. HFS was assessed by household food insecurity access scale (HFIAS). A repeated 24-h recall was used to calculate a dietary diversity score (DDS). Agricultural biodiversity (AB) was calculated by counting the number of edible plants and animals. The study was undertaken in resource-poor households in two rural areas in Kenya. Mothers/Care givers and household with children of 24–59 months of age were the main subjects. The prevalence of underweight [WAZ <−2SD] ranged between 16.7% and 21.6% and stunting [HAZ <−2SD] from 26.3% to 34.7%. Mean DDS ranged from 2.9 to 3.7 and HFIAS ranged from 9.3 to 16.2. AB was between 6.6 and 7.2 items. Households with and without children with stunted growth were significantly different in DDS (P = 0.047) after the rainy season and HFIAS (P = 0.009) in the dry season, but not with AB score (P = 0.486). The mean AB for households with children with stunted growth were lower at 6.8, compared to 7.0 for those with normal growth, however, the difference was insignificant. Data indicate that households with children with stunted growth and those without are significantly different in DDS and HFIAS but not with AB. This suggests some potential in using DDS and HFIAS as proxy measures for stunting.

Introduction

Despite strides made to reduce global hunger through, among others, increased cereal production, vulnerable people on a global scale are still hungry. The availability of cheap cereal foods has coincided with the erosion of agricultural biodiversity and reduction in dietary diversity (Frison et al. 2005). The United Nations General Assembly declared 2010 to be the International Year of Biodiversity. This provided an unprecedented opportunity to raise awareness and promote the role that agricultural biodiversity plays in the lives of people, particularly those in low income countries (Food and Agriculture Organization (FAO) 2010) Agricultural biodiversity is the basis of the food chain which contributes to food and livelihood security, especially in the developing countries which highly depend on own food supply and food-based strategies rooted in the sustainable use of biological resources to improve local diets (Wispelwey and Deckelbaum 2009).

A study in Kenya by Ekesa et al. (2008) showed a strong relationship between agricultural biodiversity and dietary diversity. The findings indicated that almost 50% of changes in dietary intake of preschool children were due to agricultural biodiversity. This implies that improving agricultural biodiversity could improve dietary diversity in this group which in turn could lead to an improvement in nutritional status (Ekesa et al. 2008). In addition, a systematic review on the contribution of edible plant and animal biodiversity to human diets by Penafiel et al. (2011) showed that there have only been a limited number of studies in this area and methods of assessing agricultural biodiversity are still uncertain. The complexity of linking agriculture and health appears to be a setback to engage in a large comprehensive study in this topic Penafiel et al. (2011) suggested a need for multidisciplinary research which incorporates appropriate biodiversity and nutritional assessment methodologies, in order to have a better understanding of dietary contributions of local food biodiversity and diets thus emphasizing the importance of this area of study.

The nutritional status of children under 5 years of age is an important indicator of household food security (Government of Kenya (GOK) 2008a). In Kenya, 1.8 million children are classified as chronically malnourished with poor breastfeeding and infant feeding practices contributing to more than 10,000 deaths per year (GOK 2008a), Reduction in undernutrition has been very slow, as trends over the past years show continuous deterioration (Food and Agriculture Organization (FAO) 2006; GOK 2007, 2008b, 2009a) Data from the Kenya Demographic and Health Survey (KDHS) 2014, however, showed that chronic malnutrition among children below 5 years had shown improvement since 2009. The prevalence of stunting and severe stunting was 26% and 8.1%, respectively. Estimates also showed that the Eastern Province recorded a high rate of stunting among children under 5 years of age (30.1% and 8.2% −2SD (Food and Agriculture Organization (FAO) 2010) and −3SD respectively) GOK 2014. In the latest national survey in Kenya, (GOK 2014) findings showed that 4% of Kenyan children under 5 years old were wasted, with 0.9% severely wasted. 11% of these children were also found to be underweight, with 2.3% being classified as severely underweight GOK 2014.

Research has shown that stunting, which is caused by long-term deprivation of food or chronic undernutrition, has long-term consequences. Stunting leads to delayed motor development, impaired immune function and generally affects cognitive development. Poor cognitive development may lead to diminished intellectual performance, decreased attention span, and poor academic achievement. Furthermore, stunting leads to reduced work capacity, increased risk of delivery complications in women, and diminished intellectual performance (Martorell 1999; Branca and Ferrari 2002; Victora et al. 2008). Stunting is also associated with a developmental delay and retarded achievement of the main child development milestones, such as walking. This might create an overall comparative disadvantage in an already difficult environment.

Interventions to correct growth and development are possible at least until the age of 5 years and are justified; although the extent to which catch-up growth is possible and the long-term implication of this remain to be clarified (Branca and Ferrari 2002). Hence, the high prevalence of stunting in Kenya needs urgent attention to reduce long-term effects on the health of the population. The link between agricultural biodiversity and nutrition is not direct because of the complex nature of food security and nutrition. There are many arguments on how human nutrition is affected by agriculture through several pathways, of which producing sufficient food is just one (Pinstrup-Andersen 2012).

The paucity of data on the relationship between agricultural biodiversity, dietary diversity, and food security with nutritional status, in Kenya, and other countries in sub-Saharan Africa, prompted this study to build on the findings of Ekesa et al. (2008) and to contextualize the associations between agricultural biodiversity, dietary diversity, food security, and anthropometric data of children. This study was carried out during two different seasons, in two areas of different agricultural biodiversity based largely on differing rainfall figures. Household food security, as measured by household food insecurity access scale (HFIAS), was included as a variable in this study. The study also used a repeated 24 h recall to assess the variability in the diet in the households and added focus group discussions to validate the data collected using the a household questionnaire.

Methods

Sample

The required sample of 500 respondents (250 in each area) was based on an effect size of 0.4 with 90% power and a significance level of 5%. Percent stunting of 35% was the principle indicator used to determine sample size calculation. Households were randomly selected by means of random number tables. Two cross-sectional studies were undertaken in resource-poor households in two rural areas in Meru in the Eastern Province of Kenya, approximately 6 months apart. The two areas were Akithii and Uringu with the latter having a marginally better rainfall and geographic assets. Phase 1 of the study was conducted during the dry season and phase 2 after the rainy season. Of the intended sample of 500, 261 were finally realized from Uringu division and 264 from Akithii division. The extra 11 and 14 for Uringu and Akithii, respectively, were allowed for the purposes of compensating incomplete questionnaires. The repeated visits were not at the same households but were randomly selected during both phases. Interviews with mothers/caregivers were used to collect data from randomly selected households and anthropometric measurements were taken for children 24–59 months old. The 24–59 month age group of children was chosen because at this age, the children are expected to be eating from the family pot and therefore their nutritional status will be a reflection of the type of diet the families are consuming. Interviews and anthropometric measures were done by trained senior nutrition students and nutrition graduates from the University of Kenyatta who were trained by an experiences dietitian.

Data collection instruments

Socio-demographic questionnaire

The socio-demographic part of the questionnaire elicited information on the socioeconomic status of the household. The questionnaire included questions on marital status, highest level of formal education for the mothers/caregivers, decision maker on the types of food bought and amount of money spent on food in the household. Other questions included: the number of people eating from one pot at least 4 days a week, the number of rooms per house (excluding bathroom/toilet), the type of toilet, and the sources of drinking water for the household. Additional questions included the fuel used for cooking, employment status of the care giver, number of contributors to the total household income, agricultural land size, and number and type of assets which have an influence on the economic status of the household which could in turn influence household food security and dietary diversity.

Dietary diversity

Dietary diversity was measured using a repeated 24-h recall with the mother/care giver. Only one child of age 24–59 months from each household participated in the survey. In cases where there was more than one child in this age bracket, one child was randomly selected. The 24-h recall was administered to each household and repeated on a separate day. The 2 days were staggered with 5 days between the recalls to take care of the variations in foods eaten over the weekend and week days. No prior notice of the repeat visit was given to mothers/caretakers in case they altered their intake. To assess the differences caused by seasonality, two recalls were conducted in the rainy season and two in the dry season in each of the sampled areas per respondent. The repeated 24-h dietary recall has been internationally used and validated (Steyn et al. 2006).

Dietary diversity was measured using unquantified data from the 24-h recalls. The dietary diversity score (DDS) was calculated for each person based on nine food groups as recommended by Food and Agriculture Organization (FAO), (2011). The groups included (1) Cereals, roots, and tubers; (2) vitamin A-rich fruits and vegetables; (3) nonrich vitamin A (other) fruit; (4) nonrich vitamin A (other) vegetables; (5) legumes and nuts; (6) meat, poultry, and fish; (7) fats and oils; (8) dairy; and (9) eggs. Other remaining items such as; tea, sugar, and sweets were not used in the DDS. DDS was calculated by summing the number of food groups consumed by the child as reported over the 24-h recall period. This was done after creating food group variables for those food groups that needed to be aggregated and by creating a new variable termed as DDS. The maximum and ideal score would be a DDS of 9 since this would mean that the child had consumed from each of the 9 food groups at least once.

Household food security

Household food security (HFS) was measured using the HFIAS developed by Coates et al. (2007) which is internationally used and validated. This assessment tool was used to estimate the prevalence of food insecurity in the area of study. It is based on the principle that the experience of food insecurity causes predictable reactions and responses that can be captured and quantified through a survey and summarized in a scale. These feelings include the following: feelings of uncertainty or anxiety over food (situation, resources, or supply); perceptions that food is of insufficient quantity (for adults and children); perceptions that food is of insufficient quality (includes aspects of dietary diversity, nutritional adequacy, preference); reported reductions of food intake (for adults and children); reported consequences of reduced food intake (for adults and children); and feelings of shame for resorting to socially unacceptable means to obtain food resources (Coates et al. 2007).

The HFIAS questionnaire consists of nine occurrence questions that represent a generally increasing level of severity of food insecurity (access) and nine "frequency-of-occurrence" questions that are asked as a follow-up to each occurrence question to determine how often the condition occurred. The frequency-of-occurrence question is skipped if the respondent reports that the condition described in the corresponding occurrence question was not experienced in the previous 4 weeks (30 days) (Coates et al. 2007). The maximum score possible on the HFIAS is 27, which would represent the highest level of food insecurity.

Agricultural biodiversity

No instrument to measure agricultural biodiversity had been developed and validated to the knowledge of the authors and hence a questionnaire was constructed using guidelines from FAO (2010) and a similar study in Kenya Ekesa et al. (2008). Agricultural biodiversity was measured by determining the variety of food plants grown, animals reared for food and food items obtained from natural habitats. A list of all food items grown, all animals reared, hunted, and other food items obtained from natural habitats through gathering or trapping was established for each household.

Anthropometric measurements

The child health card, birth certificate, or baptism card were used to ascertain and record the age of the index child. In situations where the mother/care giver did not have the documents to ascertain the age of the child, they were asked to identify a child from the neighborhood who was born almost the same time. Children were excluded if they were younger than 24 months or older than 59 months.

Height: Children were measured in a standing position, using a free standing height/length stadiometer. Before taking the reading, the field worker ensured that the child was bare feet and that the heels, buttocks, shoulders, and the back of the head touched the stadiometer. Height was measured to the nearest 0.1 mm. Each of the measurements were taken twice and an average taken to ensure accuracy Gibson (2005).

Weight

Children were weighed on an electronic scale (Camry-model EB9318) to the nearest 10 g. Children were weighed with minimum clothing, after emptying the bladder and without shoes (Gibson 2005). All the scales were calibrated by measuring a known weight to ensure that the correct measurement was achieved. Each of the measurements were taken twice and an average taken to ensure accuracy.

The children's anthropometric status was determined using the World Health Organization (2006) growth standards *Z*-scores. Children with a *Z*-score of less than -3SD for weight-for-age were categorized as being severely underweight, those with a *Z*-score of −3 to −2SD were categorized as underweight, whereas those between −2 to −1SD were categorized as being mildly underweight or at risk of being underweight (World Health Organization 2006). Children with a *Z*-score of less than −3SD for height-for-age were categorized as being severely stunted, those with a *Z*-score of −3 to −2SD were categorized as stunted, whereas those between −2 and −1SD were categorized as mildly stunted or at risk of stunting. Children with a *Z*-score <−3SD weight for-height were categorized as being severely wasted, those with a *Z* score of −3 to −2 SD were categorized as wasted, whereas those between−2 and −1SD were categorized as mildly wasted or at risk of wasting.

Data analysis

STATISTICA version 9 (StatSoft Inc. (2009) STATISTICA (data analysis software system)(www.statsoft.com), Statistical Package for Social Sciences (SPSS Version 11.5) and Food Finder 3 software were used to analyze the data collected by the 24 h recall. Dietary intake was measured during each season by conducting a repeated 24-h recall with the mother/care giver of the household. A nutrient adequacy ratio (NAR) was calculated for each nutrient as the percent of the nutrient meeting the recommended dietary intake (RDI) value for that nutrient. A mean adequacy ratio (MAR) was calculated for 11 nutrients as the mean of the NARs of these nutrients. Dietary diversity was measured using data from the 24-h recalls and classifying it into nine food groups. A DDS was calculated based on each of the food groups consumed during the period of recall up to a maximum of nine if foods had been consumed from each of the nine groups.

HFSwas measured using the HFIAS. HFIAS score was calculated for each household by summing the codes of each frequency-of-occurrence question. The agricultural biodiversity was calculated by counting the number of different crops and animals eaten either from domestic sources or from the wild. Weight and height measurements of children were taken. The following nutritional status indices were used to determine their nutritional status; Weight for age *Z* scores (WAZ), height for age *Z* scores (HAZ), and weight for height *Z* scores (WHZ) scores were determined for the children. The cut-off was<− *Z* scores based on the WHO Child Growth Standards (2006). The relationships between continuous variables and nominal input variables were analyzed using appropriate analysis of variance (ANOVA) or pooled, paired, and independent mean *T*-tests when only two groups were involved. When repeated measures were taken on the same respondents like the initial measurements and the 24-h recall, it was done with the paired *t*-test. For randomized designs the Mann–Whitney test or the Kruskal–Wallis test were used.

Ethics

The study was approved by the Committee for Human Research, Faculty of Medicine and Health Sciences, Stellenbosch University (Reference No. N11/02/037) and each participant was required to sign a consent form. Thumb prints were used for participants who could not write. The researcher also obtained permission to conduct the research from the National Council for Science, Technology and Innovations (Kenya). Written informed consent was obtained from all subjects.

Results

Demographic and socioeconomic characteristics of the study population

Overall, the majority (87.8%) of the mothers/caregivers were married, 40.6% were casual laborers, 19.5% were homemakers, whereas 18.7% had no specific occupation (Table 1). About 10.1% of the mothers/care givers were petty traders, 5.4% were unemployed, 4.5% were self-employed, and 1.2% were wage earners. The majority (84.6%) of mothers/care givers had attained a primary level of education, 5.0% had no formal education, 5.0% had some secondary education, and only 4.4% had completed secondary education. A significant difference was found to exist between the two divisions in the marital status ($P < 0.001$) and the occupation of the care giver ($P < 0.001$).

Forty-one percent of households obtained their drinking water from communal taps, 36.0% from rivers, dams or lakes, whereas 19.8% consumed water from wells or boreholes. About half (43.7%) of the households had 1–2 and 43.3% had 3–4 roomed houses, whereas a very small percentage of 1.7% had houses with seven or more rooms. Most of the households had pit latrines (91.0%) and 6.1% with ventilated improved pit latrines, whereas 2.8% did not have toilets. The majority (95.8%) of the households used wood as fuel for cooking, whereas charcoal and gas were used by 1.9% and 1.7%, respectively. A significant difference was found to exist between the two divisions in the sources of water used ($P < 0.001$) with Akithii drinking mostly from communal taps and Uringu from rivers or wells.

In the majority of households, husbands/partners (50.5%), followed by mothers/caregivers (39.9%) made the decision on how much money was spent on food. Most households in both divisions had 3–4 or 5–6 persons eating from the same pot. The number of persons contributing to household income in the slightly over half (55.7%) of households were two persons, followed by one person (40.0%) and three to four persons (3.1%). About 22.3% of the households spent Kes 1401 to Kes 2000 (~\$23.3) per week on food.

A significant difference was found to exist between the two divisions in the decision on the types of food to be purchased for a household ($P = 0.007$), the decision on the amount of money to be spent on food ($P = 0.013$), and on the amount of money spent on a weekly basis on purchasing food ($P < 0.0001$).

Anthropometric status of children 24–59 months old

Overall the percentage of children having a HAZ <−2SD, HAZ −2SD to −3SD, and HAZ <−3SD were lower in Akithii than in Uringu (Table 2). The mean HAZ scores were −1.46 and −1.44 in Akithii and −1.29 and −1.29 in Uringu during which phase 1 and 2 of data collection, respectively. The percentage of children with stunted growth (HAZ<−2SD) was 34.7 and 31.9% in Akithii for phase 1 and 2, respectively, and 26.3% and 28.2% in Uringu. The percentage of children with a WAZ <−2SD, WAZ −2 to −3SD and WAZ <−3SD were lower in Akithii than in Uringu. The mean WAZ scores were −1.19 and −1.13 in Akithii and −1.04 and −1.09 in Uringu. The percentage of children who were underweight (WAZ<−2SD) was 21.6% and 16.7% in Akithii for phases 1 and 2, respectively, and 20.3% and 20.2% in Uringu for phases 1 and 2, respectively. Overall the percentage of children having a WHZ <−2SD, WHZ −2 to −3SD, and WHZ <−3SD were similar in Akithii and Uringu. The mean WHZ scores were −0.52 and −0.43 in Akithii and −0.45 and −0.53 in Uringu for phase 1 and 2, respectively. The percentage of children with wasting (WHZ<−2SD was 7.9% and 4.6% in Akithii for phase 1 and 2, respectively, and 5.7% and 8.8% in Uringu, respectively. There were no significant differences in anthropometric variables between phases or between the two areas.

There was a positive significant relationship ($P = 0.0001$) between the number of those contributing to household income and weight status (WAZ) (Table 3). Furthermore, both WHZ ($P = 0.04$) and WAZ ($P = 0.02$) were associated with the amount of money spent on food. The number of people eating from the same pot was negatively associated with WAZ ($P = -0.03$) implying that as number of people increased weight decreased.

Dietary diversity, household food inventory assess scale, and agricultural biodiversity

Table 4 presents data on DDS, HFIAS, and AB. From this we note that about 30% more children in Akithii had a poor DDS (<4 groups) compared with Uringu (79.7% vs. 51.6%). Mean DDS in Akithii (2.9) was significantly lower than Uringu (3.7) at both phases ($P < 0.0001$). Akithii also had a significantly higher mean HFIAS (16.2 and 12.5) than Uringu (10.0 and 9.3) indicative of poorer food security($P < 0.0001$).The percentage of households with severe food insecurity was 82% and 58% in Akithii in phases 1 and 2, respectively, compared with 47% and 42% in Uringu, respectively. Mean AB was, also significantly lower in Akithii compared with Uringu (6.6 vs. 7.2 items), respectively.

Table 1. Socio-demographic characteristics of sample in Akithii and Uringu divisions of Kenya.

Demographic and socioeconomic characteristics	AKITHII	URINGU	Total for both divisions	χ^2-test
	N(%)	*N*(%)	*N*(%)	*P*-values
Education of mother/care giver				
Primary	222 (85.4)	217 (83.8)	439 (84.6)	$\chi = 5.251$
No formal education	16 (6.2)	10 (3.7)	26 (5.0)	$P = 0.263$
Some secondary	9 (3.5	17 (6.6)	26 (5.0)	
Completed secondary	10 (3.8	13 (5.0)	23 (4.4)	
Tertiary	3 (1.2)	2 (0.8)	5 (0.7)	
Marital status of mother/care giver				
Married	247 (94.3)	212 (81.2)	459 (87.8)	$\chi = 5.323$
Single	8 (3.1)	28 (10.7)	36 (6.9)	$P < 0.001$*
Divorced/separated	1 (0.4)	14 (5.4)	15 (3.0)	
Widowed	6 (2.3)	7 (2.7)	13 (2.5)	
Occupation of mother/care giver				
Casual laborer	91 (35.0)	118 (46.5)	209 (40.7)	$\chi = 31.414$
Homemaker	49 (18.9)	51 (20.1)	100 (19.5)	$P < 0.001$*
Petty trader	36 (13.8)	16 (6.3)	52 (10.1)	
Unemployed	7 (2.7)	21 (8.3)	28 (5.4)	
Self employed	15 (5.8)	8 (3.1)	23 (4.5)	
Wage-earner	1 (0.4)	5 (2.0)	6 (1.2)	
Others	61 (23.5)	45 (13.8)	96 (18.7)	
Sources of drinking water				
Communal tap	183 (70.4)	30 (11.5)	213 (41.0)	$\chi = 208.454$
River/lake/dam	49 (18.8)	138 (53.1)	187 (36.0)	$P < 0.0001$*
Well/borehole	17 (6.5)	86 (33.1)	103 (19.9)	
Own tap	11 (4.2)	3 (1.2)	14 (2.7)	
No. of rooms				
1–2 rooms	105 (40.4)	122 (46.9)	227 (43.7)	$\chi = 3.747$
3–4 room	123 (47.3)	102 (39.2)	225 (43.3)	$P = 0.290$
5–6 rooms	27 (10.4)	32 (12.3)	59 (11.3)	
7 rooms above	5 (1.9)	4 (1.5)	9 (1.7)	
Cooking fuel				
Wood	249 (95.8)	248 (95.8)	497 (95.8)	$\chi = 1.511$
Charcoal	6 (2.3)	4 (1.5)	10 (1.9)	$P = 0.825$
Gas	4 (1.5)	5 (1.9)	9 (1.7)	
Toilet type				
Pit	235 (92.2)	231 (89.9)	466 (91.0)	$\chi = 1.784$
VIP	13 (5.1)	18 (7.0)	31 (6.1)	$P = 0.618$
None	7 (2.7)	7 (2.7)	14 (2.7)	
Decision on types food purchased				
Mother/care giver	171 (65.5)	141 (54.0)	312 (59.8)	$\chi = 17.590$
Husband/partner	78 (29.9)	87 (33.3)	165 (31.6)	$P = 0.007$**
Grandmother/father	10 (3.8)	19 (7.3)	29 (5.6)	
Mother/In law	2 (0.8)	12 (4.6)	14 (2.7)	
Decision on the amount of money spent on food				
Husband/partner	133 (51.0)	130 (50.0)	263 (50.5)	$\chi = 20.997$
Mother/care giver	114 (43.7)	94 (36.2)	208 (39.9)	$P = 0.013$*
Grandmother/father	10 (3.8)	18 (6.9)	28 (5.4)	
Mother/In law	2 (0.8)	10 (3.8)	12 (2.3)	
No. of people eating from the same pot				
1–2 persons	9 (3.5)	18 (6.9)	27 (5.2)	$\chi = 26.166$
3–4 persons	62 (23.8)	100 (38.5))	162 (31.1)	$P < 0.0001$***
5–6 persons	111 (42.7)	102 (39.2)	213 (41.0)	
7–8 persons	67 (25.7)	31 (11.9)	98 (18.8)	
Above 9	11 (4.2)	9 (3.4)	20 (3.8)	

(*Continued*)

Table 1. Continued.

Demographic and socioeconomic characteristics	AKITHII N(%)	URINGU N(%)	Total for both divisions N(%)	χ^2-test P-values
No. of contributors to h/hold income				
1 Person	108 (41.7)	99 (38.4)	207 (40.0)	$\chi = 5.501$
2-Person	143 (55.2)	145 (56.2)	288 (55.7)	$P = 0.240$
3–4 Person	5 (1.9)	11 (4.3)	16 (3.1)	
More than 5 person	3 (1.2)	3 (1.2)	6 (1.2)	
Amount of money spent on food weekly (Kes)				
0–800	18 (7.0)	37 (14.3)	55 (10.7)	$\chi = 37.381$
801–1400	70 (27.2)	103 (39.9)	173 (33.6)	$P < 0.0001$***
1401–2000	56 (21.8)	59 (22.7)	115 (22.3)	
2001–2600	60 (23.3)	46 (17.8)	106 (20.6)	
2601 and above	53 (20.6)	13 (5.3)	65 (12.6)	

Significance* at $P < 0.05$; ***$P < 0.001$.

Table 2. Percentage of children in the sample in Kenya at phases 1 and 2 of the study having anthropometric values below cut-off values.

Anthropometric indices	Akithii phase 1 (n = 245) % (95%CI)	Akithii phase 2 (n = 245) % (95%CI)	Uringu phase 1 (N = 232) % (95%CI)	Uringu phase 2 (n = 232) % (95%CI)
WHZ<−2 D	7.9 (5.2–11.8)	4.6 (2.4–8.5)	5.7 (3.4–9.4)	8.8 (5.8–13.1)
WHZ−2 to −3SD	7.1 (4.5–10.9)	4.2 (2.2–7.8)	3.3 (1.7–6.3)	8.8 (5.8–13.1)
WHZ<−3SD	0.8 (0.2–2.8)	0.4 (0.2–0.8)	2.4 (1.1–5.2)	0.0 (0.0–1.6)
Mean WHZ 95% CI	−0.52 (−0.7 to −0.4)	−0.43 (−0.6–0.3)	−0.45 (−0.6 to −0.3)	−0.53 (−0.7 to −0.4)
WAZ <−2SD	21.6 (16.9–27.2)	16.7 (8.5–30.2)	20.315.6–25.9	20.2 (15.6–25.7)
WAZ<−2 to −3SD	17.1 (12.9–22.4)	11.3 (5.8–20.7)	6.0 (3.6–9.9)	16.8 (12.6–22.1)
WAZ<−3SD	4.5 (2.5–7.9)	5.4% (2.8–10.1)	3.4 (1.7–6.6)	3.4 (1.7–6.5)
Mean WAZ 95% CI	−1.19 (−1.3 to −1.3)	−1.13 (−1.3 to −1.0)	−1.04 (−1.2 to −1.1)	−1.09 (−1.2 to −1.0)
HAZ <−2SD	34.7 (29.0–40.8)	31.9 (23.4–41.7)	26.3 (21.0–32.3)	28.2 (22.8–34.2)
HAZ −2 to −3SD	25.7 (20.6–31.5)	22.3 (19.1–25.9)	20.3 (15.6–25.9)	21.4 (16.7–7.1)
HAZ<−3SD	9.0 (6.0–13.2)	9.6 (5.1–17.1)	6.0 (3.6–9.9)	6.7 (4.2–10.6)
Mean HAZ 95% CI	−1.46 (−1.6– −1.3)	−1.44 (−1.6 to−1.3)	−1.29 (−1.4 to −1.1)	−1.29 (−1.5 to −1.1)

Relationship between dietary diversity, agricultural biodiversity, household food security, and child anthropometric status

Child anthropometric indices (WAZ, HAZ, and WHZ) were correlated with DDS, AB, and HFIAS to determine the relationships between these variables (Table 5). No significant correlation was found to exist between WAZ and WHZ with DDS in this study. There was, however, a significant relationship between stunting in children (HAZ<−2SD) and dietary diversity in Phase 2 data. An increase in DDS appeared to reflect a decrease in stunting in children. No significant relationship was found to exist between AB with WAZ, HAZ, or WHZ scores or with HFIAS with WAZ, HAZ, or WHZ scores.

Table 5 also shows the relationship between HFIAS with DDS and AB. In both instances there is a significant inverse relationship ($P < 0.01$). Higher DDS and AB scores lead to better household food security. There is also a significant association between AB and DDS; as AB increases, so does DDS ($P = 0.00014$).

Relating dietary diversity, agricultural biodiversity, and household food security in households with and without children with stunted growth

The relationship between DDS, agricultural biodiversity score, and HFIAS in households with and without children with stunted growth was investigated. During Phase 1, there was a significant difference between households with and without children with stunted growth for the variable mean DDS ($P = 0.047$) and also for the variable mean HFIAS ($P = 0.009$)

Table 3. Associations between socio-demographic characteristics with child nutritional status in both phases in both divisions.

Socio-demographic characteristics	WHZ	WAZ	HAZ
No. of contributors to household income	Kruskal–Wallis $P = 0.38$	Kruskal–Wallis $P = 0.001$***	Kruskal–Wallis $P = 0.14$
Amount of money spent on food per week	Kruskal–Wallis $P = 0.04$*	Kruskal–Wallis $P = 0.02$*	Kruskal–Wallis $P = 0.55$
No. of people eating from the same pot	Spearman $r = -0.06$, $P = 0.17$	Spearman $r = -0.10$, $P = 0.03$*	Spearman $r = -0.08$, $P = 0.08$

WHZ, weight for height *Z* score; WAZ, weight for age *Z* score; HAZ, height for age *Z* score.
Significance* at $P < 0.05$; ***$P < 0.001$.

Table 4. Mean DDS, mean HFIAS, mean AB in each division over the two phases of the study.

Variables	Akithii phase 1 ($n = 245$)	Akithii phase 2 ($n = 245$)	Uringu phase 1 ($N = 232$)	Uringu phase 2 ($N = 232$)	Independent *T*-test between divisions phase 1	Independent *T*-test between divisions phase 2
Mean DDS	2.9	2.9	3.7	3.7	$P < 0.0001$	$P < 0.0001$
SD	1.10	1.0	1.12	1.11		
DDS < 4	79.7%	79.7%	51.6%	52.3%		
Mean HFIAS	16.2	12.5	10.0	9.3	$P < 0.0001$	$P < 0.0001$
SD	7.01	7.80	6.90	7.02		
Food secure	2%	11%	12%	18%		
Mild HFIS	1%	4%	7%	6%		
Moderate HFIS	14%	27%	33%	33%		
Severe HFIS	82%	58%	47%	42%		
Mean AB	6.6%	N/A	7.2	N/A	$P = 0.035$	N/A
SD	2.44	N/A	4.19	N/A		

DDS, dietary diversity; HFIAS, household food insecurity access scale; HFIS, household food insecurity; AB, agricultural biodiversity; SD, standard deviation; N/A, AB not measured in Phase 2.

in phase 2 (Table 6). Agricultural biodiversity did not show any significant differences between the two groups of households. The means for households with children presenting with stunted growth were, however, lower at 6.8, as compared to 7.0 of those with normal growth.

Discussion

In general, the prevalence of undernutrition in the study area can be classified as medium to high according to WHO standards (1997). There were marked differences in the prevalence of undernutrition in the two study areas across the two phases of data collection with Akithii being classified as an area with a high level of undernutrition, whereas Uringu was classified as presenting with a medium level of undernutrition. Uringu had a higher level of household assets (probably implying higher socioeconomic status), DDS and AB compared to Akithii may be contributing the lower undernutrition levels in this region. Akithii had higher percentages of children who presented with underweight and wasting compared to the national levels in Kenya (Kenya National Bureau of Statistics (KNBS) and ICF Macro 2010). The level of stunting was, however, the same as the national level at 35% (GOK 2009a; Kenya National Bureau of Statistics (KNBS) and ICF Macro, 2010) Uringu, in contrast, had a lower level of child undernutrition compared to the national rate. During phase 2 of the study, the percentages of children who presented with wasting, underweight, and stunting in both the study sites were generally lower compared to phase 1. This may be attributed to the effect of seasonality. During phase 2 of the study, household food security and dietary diversity improved, probably because it was during the rainy reason, unlike during phase 1 when data collection took place during the dry season.

Socio-demographic characteristics that may affect vulnerability to food insecurity and anthropometric status in children were investigated. In this study, a significant positive relationship was found between the number of contributors to household income and WAZ scores of children. The amount of money spent on food per week significantly affected WAZ and WHZ but not HAZ values. A significant inverse relationship was also found between the number of people eating from the same pot and WAZ scores, namely, the higher the number of people eating from the same pot, the lower the WAZ values.

Table 5. Association of DDS, AB, and HFIAS with each other and anthropometric variables.

Variables	Spearman *R*	*T*(*n*–2)	*P* value
Phase 1 DDS			
DDS & WAZ	−0.015	−0.335	0.73
DDS & HAZ	−0.005	−0.120	0.90
DDS & WHZ	−0.009	−0.202	0.83
Phase 2 DDS			
DDS & WAZ	0.068	1.439	0.150
DDS & HAZ	0.114	2.455	0.014
DDS & WHZ	0.021	0.454	0.649
Phase 1			
AB & WAZ	0.047	1.009	0.313
AB & HAZ	−0.005	−0.114	0.909
AB & WHZ	0.079	1.726	0.085
Phase 2			
AB & WAZ	−0.036	−0.544	0.586
AB & HAZ	−0.087	−1.311	0.191
AB & WHZ	0.088	1.359	0.175
HFIAS both phases	Pearson		
HFIAS & WAZ	−0.048	884	0.156
HFIAS & HAZ	−0.037	894	0.264
HFIAS & WHZ	−0.031	906	0.352
DDS with HFIAS	During Phase 1, the correlation using Spearman *R* was ($R = -0.158$, t (N–2) −3.565), $P = 0.0003$), whereas during Phase 2 the correlation was ($R = -0.185$, t (N–2) −3.889), $P = 0.0001$). This correlation shows that an increase in dietary diversity inversely affected HFIAS.		
AB &HFIAS	Households with higher AB more likely to be food secure; Spearman $r = -0.136$, $P = 0.002$		
AB & DDS	Households with a high AB were likely to have a high DDS; ANOVA $F(1{,}496) = 14.791$, $P = 0.00014$.		

DDS, dietary diversity; HFIAS, household food insecurity access scale; AB, agricultural biodiversity; DS, dietary diversity; HFIAS, household food insecurity access scale; HFI, household food insecurity; AB, agricultural biodiversity; SD, standard deviation; N/A, AB not measured in Phase 2.

Table 6. Relating dietary diversity, agricultural biodiversity, and household food security in households with and without children with stunted growth in both phases and divisions.

Variables	Divisions		Households with children without Stunted growth	Households with children with Stunted growth	ANOVA, *P*-value
DDS	Akithii &Uringu	Mean	3.3 (SD,1.41)	3.3 (SD, 1.22)	$P = 0.651$
	Phase 1	*N*	314	139	
	Akithii &Uringu	Mean	3.3 (SD,1.12)	3.1 (SD, 1.13)	$P = 0.047$*
	Phase 2	*N*	317	136	
	Both groups	Mean	3.3 (SD, 1.13)	3.2 (SD, 1.18)	$P = 0.090$
	(Phase 1& 2)	*N*	$N = 631$	$N = 275$	
HFIAS	Akithii &Uringu	Mean	12.4 (SD,7.38)	14.3 (SD, 7.17)	$P = 0.009$*
	Phase 1	*N*	331	145	
	Akithii &Uringu	Mean	11.1	10.1	$P = 0.232$
	Phase 2	*N*	291	127	
	Both groups	Mean	11.8 (SD,7.61)	12.4 (SD, 7.45)	$P = 0.310$
	(Phase 1& 2)	*N*	$N = 622$	$N = 272$	
AB	Both groups	Mean	7.0 (SD, 3.14)	6.8 (SD, 3.45)	$P = 0.486$
		N	$N = 317$	$N = 142$	

Significance*at $P < 0.05$.

The number of assets owned by a household also significantly influenced HAZ, scores; the higher the numbers of household assets, the higher the HAZ values were. It is important to note that the households in Akithii which is a semiarid region, (GOK 2002, 2009b) spent more money on food on a weekly basis compared to Uringu which has a high agricultural productivity (GOK 2002, 2009b)

Despite evidence from other studies showing associations between WAZ and WHZ with DDS, (Arimond and Ruel 2004; Sawadogo et al. 2006; Ekesa et al. 2008) few significant relationships were found in this study. Another recent study in Kenya also found no significant relationship between DDS, WAZ, and WHZ, (Nungo et al. 2012). There was, however, a significant positive relationship in this study between stunting in children (HAZ) with dietary diversity of the child in phase 2 of the study. A higher DDS was associated with lower stunting levels. This relationship signifies that households that had the dietary diversity score plays a significant role in child nutrition, especially HAZ. The latter finding concurs with a study in rural Bangladesh which found that reduced dietary diversity was a strong predictor of stunting in children aged 6–59 months. High dietary diversity was associated with a 31% reduced odds of being stunted among children 24–59 months, after adjusting for all potential confounders (Rah et al. 2010). Findings of other studies suggest that there is an association between child dietary diversity and nutritional status that is independent of socioeconomic factors and that dietary diversity may indeed reflect diet quality (Sawadogo et al. 2006; Penafiel et al. 2011)

In this study, there was no significant relationship between household food security and child nutritional status based on anthropometric measurements. This implies that the food security situation of the households was not related with the nutritional status of the children. While some studies have reported a positive association between household food insecurity and childhood growth indicators, (Melgar-Quinonez et al. 2009; Chaparro 2012) others have found no relationship, (Alaimo et al. 2001; Akoto et al. 2010; Kac et al. 2012). The lack of association between nutritional status indicators and the food security indicator is difficult to explain, but suggests that the relationships are more complex due to the multifaceted nature of these variables.

Due to the multifaceted nature of malnutrition, Ruel and Alderman (2013) argues that food security is necessary but not sufficient to ensure adequate nutrition and to prevent malnutrition in children because care givers also need to provide them with care, hygiene, and health-seeking practices in order for them to grow, develop, and remain healthy. Pinstrup-Andersen (2013)also emphasizes that even if household food security is achieved, malnutrition may flourish due to intrahousehold distribution, which may not correspond to individual needs or because nonfood factors that are important for nutrition such as unclean water, poor sanitation, and hygiene and inappropriate care are the most serious constraints to good nutrition. This could probably explain the lack of association between household food security status and child nutritional status based on WAZ and WHZ in this study.

Household food security in this study was significantly associated with DDS and AB, implying that a diet high in dietary diversity and agricultural biodiversity improves household food security. Dietary diversity also showed a significant positive association with agricultural biodiversity. Kenya has been described as a country rich in agricultural biodiversity with an estimated 35,000 known species of animals, plants, and microorganisms (GOK 2001). The country's agricultural biodiversity is, however, under serious threat due to among others increasing deforestation, climate change, pollution, and soil degradation (Alaimo et al. 2001). The level of agricultural biodiversity (n = 26) in Tigania west in the Eastern part of Kenya, the area of study, was found to be low and far less than the number described in an earlier study conducted in western Kenya which identified 41 different species of food in the natural habitat (Pelletier and Frongillo 2003). The improvement of agricultural biodiversity is key in ensuring diverse diets and in cushioning households from climatic shocks caused by changing weather patterns since most households depends on rain-fed agriculture. Food-based strategies have been recommended as the first priority to meet micronutrient needs (Allen 2008). A more diverse diet holds the potential to provide a more abundant supply of both macro- and micronutrients and could therefore be one of the approaches to ensure greater food and nutrition security in Kenya.

A significant difference was established between households with and without children with stunted growth in DDS during the rainy season and HFIAS in the dry season, but not with the AB score. The mean AB for households with children with stunted growth were lower compared to those with normal growth, but did not reach significant level. This suggests that DDS and household food security may have the potential of being used as proxy measures for stunting. The results of this study concur with results from an analysis based on data from five developing countries which included Bangladesh, Nepal, Pakistan, Tanzania, and Uganda (Tiwari et al. 2013). These results demonstrated that various measures of household food security significantly correlated with the nutritional status of children within a household. These results were significant even when the socioeconomic characteristics of the households were controlled. The analysis concluded that food security indicators such as food consumption and DDS can be used as proxy measures for the underlying nutritional status of children (Tiwari et al. 2013).

Conclusion

Households that have children with and without stunted growth were significantly different in individual dietary diversity and household food security levels in the dry (shortage season = Phase 1) and rainy season (after harvest season Phase 2), but not with regard to agricultural biodiversity scores. DDS influences HAZ and HFIAS, whereas households with a higher agricultural biodiversity (AB) had higher DDS. Households with a higher AB were more food secure compared to those with lower AB. DDS, HFS, and AB played a significant role in determining the levels stunting of children among children of 24–59 months. This suggests some potential in using DDS and HFIAS as proxy measures for stunting. The Interventions to improve child nutritional status in resource-poor rural households such as in the study area should therefore aim at increasing dietary diversity and/or AB in order to improve household food security.

Ethical Standards Disclosure

This study was conducted according to the guidelines laid down in the Declaration of Helsinki and all procedures involving human subjects were approved by Committee for Human Research, Faculty of Medicine and Health Sciences, Stellenbosch University (ethics reference no.N11/02/037).

Conflict of Interest

The authors declare that there is no conflict of interest.

References

Akoto, O., P. Pooja, S. David, N. Jennifer, S. Ram, T. Zaman, et al. 2010. Household food insecurity and nutritional status of children aged 6 to 23 months in Kailali District of Nepal.

Alaimo, K., C. Olson, E. Frongillo, and R. Briefel. 2001. Food insufficiency, family income, and health in US preschool and school-aged children. Am. J. Public Health 91:781–786.

Allen, L. 2008. To what extent can food-based approaches improve micronutrient status? Asia Pac. J. Clin. Nutr. 17(S1):103–105.

Arimond, M., and M. T. Ruel. 2004. Dietary diversity is associated with child nutritional status: evidence from 11 demographic and health surveys. J. Nutr. 134:2579–2585.

Branca, F., and M. Ferrari. 2002. Impact of micronutrient deficiencies on growth: the stunting syndrome. INRAN (National Institute for Food Nutrition Research), Rome.

Chaparro, C. 2012. Household food health, infectious diseases, and nutrition, insecurity and nutritional status of women of bureau for global health, United States Agency, reproductive age and children under 5 years of for International Development (USAID), under age in five departments of the Western terms of Cooperative Agreement No. AID- OAA-Highlands of Guatemala: An Analysis of Data A-11-00014, through the FANTA-2 Bridge, from the national maternal-infant health survey managed by FHI 360. 2008–09 of Guatemala. Washington, DC: FHI 360/FANTA-2 Bridge.

Coates, J., A. Swindale, and P. Bilinsky. 2007. Household Food Insecurity Access Scale (HFIAS) for Measurement of Household Food Access: Indicator Guide (v3). Washington, DC: Food and Nutrition Technical Assistance II Project (FANTA-II Project). Academy for Educational Development (AED), Washington DC.

Ekesa, B. N., M. K. Walingo, and M. O. Onyango. 2008. Role of agricultural biodiversity on dietary intake and nutritional status of preschool children in Matungu division, Western Kenya. Afr. J. Food Sci. 2:026–032.

Food and Agriculture Organization (FAO). 2006. Food security committee report. Food and Agriculture Organization of the United Nations, Rome.

Food and Agriculture Organization (FAO). 2010. Expert Consultation on Nutrition Indicators for Biodiversity – 2. Food consumption. Food and Agriculture Organization of the United Nations, Rome.

Food and Agriculture Organization (FAO). 2011. Guidelines for measuring household and individual dietary diversity. Food and Agriculture Organization of the United Nations, Rome.

Frison, E., I. F. Smith, T. Johns, J. Cherfas, and P. Eyzaguirre. 2005. Using biodiversity for food, dietary diversity, better nutrition and health. South Afr. J. Cli. Nutr. 18:112–114.

Gibson, R. S. 2005. Principles of nutritional assessment, 2nd ed. Oxford University Press, New York.

Government of Kenya (GOK). 2001. Natural resource aspects of sustainable development in Kenya. Government Printers, Nairobi.

Government of Kenya (GOK). 2002. National development plan (2002–2008). Nairobi, Government Press, Ministry of Planning and National Development.

Government of Kenya (GOK). 2007. Kenya integrated household budget survey (KIHBS). Government Press, Nairobi.

Government of Kenya (GOK). 2008a. Economic survey. Government Press, Central Bureau of Statistics, Ministry of Planning and National Development, Nairobi.

Government of Kenya (GOK). 2008b. Food insecurity assessment in Kenya. Based on Kenya integrated household budget survey 2005/06. Government Press, Nairobi.

Government of Kenya (GOK). 2009a. Kenya demographic and health survey 2008/9 government press. Government Press, Nairobi.

Government of Kenya (GOK). 2009b. Drought Monthly EWS Bulletin -Meru North District. (accessed May 30 2009).

Government of Kenya (GOK). 2014. Kenya Demographic and Health Survey 2014 Government Press. Government Press, Nairobi.

Kac, G., M. M. Schlüssel, R. Pérez-Escamilla, G. Velásquez-Melendez, and A. A. M. da Silva. 2012. Household food insecurity is not associated with BMI for age or weight for height among Brazilian children aged 0–60 months. PLoS ONE 7:e45747. doi:10.1371/journal.pone.0045747.

Kenya National Bureau of Statistics (KNBS) and ICF Macro. 2010. Kenya Demographic and Health Survey 2008-09. KNBS and ICF Macro, Calverton, Maryland.

Martorell, R. 1999. The nature of child malnutrition and its long-term implications. Food Nutr. Bull. 20:288–292.

Melgar-Quinonez, H., M. Hackett, and M. Alvarez. 2009. Household food insecurity associated with stunting and underweight among preschool children in Antioquia, Colombia. Pan Am. J. Public Health 25:506–510.

Nungo, R. A., M. W. Okoth, and S. K. Mbugua. 2012. Nutrition status of children under-five years in cassava consuming communities in Nambale, Busia of Western Kenya. Food Nutr. Sci. 3: 796–801. doi:10.4236/fns.2012.36107; Available at: http://www.SciRP.org/journal/fns (accessed 15 October 2013).

Pelletier, D. L., and E. A. Jr Frongillo. 2003. Changes in child survival are strongly associated with changes in malnutrition in developing countries. J. Nutr. 133:107–119.

Penafiel, D., C. Lachat, R. Espinel, P. Van Damme, and P. Kolsteren. 2011. A systematic review on the contributions of edible plant and animal biodiversity to human diets. EcoHealth 8:1–19.

Pinstrup-Andersen, P. 2012. Food systems and human health and nutrition: an economic policy perspective with a focus on Africa. Available at: http://iis-db.stanford.edu/evnts/6697/Pinstrup-Andersen_10_11_12.pdf (accessed October 24, 2013).

Pinstrup-Andersen, P. 2013. Can agriculture meet future nutrition challenges? Eur. J. Dev. Res. 25:5–12.

Rah, J. H., N. Akhter, R. D. Semba, S. de Pee, M. W. Bloem, A. A. Campbell, et al. 2010. Low dietary diversity is a predictor of child stunting in rural Bangladesh. Eur. J. Clin. Nutr. 64:1393–1398,Macmillan publishers.

Ruel, M. T., and H. Alderman. 2013. Nutrition-sensitive interventions and programmes: how can they help to accelerate progress in improving maternal and child nutrition? Lancet 382: Pp.536. Available at: http://dx.doi.org/10.1016/S0140-6736(13)60843-0 (accessed October, 12 2013).

Sawadogo, P. S., Y. Martin-Prevel, M. Savy, Y. Kameli, P. Traissac, A. S. Traore, et al. 2006. An infant and child feeding index is associated with the nutritional status of 6 to 23 month-old children in rural Burkina Faso. J. Nutr. 136:656–663.

Steyn, N. P., J. H. Nel, G. Nantel, G. Kennedy, and D. Labadarios. 2006. Food variety and dietary diversity scores in children: are they good indicators of dietary adequacy? Public Health Nutr. 5:644–650.

Tiwari, S., E. Skoufias, and M. Sherpa. 2013. Linking measures of household food security to nutritional outcomes in Bangladesh, Nepal, Pakistan, Uganda, and Tanzania. A World Bank policy research working paper 6584. Washington DC.

Victora, C. G., L. Adair, C. Fall, C. Pedro, P. C. Hallal, R. Martorell, et al. 2008. Maternal and child undernutrition: consequences for adult health and human capital. Lancet 371:340–357.

Wispelwey, P. B., and R. J. Deckelbaum. 2009. Preventive nutrition, eco-nutrition: prevention malnutrition with agro diversity. Humana Press, New York.

World Health Organization (WHO). 1997. Global database on child growth and malnutrition. World health organization, Geneva.

World Health Organization (WHO). 2006. New child growth standards. Geneva, WHO; Available at: http://www.who.int/childgrowth (accessed 11 December 2012).

8

Safety of micronized palmitoylethanolamide (microPEA): lack of toxicity and genotoxic potential

Earle R. Nestmann

Health Science Consultants Inc., Mississauga, Ontario L5N 7S2, Canada

Keywords
Acute, Ames test, micronized, micronucleus, mutagenicity, palmitoylethanolamide, subchronic toxicity

Correspondence
Earle R. Nestmann, Health Science Consultants Inc., Mississauga, ON L5N 7S2, Canada. E-mail: enestmann@healthscienceconsultants.com

Funding Information
Earle Nestmann acknowledges the financial support from Prismic Pharmaceuticals, Inc. to Health Science Consultants Inc., to compensate for the time required to prepare this paper.

Abstract

Palmitoylethanolamide (PEA) is a natural fatty acid amide found in a variety of foods, which was initially identified in egg yolk. MicroPEA of defined particle size (0.5–10 μm) was evaluated for mutagenicity in *Salmonella typhimurium*, for clastogenicity/aneuploidy in cultured human lymphocytes, and for acute and subchronic rodent toxicity in the rat, following standard OECD test protocols, in accordance with Good Laboratory Practice (GLP). PEA did not induce mutations in the bacterial assay using strains TA1535, TA97a, TA98, TA100, and TA102, with or without metabolic activation, in either the plate incorporation or liquid preincubation methods. Similarly, PEA did not induce genotoxic effects in human cells treated for 3 or 24 h without metabolic activation, or for 3 h with metabolic activation. PEA was found to have an LD50 greater than the limit dose of 2000 mg/kg body weight (bw), using the OECD Acute Oral Up and Down Procedure. Doses for the 90-day rat oral toxicity study were based on results from the preliminary 14-day study, that is, 250, 500, and 1000 mg/kg bw/day. The No Effect Level (NOEL) in both subchronic studies was the highest dose tested.

Introduction

The history of PEA as a natural food ingredient with medicinal properties has been described by Masek and Raskova (1967). The initial observation was in 1943 by Coburn et al. (1943), as part of an epidemiological study focused on childhood rheumatic fever, the incidence of which was higher in those children consuming diets low in eggs. These investigators noted that occurrence was reduced in children fed egg yolk powder, and subsequently they demonstrated antianaphylactic properties in guinea pig with a lipid extract from egg yolk (Coburn et al. 1954).

Subsequently, a crystalline anti-inflammatory agent was isolated from egg yolk as well as from soybean lecithin (Kuehl et al. 1957). They identified the chemical structure to be N-2 hydroxyethyl palmitamide, or PEA. Further studies on the anti-inflammatory, antianaphylactic, antiserotonin, and antihistamine effects of PEA were conducted by Ganley et al. (1958) and Ganley and Robinson (1959). It was later found that PEA is an endogenous compound, locally synthesized in animal and human tissues and body fluids, to protect against perturbing inflammation (Skaper et al. 2013, 2014).

The purpose of this study is to review the safety of PEA, in addition to publishing new toxicology data, to establish a robust safety profile for the use of this substance in health products intended for human and veterinary consumption. Background information stems from the early recognition of PEA as a potential therapeutic agent. A wide-ranging drug development program was initiated by the Institute of Pharmacology of the Czechoslovak Academy of Sciences, whose efforts are documented in a comprehensive, unpublished English summary by Professor Karel Masek, M.D., Dr. Sc., Head of the Institute (Masek 1980). These and many other pharmacological and clinical studies were conducted in support of the clinical development of PEA as a pharmaceutical agent named IMPULSIN® (Spofa) and also marketed in Spain under the name Palmidrol (Laboratorie Prodes, S.A.). The studies have been summarized in three lengthy appendices: (1) background, safety studies, and pharmacology, (2) clinical studies, and (3) references and approval of manufacturing in 1970 by the Czech Ministry of Health (Masek 1980).

In light of the fact that these previous studies are not well documented or published, new GLP studies as described in this study have been performed to establish a more robust safety profile for PEA. The results of genetox assays as well as acute and repeat dose, oral toxicity studies in the rat will be described. The new studies have been performed using a PEA preparation of defined purity and particle size, on the basis of recent evidence suggesting that particle size is a relevant issue in defining biological consequences of PEA oral administration (Skaper et al. 2013; Impellizzeri et al. 2014).

Materials and Methods

Laboratory

GLP (Good Laboratory Practice) tests (Intox, 2015a,b,c,d,e, 2016) were carried out in the test facility of INTOX Pvt. Ltd. in Maharashtra, India (Intox), on behalf of study sponsor Prismic Pharmaceuticals of Scottsdale, Arizona (Prismic). Intox has been certified as a GLP compliant laboratory both by the National GLP Compliance Monitoring Authority of India and by the Food and Consumer Product Safety Authority of the OECD. All studies described in this study were audited and verified by the laboratory's Quality Assurance Unit.

Test material

The test material, micronized PEA (particle size 0.5–10 μm; purity 99%; microPEA), was manufactured by Epitech Group Srl, Milano Italy, supplied by Prismic, and met all specifications as outlined in the required Certificate of Analysis. The term microPEA in this paper includes both micronized and ultramicronized PEA, as the particle size distribution of 0.5-10 μm includes both fractions. The analytical method was validated in a GLP study which also verified the homogeneity of microPEA in the dosing matrix used in the animal studies as well as its stability over the period from preparation to dosing (Intox, 2015e). The test article was characterized by the sponsor who provided an authorized "Certificate of Analysis" for each study described in this study.

In vitro studies

Metabolic activation

As suggested by Maron and Ames (1983), some degree of mammalian metabolism was introduced into the in vitro test systems by using a fraction of rat liver, referred to as S9. S9 was prepared on site at Intox after inducing metabolizing enzymes by injection of rats with phenobarbitone and β-naphthoflavone (OECD, 1997).

Bacterial reverse mutation test

The Salmonella mammalian microsome reverse mutation test protocol conformed to the appropriate OECD Guideline (OECD, 1997), which is based on the 'Ames' test as described by Maron and Ames (1983), and was found to be compliant with GLP (Intox, 2015a).

Bacterial strains

The tester strains TA1535, TA97a, TA98, TA100, and TA102, as recommended (OECD, 1997), were obtained from Moltox of Boone, North Carolina. Their identity and characteristics were verified prior to testing (Intox, 2015a).

Preliminary range-finding experiments

MicroPEA was found to be uniformly suspended in Pluronic F68 at the concentration of 50 mg/mL. It was shown to precipitate when incorporated into agar plates at the levels of 4000 and 5000 but not at 3000 μg/plate, chosen as the highest test dose as recommended by OECD (1997). The doses of 3000, 2000, 1000, 500, and 250 μg/plate were selected to evaluate toxicity in strain TA100 with the presence and absence of S9. Slight cytotoxicity was found at 3000 μg/plate (-S9), the maximum dose for both the plate incorporation test and preincubation assay (Intox, 2015a).

Controls

Negative, including blank sterility controls, and positive controls were included in the testing of microPEA, both in the presence and absence of S9 to verify spontaneous mutation frequencies and strain-specific responses to known mutagens. Positive control compounds without S9 mix were as follows: sodium azide (Sigma Aldrich St. Louis, MO, USA) for TA1535, ICR 191 (Sigma Aldrich) for TA97a; 3-methylmethane sulfonate (Sigma Aldrich) for TA100 and TA102; and, 4-nitroquinoline-N-oxide (Acros Organics, Geel, Belgium) for TA98. Positive controls with S9 mix were as follows: 2-aminoanthracene (Sigma

Aldrich) for TA1535; 2-aminofluorene (Sigma Aldrich) for TA97a, TA98, and TA100; and, danthron (Sigma Aldrich) for TA102.

Media

Test strains were grown overnight in Oxoid nutrient broth No. 2, combined with test chemical and S9 in soft overlay agar containing 0.6% agar, 0.5% NaCl, and 0.05 mmol/L histidine–biotin, then plated on agar (2%) containing Vogel–Bonner minimal medium E and 2% glucose, as previously described (Maron and Ames 1983).

Test method

Both plate incorporation and preincubation methods (OECD, 1997) were employed, both in the absence and presence of S9. For preincubation, the treatment mixtures were incubated at 37C for 20 min prior to plating. Test plates in triplicate were incubated at 37°C for 68–72 h at which time revertant colonies were counted and the plates were examined for extent of background growth as an indicator of cytotoxicity.

In vitro mammalian cell micronucleus test

The test protocol conformed to the appropriate OECD Guideline (OECD, 2014) and was performed according to GLP (Intox, 2015b), using cultured lymphocytes from healthy human volunteers.

Preliminary range-finding experiments

MicroPEA was found to be sufficiently suspended in Pluronic F68 at the concentration 1000 μg/mL, with minimum precipitation and no cytotoxicity as measured by the cytokinesis-block proliferation index (CBPI). Based on these results, the tests were performed with 250, 500, and 1000 μg/mL (Intox, 2015b).

Controls

Controls included negative (NaCl) and vehicle (Pluronic F68) controls, ±S9. Positive controls –S9 included the aneugenic compound vinblastine, and clastogenic agent mitomycin C. Cyclophosphamide was the positive control to show that the S9 metabolic fraction was active.

Test method (OECD, 2014)

Experiments 1 and 2 were conducted in the absence of S9, with exposure of the cells to microPEA for 3 h and 24 h, respectively. Experiment 3 involved exposure for 3 h in the presence of S9. All experiments were conducted with duplicate cultures of cells, after growing exponentially for 48 h from culture initiation. Cytochalasin B was added after termination of treatment in Experiments 1 and 3, and added with treatment in Experiment 2. Cell harvesting was done 72 h after culture initiation, slides were prepared, and the cells were stained with 5% Giemsa. Microscopic examination of 2000 cells determined the percent incidence of micronuclei in binucleated cells (BNCs).

In vivo studies

Delivery of test article

Preliminary tests found that microPEA was suitable for oral gavage by suspension in water with Tween 80 (0.5% w/v) as a surfactant and carboxymethyl cellulose (1% w/v) as a suspending agent (Intox, 2015c,d, 2016). Analyses performed to verify the concentrations of microPEA in dosing formulations in the 90-day study showed that they were within an acceptable range compared to their respective nominal concentrations (Intox, 2016).

Acute oral toxicity

Study design

MicroPEA was tested, in accordance with GLP, in the female rat to determine its potential to cause acute lethality (Intox, 2015c), using the "Up and Down Procedure" described in Guideline 425 of OECD (2008a). To minimize the number of animals, the up and down procedure adopted by OECD (2008a) for acute toxicity testing strives to use a maximum of five animals, starting with a single dose to a single rat. After a period of observation, the dose may or may not be adjusted up or down before dosing the next animal. As microPEA is not expected to have potent toxicity, the intent of this study was to test at the maximum dose of 2000 mg/kg bw. Thus, this test is characterized as a limit test, using Sprague-Dawley rats (Vivo Bio Tech Ltd, Telangana, India).

Test method (OECD, 2008a)

The rat is the preferred rodent species for this test, and the female is recommended for testing since in cases where differences are found between male and female rats, the female is usually the more sensitive sex. Administration of the test material is by gavage. A limit test is suggested for materials suspected to be relatively nontoxic, as is the case for microPEA. A stepwise progression begins with dosing one animal with the limit dose. The main LD50 study is conducted if the animal dies within 48 h, but if not, then four additional animals are dosed sequentially at a minimum of 48 h intervals. The resulting LD50 is >2000 mg/kg bw when three or more animals survive after 14 days. Results to be recorded include body weight, observations of any sign(s) of toxicity, and any gross pathological changes.

14-day study

Study design

Sprague-Dawley rats (Vivo Bio Tech Ltd), age 6–7 weeks, in groups of five of each sex, were gavaged with a vehicle control and with microPEA at doses of 100, 300, and 1000 mg/kg bw/day (Intox, 2015c). This study was conducted according to GLP.

Test method (OECD, 2008b)

This study, intended to be a dose-ranging study to identify doses to be used in a subsequent 90-day study, was based on recommendations in the OECD Guideline for the Repeated Dose 28-day Oral Toxicity Study in Rodents (OECD, 2008b). The preferred species is the rat, and administration by gavage is a recommended method of dose delivery. Ten animals, five of each sex, are used for each dose delivered daily for the duration of the study. Three dose levels set at two to four times intervals plus control are used, with 1000 mg/kg bw considered a maximum dose. Dosage is daily for the duration of the study with daily observation for mortality and clinical signs. Body weight and food consumption should be recorded weekly at a minimum. Samples for hematology and clinical chemistry analysis are taken just prior to sacrifice, and gross necropsy was performed, recording any gross pathological observations and organ weights.

90-day study

Study design

Rats (Sprague-Dawley, as above) were divided into six groups. Four groups of 20 (10 males and 10 females) were treated for 90 days by oral gavage with the vehicle control (G1), the low dose of 250 mg/kg bw/day (G2), the mid dose of 500 mg/kg bw/day (G3), or the high dose of 1000 mg/kg bw/day (G4). An additional 10 animals (five males and five females) in the control [G1(R)] and in the high-dose [G4(R)] groups were allowed to recover for an additional 28 days (Intox, 2016). This study was conducted according to GLP.

Test method (OECD, 1998)

The rat is the preferred rodent according to the OECD Guideline for the Repeated Dose 90-Day Oral Toxicity Study in Rodents (OECD, 1998), and dosing every day for 90 consecutive days should begin as soon as possible after weaning. At least 20 animals (10 males and 10 females) are used for each dose level and control. It is recommended that groups of 10 control animals (five males and five females) and 10 animals (five males and five females) treated at the highest dose be maintained after the treatment period to see whether treated animals recover from toxic effects or if they persist. Three dose levels set at two to four times intervals plus control are used, with 1000 mg/kg bw considered a maximum dose. Dosage is daily for the duration of the study with twice daily observation for mortality and weekly for clinical signs. Ophthalmological examinations are performed before study initiation and at study termination. Neurological parameters include qualitative and quantitative assessment of sensory reactivity, grip strength, motor activity, frequency of urination, defecation, rearing, and landing foot splay. Body weight and food consumption are recorded weekly at a minimum. Samples for hematology and clinical chemistry analysis are taken just prior to sacrifice. Hematological parameters include hematocrit, hemoglobin concentration, erythrocyte count, total and differential leukocyte count, platelet count, and blood clotting time. Clinical chemistry determinations include sodium, potassium, glucose, total cholesterol, urea, blood urea nitrogen, creatinine, total protein and albumin, and two or more enzymes that indicate hepatocellular effects. Urine samples taken during the last week before sacrifice are examined for appearance, volume, osmolality or specific gravity, pH, protein, glucose, and presence of blood or blood cells. At study termination, gross necropsy is performed including complete external body examination and organ weights recorded for liver, kidneys, adrenals, testes, epididymides, uterus, ovaries thymus, spleen, brain, and heart. Histopathological examination is performed on tissue samples from: all gross lesions, representative brain regions, spinal cord at three levels, pituitary, thyroid, parathyroid, thymus, esophagus, salivary glands, stomach, small and large intestines (including Peyer's patches), liver, pancreas, kidneys, adrenals, spleen, heart, trachea, lungs, aorta, gonads, uterus, accessory sex organs, female mammary gland, prostate, urinary bladder, lymph nodes, peripheral nerve, bone marrow section, skin, and eyes if changes were observed upon examination. Tissue samples are fixed in 10% neutral buffered formalin before embedding in paraffin wax. Sections of 5 μm thickness are stained with hematoxylin and eosin for microscopic examination.

The results were analyzed statistically with IBM SPSS Statistical Software (version 23). Following assessment of homogeneity, using Levene's test, of body weight, food consumption, hematology, clinical chemistry, organ weight, and neurological examination data, different groups were subjected to one-way analysis of variance (ANOVA). Comparisons between treated and control groups were analyzed by *t* tests with variance evaluated at the 5% level of significance.

Results

Ames test

Results from triplicate cultures in Experiment 1 using the plate incorporation test, and in Experiment 2 using the preincubation assay show that microPEA did not induce a dose-dependent or 2-fold increase in revertant colonies at doses of 30, 90, 300, 900, and 3000 μg/plate, without and with S9 for metabolic activation (Tables 1 and 2). Neither were there any cytotoxic effects. All negative and positive control values were within expected and normal ranges. Thus, it is concluded that microPEA is not mutagenic in the Ames test (Intox, 2015a).

In vitro mammalian cell micronucleus test

MicroPEA did not induce a biologically significant, dose-related increase in the percent incidence of micronuclei in binucleated cells (BNCs) at any dose in any of the three experiments, either in the absence or presence of S9 for mammalian metabolism (Tables 3–5). In addition, microPEA did not produce cytotoxicity as assessed by the cytokinesis-block proliferation index (CBPI) in either the preliminary cytotoxicity screen or in the three experiments as described above (Intox, 2015b).

Acute oral toxicity study

MicroPEA did not induce any mortality at the limit dose of 2000 mg/kg bw or abnormal clinical signs in any of the five test animals observed at 10 and 30 min, 1, 2, and 4 h, and thereafter daily until day 15 postdosing. Each animal was subjected to gross necropsy, and no gross pathological abnormalities were found. Microscopic pathology was not conducted in the absence of any gross pathological changes. The LD50 was reported to be >2000 mg/kg bw (Intox, 2015c).

14-day oral toxicity study

No incidence of clinical signs or death was found following 14 days of treatment with microPEA at 0, 100, 300, or 1000 mg/kg bw/day. Furthermore, no adverse effects were observed on body weight gain, food consumption, hematological parameters, clinical chemistry, gross pathology, or on absolute or relative organ weights (data not shown). Thus, the No Observed Effect Level (NOEL) from this study is >1000 mg/kg bw/day (Intox, 2015c).

90-day oral toxicity study

No treatment-related adverse effects were found in this subchronic study, and the NOEL is considered to be the highest dose level of 1000 mg/kg bw/d. There were some incidental findings, described below, that are concluded to be unrelated to treatment and of no toxicological significance.

Survival was 100%, for both male and female rats, in all control, treatment, and recovery groups. No clinical signs were found in any group other than respiratory rales in one control male (day 84 until termination at day 91) and one treated, mid-dose (500 mg/kg bw/d) male from day 80 until day 91; these observations were incidental, not dose-related, and of no toxicological significance. No ophthalmological effects were found in any control or treated animal, either before or after dosing, and neurological observations made during the 12th week were the same in control and treated, male and female rats. Similarly, urine samples taken on day 88 of the study showed no significant differences in urinalysis parameters between high-dose males and females compared to their respective control groups.

There was no difference in average body weights between the control and any of the three treatment groups after 90 days (Table 6). The average weight of male animals in the high treatment recovery group [G4(R)], however, was less than the average of males in the control recovery group [G1(R)], a difference that was statistically significant ($P < 0.05$). Although this comparison makes it appear that the G4(R) male animals lost weight between Day 90 and Day 97 while G1(R) control males gained weight over that week, this was not the case. Further analysis reveals that the subset of 5 G4(R) male animals was smaller from early in the study and gained weight as normally as the other 10 G4 males over the full course of the treatment and recovery periods. The individual animal data show that the subset of 5 G4(R) treated males weighed slightly less than the G1(R) control males from Day 7 of the study, but not enough to skew the combined average weights of all 15 treated [G4/G4(R)] male animals compared to the combined average weights of all 15 male control [G1/G1(R)] animals. The average body weights for both combined [G1/G1(R)] and combined [G4/Gr(R)] males at day 90 are identical (475 g). Although the average weights of the 15 animals in the combined groups are the same, there is a difference in average weights between the subsets of five G1(R) males and five G4(R) males at day 90 (484 and 437 g, respectively). This difference between these subsets of five animals is not a result of an adverse effect on weight gain which was normal for all test animals. Furthermore, weekly measurements of food consumption showed no differences between

Table 1. Summary data on histidine revertant colonies (plate incorporation method).

Treatment	Concentration		TA1535		TA97a		TA98		TA100		TA102	
	(μg/plate)	S9	Mean	±SD	Mean	±SD	Mean	±SD	Mean	±SD	Mean	±SD
Micronized Palmitoylethanolamide	3000	–	17.67	1.53	111.33	13.32	18.33	3.06	120.00	5.29	264.00	10.58
(particle size 0.5–10 μm)	900		20.00	4.36	128.67	8.33	22.00	1.00	124.00	5.29	230.67	16.65
	300		16.00	2.65	146.00	4.00	29.67	5.03	124.67	2.31	246.67	16.65
	90		9.67	3.06	102.67	15.53	32.67	3.79	128.00	2.00	265.33	10.07
	30		16.67	3.79	92.67	3.06	30.67	6.66	124.00	5.29	272.00	28.00
Negative control	0	+	6.00	2.65	115.33	15.14	19.67	3.06	130.00	6.93	258.67	18.04
Vehicle control (pluronic F68)	100 μL		13.33	3.51	97.33	8.08	21.33	2.52	124.00	5.29	256.00	10.58
Micronized palmitoylethanolamide	3000		17.00	1.00	112.67	12.22	32.33	1.53	125.33	3.06	254.67	12.22
(particle size 0.5–10 μm)	900		17.67	3.06	106.67	9.02	36.67	2.08	129.33	7.02	274.67	18.04
	300		22.33	2.08	109.33	7.02	41.33	1.53	120.00	5.29	260.00	16.00
	90		25.67	5.86	107.33	11.02	26.67	2.08	128.00	5.29	256.00	17.44
	30		18.00	2.65	122.67	1.15	26.00	4.36	136.00	2.00	250.67	6.11
Negative control	0		10.67	3.79	100.00	16.37	29.00	4.36	131.00	6.11	258.67	16.17
Vehicle control (Pluronic F68)	100 μL		13.00	1.00	105.33	9.45	26.67	2.08	128.67	8.33	258.67	6.11
Positive controls												
Sodium azide	2	–	261.33	40.07	–	–	–	–	–	–	–	–
ICR 191	1		–	–	674.67	153.74	–	–	–	–	–	–
4-Nitroquinoline-N-oxide	0.5		–	–	–	–	653.33	106.53	–	–	–	–
3-Methylmethane sulfonate	1 μL		–	–	–	–	–	–	1272.00	115.38	1360.00	21.17
2-Aminoanthracene	10	+	256.00	18.33	–	–	–	–	–	–	–	–
2-Aminofluorene	20		–	–	743.00	41.80	1445.33	41.05	1432.00	127.00	–	–
Danthron	30		–	–	–	–	–	–	–	–	1664.00	170.27

S9: (–) Without S9, (+) With S9.

Table 2. Summary data on histidine revertant colonies (preincubation method).

Treatment	Concentration (μg/plate)	S9	TA1535 Mean	TA1535 ±SD	TA97a Mean	TA97a ±SD	TA98 Mean	TA98 ±SD	TA100 Mean	TA100 ±SD	TA102 Mean	TA102 ±SD
Micronized palmitoylethanolamide	3000	–	14.00	3.61	110.67	13.61	38.33	3.79	138.00	10.58	234.67	22.03
(particle size 0.5–10 μm)	900		10.33	1.53	129.33	8.08	28.33	8.02	154.00	5.29	289.33	28.10
	300		11.00	1.73	111.33	6.11	24.00	2.65	146.00	14.42	328.00	30.20
	90		17.33	5.51	124.00	5.29	24.67	1.15	154.67	6.43	280.00	26.23
	30		13.33	1.15	125.33	3.06	30.00	2.65	148.00	2.00	264.00	10.58
Negative control	0		14.33	3.51	101.33	4.16	25.33	6.81	128.00	5.29	282.67	30.02
Vehicle control (Pluronic F68)	100 μL		19.00	4.36	108.00	5.29	38.67	4.51	129.33	3.06	250.67	8.33
Micronized palmitoylethanolamide	3000	+	11.33	5.86	114.67	6.43	39.33	1.53	158.00	24.33	256.00	4.00
(particle size 0.5–10 μm)	900		7.33	2.52	124.00	3.46	42.00	2.65	136.00	12.17	245.33	6.11
	300		16.67	3.79	128.00	5.29	40.00	2.65	146.00	2.00	253.33	8.33
	90		11.67	0.58	104.67	4.16	37.67	4.73	121.33	8.33	249.33	8.33
	30		15.00	4.58	110.67	6.43	25.67	3.06	124.67	7.57	248.00	10.58
Negative control	0		15.67	2.52	96.67	10.07	22.00	7.94	117.33	6.43	282.67	38.85
Vehicle control (Pluronic F68)	100 μL		25.00	2.65	108.00	5.29	31.67	3.06	158.67	34.08	254.67	9.24
Positive controls												
Sodium azide	2	–	650.67	57.87	–	–	–	–	–	–	–	–
ICR 191	1		–	–	765.33	60.04	–	–	–	–	–	–
4-Nitroquinoline-N-oxide	0.5		–	–	–	–	1421.33	124.02	–	–	–	–
3-Methylmethane sulfonate	1 μL		–	–	–	–	–	–	770.67	56.19	1533.33	53.27
2-Aminoanthracene	10	+	693.33	113.23	–	–	–	–	–	–	–	–
2-Aminofluorene	20		–	–	564.00	90.60	608.00	152.63	518.67	232.91	–	–
Danthron	30		–	–	–	–	–	–	–	–	1210.67	162.45

S9: (–) Without S9, (+) With S9.

Table 3. Summary of incidence of micronucleated BNCs and cytotoxicity.

Cultured lymphocytes treated for 3 h without metabolic activation – Experiment no. 1

Test/control article & dose (μg/mL)	Dose μg/mL	No. of cells analyzed	No. of BNC with MN	% of BNC with MN	CBPI	% Cytostasis
Negative control 0.9% Saline w/v	–	2008	3	0.15	1.87	–
Vehicle control pluronic F68	–	2005	5	0.25	1.85	–
Positive control MMC	0.8	2000	31	1.55[1]	1.55	35.65
Positive control VBL	0.08	2000	31	1.55[1]	1.56	34.38
Micronized palmitoylethanolamide	1000	2000	6	0.30	1.71	16.95
(particle size 0.5–10 μm)	500	2013	4	0.20	1.75	11.86
	250	2000	5	0.25	1.74	13.27

[1] $P < 0.05$.

Table 4. Summary of incidence of micronucleated BNCs and cytotoxicity.

Cultured lymphocytes treated for 24 h without metabolic activation – Experiment no. 2

Test/control article & dose (μg/mL)	Dose μg/mL	No. of cells analyzed	No. of BNC with MN	% of BNC with MN	CBPI	% Cytostasis
Negative control 0.9% saline w/v	–	2006	3	0.15	1.76	–
Vehicle control pluronic F68	–	2010	4	0.20	1.77	–
Positive control MMC	0.8	2000	34	1.70[1]	1.58	24.51
Positive control VBL	0.08	2000	29	1.45[1]	1.59	23.97
Micronized palmitoylethanolamide	1000	2000	7	0.35	1.62	19.72
(particle size 0.5–10 μm)	500	2000	6	0.30	1.64	17.40
	250	2000	5	0.25	1.75	3.66

[1] $P < 0.05$.

Table 5. Summary of incidence of micronucleated BNCs and cytotoxicity.

Cultured lymphocytes treated for 3 h with metabolic activation – Experiment no. 3

Test/control article & dose (μg/mL)	Dose μg/mL	No. of cells analyzed	No. of BNC with MN	% of BNC with MN	CBPI	% Cytostasis
Negative control 0.9% saline w/v	–	2007	2	0.10	1.79	–
Vehicle control pluronic F68	–	2007	4	0.20	1.78	–
Positive control CPM	6.25	2000	36	1.80[1]	1.68	13.82
Micronized palmitoylethanolamide	1000	2006	2	0.10	1.74	5.38
(particle size 0.5–10 μm)	500	2021	3	0.15	1.76	3.35
	250	2000	4	0.20	1.75	4.20

[1] $P < 0.05$.

treated and control groups over the course of the 90-day study and recovery period. Based on these observations and the analysis described above, it is concluded that consumption of microPEA did not have an adverse effect on body weight or body weight gain.

Table 7 shows a summary of hematology data for all animals, male and female, control, treated, and recovery. The results are normal with no differences between control and treated groups except for elevated total WBC counts for the high-dose group at the end of the recovery period. Although statistically higher than concurrent controls, the value $10.08 \times 10^3/cm^2$ is well within the historical range (8.3 to $18.5 \times 10^3/cm^2$) for control rats in 90-day studies at the test facility. Furthermore, no correlating adverse effects were observed in this test group with regard to clinical signs, blood chemistry, organ weights, and gross or microscopic pathology, indicating no toxicological significance for this incidental finding.

Clinical chemistry findings are shown in Table 8. A few isolated measurements were statistically different from controls, but are considered to be incidental and without biological significance due to lack of any dose dependency as well as their values falling within ranges of the laboratory's historical controls.

Table 6. Summary of body weights (g).

Male rats

Group	Dose mg/kg/day		Study days 1	7	14	21	28	35	42	49	56	63	70	77	84	90	97	104	111	118
Vehicle control: analytical grade water with Tween 80 (about 0.5% w/v) and carboxymethyl cellulose (1% w/v)																				
G1 &	0	Mean	253.13	286.60	315.20	341.67	371.33	383.53	402.13	419.93	432.20	445.27	457.07	468.53	473.47	474.67	490.20	494.40	498.00	500.80
G1 (R)		±SD	14.16	17.26	22.68	23.88	23.44	25.58	29.44	32.04	33.13	34.01	33.71	36.10	37.75	41.83	35.15	36.21	35.12	35.37
		n	15	15	15	15	15	15	15	15	15	15	15	15	15	15	5	5	5	5
Test article: micronized palmitoylethanolamide (particle size 0.5–10 μm)																				
G2	250	Mean	254.10	287.80	312.60	337.60	358.60	371.10	390.70	408.00	419.90	432.20	439.70	449.00	454.30	459.30	–	–	–	–
n = 10		±SD	15.01	14.43	16.32	17.63	17.21	17.63	18.49	23.95	26.87	25.40	26.22	25.77	25.92	26.07	–	–	–	–
G3	500	Mean	252.90	292.40	325.10[1]	349.00	372.90	386.50	405.60	422.10	436.50	449.40	456.70	469.80	472.20	475.30	–	–	–	–
n = 10		±SD	17.70	15.37	14.23	15.08	20.58	21.40	24.61	26.48	28.78	30.03	29.41	27.45	23.18	22.55	–	–	–	–
G4 & G4	1000	Mean	253.87	290.27	317.20	354.13	377.47	390.07	406.33	421.73	433.80	443.67	453.07	463.27	470.40	475.00	439.80[1]	445.40[1]	448.60[1]	451.20[1]
(R)		±SD	12.89	16.39	28.55	25.14	27.69	31.47	32.04	34.07	35.46	35.66	35.62	38.62	40.44	42.03	16.62	17.17	16.91	17.54
		n	15	15	15	15	15	15	15	15	15	15	15	15	15	15	5	5	5	5

Female rats

Group	Dose mg/kg/day		Study days 1	7	14	21	28	35	42	49	56	63	70	77	84	90	97	104	111	118
Vehicle control: analytical grade water with Tween 80 (about 0.5% w/v) and carboxymethyl cellulose (1% w/v)																				
G1 & G1	0	Mean	194.20	210.60	222.73	238.60	247.60	255.53	263.67	268.67	271.93	274.47	281.20	285.20	289.07	292.07	295.80	297.60	299.60	300.40
(R)		±SD	7.63	8.42	9.32	13.34	12.19	13.64	15.14	15.74	16.37	17.15	19.42	20.15	21.05	21.26	30.86	30.64	30.65	30.75
		n	15	15	15	15	15	15	15	15	15	15	15	15	15	15	5	5	5	5
Test article: micronized palmitoylethanolamide (particle size 0.5–10 μm)																				
G2	250	Mean	194.50	212.30	224.20	242.60	253.60	260.00	267.80	272.60	277.50	280.90	285.00	290.70	294.20	297.30	–	–	–	–
n = 10		±SD	12.11	13.69	13.09	13.44	16.42	16.83	16.59	17.94	19.61	20.58	20.55	20.90	20.75	21.11	–	–	–	–
G3	500	Mean	193.40	211.40	224.80	237.30	246.40	254.00	262.80	264.50	272.10	274.90	281.00	286.30	290.10	292.40	–	–	–	–
n = 10		±SD	8.33	11.57	9.75	9.36	9.31	10.04	10.85	9.66	12.90	13.59	14.45	14.19	14.69	14.77	–	–	–	–
G4 & G4	1000	Mean	193.60	211.40	225.73	236.20	245.40	253.27	262.07	266.27	270.73	273.47	278.33	283.13	289.53	291.80	286.80	289.40	291.40	292.20
(R)		±SD	7.31	9.15	11.41	11.87	11.69	11.96	13.07	14.72	14.35	14.52	15.69	15.68	17.22	17.90	10.18	8.56	8.05	7.66
		n	15	15	15	15	15	15	15	15	15	15	15	15	15	15	5	5	5	5

[1]Significantly different from control group ($P < 0.05$).

Table 7. Summary of hematology data.

Male rats

End of treatment period (Day 91)

Group	Dose (mg/kg/day)		Hb (g/dL)	PCV (%)	Total RBC (×10^6/cmm)	RBC indices: MCH (pg)	MCV (fL)	MCHC (g/dL)	Total WBC (×10^3/cmm)	Differential WBC count (%): N	L	M	E	B	Platelets (×10^3/cmm)	Prothrombin time (s)	APTT (s)	Reticulocyte count (%)	General blood picture
Vehicle control: analytical grade water with Tween 80 (about 0.5% w/v) and carboxymethyl cellulose (1% w/v)																			
G1	0	Mean	15.23	41.82	8.57	17.81	48.87	36.45	5.79	29.71	67.00	0.898	2.368	0.003	890.50	16.05	15.29	1.77	NAD
n = 10		±SD	0.68	2.43	0.62	0.91	2.08	0.74	1.60	13.19	12.49	0.402	0.882	0.010	220.47	1.10	2.33	0.43	–
Test article: micronized palmitoylethanolamide (particle size 0.5–10 *μ*m)																			
G2	250	Mean	15.21	41.60	8.54	17.85	48.86	36.57	5.85	31.34	65.39	0.570	2.700	0.000	890.10	15.74	15.84	1.83	NAD
n = 10		±SD	0.68	1.99	0.51	1.15	3.64	0.48	1.05	12.86	11.74	0.354	1.483	0.000	290.86	0.65	2.06	0.41	–
G3	500	Mean	15.03	41.31	8.55	17.59	48.34	36.41	6.17	35.28	61.26	0.660	2.759	0.000	865.80	16.46	15.29	2.22	NAD
n = 10		±SD	0.64	2.15	0.40	0.71	2.39	0.83	1.06	7.58	7.09	0.289	1.286	0.000	269.06	1.40	2.37	0.59	–
G4	1000	Mean	15.59	42.79	8.68	18.02	49.46	36.44	6.48	29.45	67.38	0.719	2.436	0.000	846.20	15.85	15.66	2.23	NAD
n = 10		±SD	0.54	1.64	0.55	1.16	3.03	0.45	1.48	3.81	3.71	0.443	0.667	0.000	217.04	1.00	2.28	0.70	–

Female rats

End of treatment period (Day 91)

Group	Dose (mg/kg/day)		Hb (g/dL)	PCV (%)	Total RBC (×10^6/cmm)	RBC indices: MCH (pg)	MCV (fL)	MCHC (g/dL)	Total WBC (×10^3/cmm)	Differential WBC count (%): N	L	M	E	B	Platelets (×10^3/cmm)	Prothrombin time (s)	APTT (s)	Reticulocyte count (%)	General blood picture
Vehicle Control: Analytical grade water with Tween 80 (about 0.5% w/v) and carboxymethyl cellulose (1% w/v)																			
G1	0	Mean	14.68	40.44	7.72	19.06	52.48	36.32	3.55	20.83	74.46	0.795	3.922	0.004	748.20	13.68	12.62	2.93	NAD
n = 10		±SD	0.50	1.65	0.45	0.81	1.63	0.76	1.78	5.91	5.75	0.244	0.906	0.014	331.40	1.24	1.61	0.77	–
Test article: micronized palmitoylethanolamide (particle size 0.5–10 *μ*m)																			
G2	250	Mean	14.57	40.23	7.79	18.76	51.81	36.23	5.59	26.36	68.31	2.863	2.372	0.129	879.20	14.55	13.61	2.76	NAD
n = 10		±SD	0.86	2.59	0.49	1.45	4.29	0.64	2.66	14.15	15.39	3.100	1.273	0.255	270.69	2.20	1.72	0.73	–
G3	500	Mean	14.99	42.15	7.91	18.97	53.33	35.57	3.68	28.64	67.20	0.840	3.304	0.006	823.30	14.97	13.45	2.53	NAD
n = 10		±SD	0.57	1.65	0.38	0.43	1.21	0.59	1.00	9.17	8.60	0.275	1.856	0.013	365.14	1.62	1.49	0.71	–
G4	1000	Mean	15.10	41.96	7.94	19.03	52.87	36.00	4.42	27.48	67.40	2.140	2.984	0.003	802.30	12.86	14.23	2.66	NAD
n = 10		±SD	0.55	1.92	0.38	0.49	1.80	0.64	1.44	9.67	10.44	2.663	0.792	0.009	254.75	1.25	1.03	1.06	–

Table 7. Continued.

Male rats

Termination of recovery period (Day 119)

Group	Dose (mg/kg/day)		Hb (g/dL)	PCV (%)	Total RBC (×10^6/cmm)	RBC indices: MCH (pg)	MCV (fL)	MCHC (g/dL)	Total WBC (×10^3/cmm)	Differential WBC count (%): N	L	M	E	B	Platelets (×10^3/cmm)	Prothrombin time (s)	APTT (s)	Reticulocyte count (%)	General blood picture
Vehicle control: analytical grade water with Tween 80 (about 0.5% w/v) and carboxymethyl cellulose (1% w/v)																			
G1 (R)	0	Mean	15.20	42.66	8.75	17.38	48.78	35.62	6.56	30.32	66.96	0.697	2.024	0.000	931.20	18.00	14.86	1.91	NAD
n = 5		±SD	0.80	2.01	0.41	0.32	1.02	0.27	1.17	6.25	5.66	0.380	0.766	0.000	189.98	1.26	1.27	0.47	–
Test article: micronized palmitoylethanolamide (particle size 0.5–10 μm)																			
G4 (R)	1000	Mean	13.70	39.32	7.20	19.39	55.98	34.80	10.08[1]	25.64	68.18	3.718	2.456	0.022	888.40	18.62	14.92	2.13	NAD
n = 5		±SD	1.94	4.93	1.62	2.47	9.31	1.24	2.12	7.70	11.26	5.311	0.697	0.041	60.01	0.74	1.80	0.32	–

Female rats

Termination of recovery period (Day 119)

Group	Dose (mg/kg/day)		Hb (g/dL)	PCV (%)	Total RBC (×10^6/cmm)	RBC indices: MCH (pg)	MCV (fL)	MCHC (g/dL)	Total WBC (×10^3/cmm)	Differential WBC count (%): N	L	M	E	B	Platelets (×10^3/cmm)	Prothrombin time (s)	APTT (s)	Reticulocyte count (%)	General blood picture
Vehicle control: analytical grade water with Tween 80 (about 0.5% w/v) and carboxymethyl cellulose (1% w/v)																			
G1 (R)	0	Mean	14.88	40.34	7.93	18.80	50.95	36.90	4.07	31.76	64.72	0.990	2.434	0.068	785.00	17.22	11.94	1.67	NAD
n = 5		±SD	0.53	1.84	0.52	0.74	1.58	0.46	1.32	9.56	9.51	0.365	0.884	0.132	233.93	0.42	1.64	0.34	–
Test article: micronized palmitoylethanolamide (particle size 0.5–10 μm)																			
G4 (R)	1000	Mean	14.98	40.36	7.82	19.23	51.80	37.12	8.01	23.14	73.76	0.466	2.618	0.033	906.60	17.98	12.08	2.70	NAD
n = 5		±SD	0.24	1.00	0.60	1.41	3.64	0.53	3.75	5.95	5.70	0.341	0.890	0.063	89.16	1.91	0.51	1.08	–

Hemoglobin, hematocrit (PCV), total erythrocyte count (total RBC), total leukocyte count (total WBC), differential leukocyte (WBC) counts, erythrocyte indices, namely, mean corpuscular volume (MCV), mean corpuscular hemoglobin (MCH), mean corpuscular hemoglobin concentration (MCHC), total platelet count, reticulocyte count, and coagulation parameters namely. prothrombin time (PT) and activated partial thromboplastin time (APTT).

[1]Significantly different from control group ($P < 0.05$).

Table 8. Summary of clinical chemistry data.

Male rats

End of treatment period (Day 91)

Group	Dose (mg/kg/day)		TP (g/dL)	ALB (g/dL)	ALT (IU/L)	AST (IU/L)	ALP (IU/L)	TBIL (mg/dL)	GLU (mg/dL)	CHOL (mg/dL)	BUN (mg/dL)	UREA (mg/dL)	CRE (mg/dL)	GGT (IU/L)	TG (mg/dL)	Na (mmol/L)	K (mmol/L)	Ca (mg/dL)	PHO (mg/dL)	Globulin (g/dL)	A/G Ratio (g/dL)
Vehicle: analytical grade water with Tween 80 (about 0.5% w/v) and carboxymethyl cellulose (1% w/v)																					
G1	0	Mean	6.70	1.14	38.50	73.80	98.90	0.10	108.40	99.30	15.70	22.61	0.40	4.40	81.40	151.50	5.12	9.66	6.80	5.56	0.21
$n = 10$		±SD	0.33	0.12	10.22	9.90	13.92	0.00	26.73	13.47	2.98	4.30	0.07	1.07	32.85	4.43	0.29	0.25	0.67	0.29	0.02
Test article: micronized palmitoylethanolmide (particle size 0.5–10 μm)																					
G2	250	Mean	6.93	1.18	43.80	120.80	99.00	0.09	103.80	92.70	14.30	20.59	0.40	3.90	95.50	151.00	5.10	9.82	6.79	5.75	0.21
$n = 10$		±SD	0.25	0.28	19.31	45.94	46.48	0.03	9.38	18.11	1.95	2.80	0.08	0.88	35.68	3.13	0.22	0.22	0.53	0.39	0.06
G3	500	Mean	6.78	1.05	56.60	105.30[1]	122.60	0.10	111.50	86.70	15.90	22.90	0.42	4.60	90.50	149.50	5.26	9.37	7.58[1]	5.73	0.19
$n = 10$		±SD	0.31	0.31	31.02	25.74	45.41	0.00	16.69	14.00	2.23	3.22	0.04	1.26	39.93	4.43	0.30	0.43	0.75	0.37	0.06
G4	1000	Mean	7.19[1]	1.33	45.50	90.60	97.80	0.09	108.00	98.80	15.60	22.46	0.41	4.50	103.30	152.00	5.20	9.66	6.86	5.86	0.23
$n = 10$		±SD	0.28	0.08	15.28	18.46	8.77	0.03	4.37	17.40	2.22	3.20	0.09	0.71	20.62	1.94	0.30	0.23	0.44	0.30	0.02

Female rats

End of treatment period (Day 91)

Group	Dose (mg/kg/day)		TP (g/dL)	ALB (g/dL)	ALT (IU/L)	AST (IU/L)	ALP (IU/L)	TBIL (mg/dL)	GLU (mg/dL)	CHOL (mg/dL)	BUN (mg/dL)	UREA (mg/dL)	CRE (mg/dL)	GGT (IU/L)	TG (mg/dL)	Na (mmol/L)	K (mmol/L)	Ca (mg/dL)	PHO (mg/dL)	Globulin (g/dL)	A/G Ratio (g/dL)
Vehicle: analytical grade water with Tween 80 (about 0.5% w/v) and carboxymethyl cellulose (1% w/v)																					
G1	0	Mean	6.70	1.14	38.50	73.80	98.90	0.10	108.40	99.30	15.70	22.61	0.40	4.40	81.40	151.50	5.12	9.66	6.80	5.56	0.21
$n = 10$		±SD	0.33	0.12	10.22	9.90	13.92	0.00	26.73	13.47	2.98	4.30	0.07	1.07	32.85	4.43	0.29	0.25	0.67	0.29	0.02
Test article: micronized palmitoylethanolmide (particle size 0.5–10 μm)																					
G2	250	Mean	7.29[1]	1.44	31.80	87.30	80.70[1]	0.10	95.80	113.80	15.80	22.75	0.44	5.20	48.60	144.80	4.59	10.19	5.86	5.85	0.25
$n = 10$		±SD	0.42	0.28	4.96	10.71	43.69	0.00	3.99	29.98	2.57	3.71	0.12	0.79	10.84	6.37	0.26	0.22	0.93	0.50	0.06
G3	500	Mean	6.98	1.44	27.80	83.80	57.00	0.10	100.90	110.30	15.30	22.03	0.33	4.50	58.50	142.50	4.48	10.16	6.21	5.54	0.26
$n = 10$		±SD	0.41	0.16	4.02	6.49	14.09	0.00	17.68	17.86	1.57	2.26	0.16	0.71	27.37	9.86	0.29	0.26	0.69	0.43	0.04
G4	1000	Mean	7.12[1]	1.48	31.60	86.10	52.70	0.10	97.60	119.00	15.40	22.18	0.41	4.30	65.50	148.30	4.66	10.04	6.04	5.64	0.26
$n = 10$		±SD	0.16	0.16	5.21	6.79	8.15	0.00	6.65	21.99	1.71	2.47	0.13	0.67	33.69	4.57	0.46	0.46	0.55	0.15	0.03

Table 8. Continued.

Male rats

End of recovery period (Day 119)

Group	Dose (mg/kg/day)		TP (g/dL)	ALB (g/dL)	ALT (IU/L)	AST (IU/L)	ALP (IU/L)	TBIL (mg/dL)	GLU (mg/dL)	CHOL (mg/dL)	BUN (mg/dL)	UREA (mg/dL)	CRE (mg/dL)	GGT (IU/L)	TG (mg/dL)	Na (mmol/L)	K (mmol/L)	Ca (mg/dL)	PHO (mg/dL)	Globulin (g/dL)	A/G Ratio (g/dL)
Vehicle control: analytical grade water with Tween 80 (about 0.5% w/v) and carboxymethyl cellulose (1% w/v)																					
G1 (R)	0	Mean	6.42	1.04	39.60	85.80	73.20	0.20	91.00	93.80	14.40	20.74	0.30	4.60	109.00	142.60	5.00	9.22	6.66	5.38	0.19
$n = 5$		±SD	0.16	0.05	9.13	15.39	20.45	0.00	11.85	12.38	3.05	4.39	0.00	1.14	29.55	2.07	0.37	0.23	0.53	0.13	0.01
Test article: micronized palmitoylethanolamide (particle size 0.5–10 μm)																					
G4 (R)	1000	Mean	6.36	1.04	58.80[1]	102.8	97.00	0.24	83.00	71.20[1]	15.80	22.75	0.28	5.40	108.20	143.00	5.20	9.02	6.38	5.32	0.20
$n = 5$		±SD	0.44	0.09	7.79	10.64	12.79	0.05	7.58	7.05	1.48	2.14	0.11	1.14	55.28	1.58	0.66	0.68	0.52	0.42	0.02

Female rats

End of recovery period (Day 119)

Group	Dose (mg/kg/day)		TP (g/dL)	ALB (g/dL)	ALT (IU/L)	AST (IU/L)	ALP (IU/L)	TBIL (mg/dL)	GLU (mg/dL)	CHOL (mg/dL)	BUN (mg/dL)	UREA (mg/dL)	CRE (mg/dL)	GGT (IU/L)	TG (mg/dL)	Na (mmol/L)	K (mmol/L)	Ca (mg/dL)	PHO (mg/dL)	Globulin (g/dL)	A/G Ratio (g/dL)
Vehicle control: analytical grade water with Tween 80 (about 0.5% w/v) and carboxymethyl cellulose (1% w/v)																					
G1 (R)	0	Mean	7.18	1.36	25.40	70.60	66.20	0.30	98.80	128.60	12.40	17.86	0.40	3.80	38.80	148.80	4.72	9.58	5.60	5.82	0.24
$n = 5$		±SD	0.46	0.29	4.83	6.23	18.53	0.00	9.50	40.32	2.61	3.76	0.07	0.84	6.14	6.06	0.33	0.30	0.48	0.54	0.06
Test article: micronized palmitoylethanolamide (particle size 0.5–10 μm)																					
G4 (R)	1000	Mean	7.28	1.40	46.00[1]	103.40[1]	94.20	0.30	97.20	98.00	17.60[1]	25.34[1]	0.42	4.80	51.80	145.00	4.68	9.76[1]	5.42	5.88	0.24
$n = 5$		±SD	0.54	0.16	8.12	7.96	33.79	0.00	9.31	15.95	2.88	4.15	0.04	0.45	14.89	1.22	0.26	0.17	0.78	0.43	0.02

TP, total protein; ALB, albumin; ALT, alanine aminotransferase; AST aspartate aminotransferase; ALP, alkaline phosphatase, TBIL, total bilirubin, GLU, glucose; CHOL, total cholesterol; BUN, blood urea nitrogen; UREA, urea, calculated; CRE, creatinine; GGT, gamma glutamyltranspeptidase; TG, triglycerides; Na, sodium; K, potassium; Ca, calcium; PHO, phosphorus; A/G ratio, globulin, albumin/globulin ratio (calculated).

[1]Significantly different from control group ($P < 0.05$).

There were no differences in organ or tissue weights attributable to 90 days of treatment with microPEA. The only statistically significant difference in mean organ weights noted at end of the 90-day treatment was that of the relative, but not absolute, heart weight in females being lesser than the control, which in absence of dose dependence, was considered to be incidental. At the end of the 28-day recovery period, absolute and relative adrenal weights only in male rats were statistically higher in G4(R) as compared to G1(R) controls (Tables 9 and 10), and absolute liver weights were significantly lower in G4(R) females only than in G1(R) control rats (Table 9). These results appear to be incidental due to the lack of any changes in other correlated parameters, such as necropsy findings, histopathology findings, clinical hematology, and clinical chemistry.

Gross necropsy revealed an absence of any remarkable gross abnormalities in all but two male animals at the end of the 90-day treatment period and two males at the end of the 28-day recovery phase. One G3 rat had multiple abscesses in the lungs and another G3 animal had underweight testes and epididymides following 90 days of treatment. These incidental findings were found only in the mid-dose group and are concluded to be unrelated to dosing with microPEA. Moderate splenic enlargement was found in two G4(R) males at the end of the recovery period, but subsequent histopathologic examination showed this to be due to splenic congestion, a common condition considered to be incidental in this case (Intox, 2016) in the absence of any other causal factors (Cesta et al., 2014).

Histopathological evaluation of tissues and organs listed above, from control (G1) and high-dose (G4) groups, showed no incidence of any remarkable findings that could be related to treatment due to lack of any dose dependency as well as their values falling within ranges of the laboratory's historical controls. Single animals in different groups showed the following isolated (1 in 20 animals) findings in the kidney, known to be common background lesions: tubular dilatation (G1 female); focal tubular regeneration (G4 male) or degeneration (G4 female); and lymphocytic infiltration (G1 male). Two high-dose females showed a low incidence of renal tubular hyaline casts which was not associated with any other pathology in the kidney or kidney weight, or were there any associated effects in clinical chemistry or hematology parameters, body weight, or food consumption. These findings are considered to be incidental and of no biological significance. Microscopic changes in the lungs, thought to be due to accidental aspiration of control or test formulations during gavage administration, and thus not treatment related, including: minimal-to-mild perivascular aggregation of lymphocytes in 8 of 20 control animals (G1) and in 6 of 20 high-dose animals (G4); mild peribronchial lymphoid tissue hyperplasia (3 in G1 compared to 4 in G4); alveolar macrophages in two animals each in G1 and G4; and minimal suppurative pneumonia (2 G1 males and 1 G4 male). Intestinal findings included isolated instances of minimal submucosal lymphoid hyperplasia in the terminal ileum (1 G1 male), colon (2 G1 males and 1 G4 male), and rectum (1 G1 male and 2 G4 females). Ectopic thymus, a developmental abnormality occasionally found in rodents that is generally unrelated to treatment, was observed in one control female (G1) and in two treated females (G4). The only other histopathological findings were in single control animals. Overall the histopathological evaluation showed no treatment-related effects of any biological significance.

Table 9. Summary of absolute organ weights (end of recovery period) (g).

Male rats

Group	Dose mg/kg/day		Fasting body Wt. (g)	Adrenals	Testes	Kidneys	Liver	Brain	Thymus	Heart	Spleen	Epididymides
G1 (R)	0	Mean	483.60	0.044	3.77	4.10	14.87	2.44	0.55	1.64	0.84	1.41
$n = 5$		±SD	34.09	0.006	0.40	0.58	1.89	0.20	0.08	0.32	0.14	0.18
G4 (R)	1000	Mean	434.60	0.057[1]	3.66	3.35	12.45	2.31	0.46	1.50	2.02	1.31
$n = 5$		±SD	19.27	0.006	0.30	0.50	1.91	0.17	0.14	0.24	1.23	0.16

Female rats

Group	Dose mg/kg/day		Fasting body Wt.	Adrenals	Ovaries	Kidneys	Liver	Brain	Thymus	Heart	Spleen	Uterus
G1 (R)	0	Mean	288.00	0.076	0.154	2.19	8.46	2.27	0.36	1.22	0.87	1.33
$n = 5$		±SD	31.96	0.016	0.029	0.09	0.40	0.12	0.08	0.12	0.47	0.84
G4 (R)	1000	Mean	279.40	0.064	0.138	2.04	7.44[1]	2.10	0.29	1.09	0.93	1.08
$n = 5$		±SD	7.64	0.008	0.013	0.37	0.68	0.15	0.03	0.07	0.44	0.51

[1]Organ weights of treated rats differ significantly ($P > 0.05$) from those of the control group.

Table 10. Summary of relative organ weights at end of recovery period (%).

Male rats

Group	Dose mg/kg/day		Fasting body Wt. (g)	Adrenals	Testes	Kidneys	Liver	Brain	Thymus	Heart	Spleen	Epididymides
G1 (R)	0	Mean	483.60	0.009	0.78	0.85	3.07	0.51	0.11	0.34	0.17	0.29
n = 5		±SD	34.09	0.001	0.04	0.10	0.29	0.03	0.02	0.06	0.02	0.03
G4 (R)	1000	Mean	434.60	0.013[1]	0.84	0.77	2.86	0.53	0.11	0.34	0.46	0.30
n = 5		±SD	19.27	0.001	0.07	0.12	0.37	0.05	0.03	0.05	0.28	0.04

Female rats

Group	Dose mg/kg/day		Fasting body Wt.	Adrenals	Ovaries	Kidneys	Liver	Brain	Thymus	Heart	Spleen	Uterus
G1 (R)	0	Mean	288.00	0.026	0.054	0.77	2.97	0.80	0.12	0.43	0.30	0.45
n = 5		±SD	31.96	0.005	0.012	0.09	0.40	0.08	0.03	0.06	0.17	0.23
G4 (R)	1000	Mean	279.40	0.023	0.049	0.73	2.67	0.75	0.10	0.39	0.34	0.39
n = 5		±SD	7.64	0.003	0.006	0.15	0.27	0.07	0.01	0.03	0.17	0.19

[1]Organ weights of treated rats differ significantly ($P > 0.05$) from those of the control group.

Discussion

The results of the new toxicological studies described in this study show that microPEA has a favorable safety profile for its use in health products intended for human and companion animal consumption, with a no effect level in repeated dose studies that is >1000 mg/kg bw. These results are in agreement with earlier studies done with PEA by the then Czechoslovakia Academy of Sciences that were not published but are described in the review by Masek (1980). The first was an acute oral LD50 study using 1, 2, and 4 g/kg bw in the mouse. No deaths occurred in this acute toxicity study (Masek 1980). The second study was a chronic toxicity study in the mouse in which 0, 100, or 500 mg PEA per kg bw was administered to 50 mice in each group for 6 months (Masek 1980). At interim and terminal sacrifice, histological examination of lymph nodes, spleen, liver, lungs, and kidneys revealed some incidence of various lesions, but no difference in occurrence between treated and control groups. In the third study, a 6-month chronic toxicity study in the rat, groups of 10 animals were exposed to 0, 100, and 500 mg PEA per kg bw (Masek 1980). Histological examination of kidneys, lymph nodes, liver, lungs, and spleen showed no differences in the incidence of adverse effects between the treated groups and the control. The fourth study examined embryotoxicity in pregnant mice that were given PEA at the dose 50 mg/kg bw for 12 days. No teratogenic or embryotoxic effects were found (Masek 1980). Finally, a 2-month study was attempted in the dog (Masek 1980), but it suffered from too many deficiencies (e.g., a total of only seven animals, two dogs per treatment group, three dogs in the control group, background disease) to be considered as adequate for evaluation and no conclusions can be drawn. More recently, in an unpublished genetic toxicology study using the Salmonella bacteria reverse mutation assay (i.e., Ames Test), the results showed that PEA has no mutagenic activity in any of the five standard tester strains, either in the absence or with the presence of a mammalian metabolic activation system (Biolabs, 1992a). In additional unpublished toxicology studies by the same laboratory, all conducted in accordance with Good Laboratory Practice (GLP), PEA was shown to have low acute oral toxicity with an LD50 >5000 mg/kg body weight (bw) in the rat (Biolabs, 1992b), and was not sensitizing in a standard study using the guinea pig (Biolabs, 1992c). These studies are interpreted to mean that PEA (1) is not expected to show any genotoxic or carcinogenic potential, (2) has low oral toxicity, and (3) has no allergic sensitization potential.

These results of the GLP genotoxicity and rodent toxicology studies (Intox, 2015a,b,c,d, 2016) are in agreement with the aforementioned previous unpublished studies (Masek 1980, Biolabs, 1992a,b,c).

1. The genetox studies show a complete absence of mutagenic potential in Salmonella bacteria, interpreted to mean that the test substance is not likely to be a genotoxic carcinogen (OECD, 1997). The conclusion that microPEA is unlikely to be a genotoxic carcinogen is strengthened by the negative results of the micronucleus test, performed using human lymphocytes (Intox, 2015b). This test battery of two in vitro assays (i.e., the Ames and micronucleus tests) is either recommended or required by regulatory agencies worldwide, to investigate the carcinogenic potential of new substances during the premarket review and approval process.

2. The results from rodent studies show that the previous and present acute oral toxicity studies are in agreement (Masek 1980; Biolabs, 1992b; Intox, 2015c), and repeat oral toxicity studies consistently show an absence of adverse effects at the highest doses tested (Masek 1980, Intox, 2015d, 2016).

Although it is not the objective of this study to describe any aspect of the efficacy endpoints or findings of clinical studies, many human studies have been reported on the possible uses of PEA in the treatment and prevention of many types of illness and disorder. Initial tolerance studies were performed and described in the summary by Masek (1980). In one study, for example, five hospitalized children were given 50 mg PEA per kg bw for 2 weeks, and no side effects were observed. In another, 15 adults were given 100 mg PEA per kg bw for 3 weeks, and 12 biochemical parameters were examined before and after exposure to PEA. No adverse effects were found. Subsequently, two large studies were used to provide documentation for the approval of PEA as a drug (i.e., IMPULSIN®). In one featuring two trials (Masek et al. 1974), 1300 subjects were involved, about half receiving 30 mg/kg bw of PEA, and the other half a placebo, for a period of 12 consecutive days. Another study, using the same dosing regimen, involved more than 1800 subjects divided into three separate trials (Kahlich et al. 1979). No adverse side effects were reported in these studies.

It is noted, however, that most human studies have been done to examine the efficacy of PEA rather than its safety. It is also noted that the studies were short term, in the order of 2 weeks of consumption. Dozens of such studies have been done over a period of 40 years, which provides some indication of the safety of PEA. A reasonable number of recent human studies have been conducted by Italian investigators in the last few years, using a daily intake of 600 to 1200 mg, usually in two 300 mg installments. The test material in these studies mostly was identified as microPEA by the tradenames Normast®, Visimast®, or Pelvilen® that are commercially available from the company Epitech in Saccolongo, Italy. Epitech is also the supplier of the microPEA used for the toxicity testing in this study. A study by Canteri et al. (2010) used three groups of subjects, including a placebo group, over a period of 21 days. This was a randomized double-blind study with over 100 subjects: 35 in the placebo group, 38 receiving 300 mg/day, and 38 administered 600 mg of microPEA (Normast® 300) per day. No adverse effects were observed. In a similar randomized, double-blind study using Normast® 300 and Normast® 600 for 21 days, 209 volunteers (placebo group), 212 individuals (300 mg microPEA per day), and 215 others (600 mg microPEA/day), showed no adverse effects (Guida et al. 2010). In an open study without controls, Schifilliti et al. (2014) reported no adverse effects after 60 days in 30 subjects who were given 300 mg microPEA (Normast® 300) twice a day. Bacci et al. (2011) conducted a 15-day study with subjects acting as their own control. One adverse event was reported and considered to be irrelevant to microPEA (Normast® 300) exposure of 300 mg, twice a day; 26 subjects completed the study. Pescosolido et al. (2011) administered 600 mg of microPEA (Visimast®) per day for 15 days. Subjects acted as their own controls, and no comment was made about possible side effects. Over a period of 2 months, 20 patients (10 males and 10 females) were given 300 mg of PEA (form and source not provided) twice a day in an observational study that did not report whether or not adverse events occurred (Truini et al. 2011). In a 6-month study in 16 patients and in 16 nonblinded controls, side effects were reported not to have occurred following consumption of 300 mg of microPEA (Visimast®) twice a day (Costagliola et al. 2014). Additional studies have been published that use amounts in excess of 600 mg/day, including Marini et al. (2012) in which 12 subjects received 300 mg of microPEA (Epitech) twice a day for 7 days, and then 300 and 600 mg (total 900 mg) for 7 days. There was no placebo control, but another group of 12 subjects received ibuprofen, and it was reported that there were no side effects. Indraccolo and Barbieri (2010) administered 400 mg microPEA (Pelvilen®) twice a day (total 800 mg) to four subjects for 90 days. There were no controls, and the authors considered it "anecdotal" with a "total lack of side effects". Calabro et al. (2010) reported a single case study, with no further details, in which the subject was given 1200 mg of PEA (form and source not reported) for 2 weeks. In a 30-day trial, 12 (0 mg, but not placebo), 6 (600 mg microPEA), and 8 (1200 mg microPEA) subjects were reported to have no adverse effects after treatment with Normast® 300 (Conigliaro et al. 2011). Assini et al. (2010), in a published note with no details or comments about safety, treated 25 subjects and 25 controls, with 600 mg PEA (form and source not provided) twice a day or 0 treatment (not placebo) for 60 days. Desio (2010) conducted an observational study with no control using 600 mg PEA (form and source not reported) twice a day for 45 days in 16 males and 14 females. There were no side effects.

As summarized above, a number of studies have been conducted with varying numbers of subjects and varying durations of daily microPEA consumption. Reviews of these (Skaper et al. 2014; Paladini et al. 2016) provide useful summaries of the efficacy of micronized PEA, as well as favorable comments on its safety. A common observation from the totality of the evidence described is the lack of adverse effects of doses as high as 1200 mg of microPEA per day. The most common regimen was 300 mg twice a day, although a sizeable body of evidence is accumulating on amounts 1200 mg/day. Adverse effects have been reported to be absent (Gatti et al. 2012; Skaper et al. 2014; Paladini et al. 2016).

In summary, available data from rodent and human studies support the safety of PEA in general, and of microPEA specifically, in products intended for human and companion animal consumption.

Acknowledgments

Earle Nestmann acknowledges the financial support from Prismic Pharmaceuticals, Inc. to Health Science Consultants Inc., to compensate for the time required to prepare this study.

Conflict of Interest

None declared.

References

Assini, A., D. Laricchia, R. Pizzo, L. Pandolfini, M. Belletti, M. Colucci, et al. 2010. The carpal tunnel syndrome in diabetes: clinical and electrophysiological improvement after treatment with PEA. Eur. Feder. Neurol. Soc. 17:72–350.

Bacci, C., G. Cassetta, B. Emanuele, and M. Berengo. 2011. Randomized split-mouth study on postoperative effects of PEA for impacted lower third molar surgery. International scholarly research notices ISRN surgery.

Biolabs SGS srl. 1992a. Prove di mutagenesis-test della Salmonella typhimurium. Rapporto N. 91/4755 (in Italian).

Biolabs SGS srl. 1992b. Tossicita' orale acute nel ratto (dose limite). Rapporto N. 91/4892 (in Italian).

Biolabs SGS srl. 1992c. Sensibilizzazione allergica nella cavia. Rapporto N. 91/4894 (in Italian).

Calabro, R. S., G. Gervasi, S. Marina, P. N. Mondo, and P. Bramanti. 2010. Misdiagnosed chronic pelvic pain - pudenal neuralgia responding to a novel use of PEA. Pain Med. 11:781–784.

Canteri, L., S. Petrosino, and G. Guida. 2010. Reduction in the consumption of anti-inflammatory and analgesic agents during the treatment of chronic neuropathic pain in patients with compression lumbosciatalgia and treated with Normast 300 mg. DOLOR 25:227–234.

Cesta, M. F., R. A. Herbert, A. Brix, D. E. Malarkey, and R. C. Sills, eds. 2014. National Toxicology Program Nonneoplastic Lesion Atlas. Available at: http://ntp.niehs.nih.gov/nnl/hematopoietic/bone_marrow/fibrosis/index.cfm

Coburn, A. F., L. V. Moore. 1943. Nutrition as conditioning factor in the rheumatic state. Am. J. Dis. Child. 65:744–756, cited in Kuehl et al., 1957.

Coburn, A. F., C. E. Graham, and J. Haninger. 1954. The effect of egg yolk in diets on anaphylactic arthritis (passive Arthus phenomenon) in guinea pig. J. Exp. Med. 100:425, cited in Masek and Raskova, 1967.

Conigliaro, R., V. Drago, P. S. Foster, C. Schievano, and V. Di Marzo. 2011. Use of PEA in the entrapment neuropathy of the median in the wrist. Minerva Med. 102:141–147.

Costagliola, C., et al. 2014. Effect of palmitoylethanolamide on visual field damage progression in normal tension glaucoma patients: results of an open-label 6 month follow up. J. Med. Food 17:949–954.

Desio, P. 2010. Combination of pregabalin and PEA for neuropathic pain treatment. Pathos 17:9–14.

Ganley, O. H., and H. J. Robinson. 1959. Antianaphylactic and antiserotonin activity of a compound obtained from egg York, peanut oil, and soybean lecithin. J. Allergy 30:415, cited in Masek, 1980.

Ganley, O. H., O. E. Graessle, and H. J. Robinson. 1958. Anti-inflammatory activity of compounds obtained from egg yolks, peanut oil and soybean lecithin. J. Lab. Clin. Med. 51:708, cited in Masek, 1980.

Gatti, A., M. Lazzari, V. Gianfelice, A. DiPaolo, E. Sabato, and A. F. Sabato. 2012. Palmitoylethanolamide in the treatment of chronic pain caused by different etiopathogenesis. Pain Med. 13:1121–1130.

Guida, G., M. De Martino, A. De Fabiani, L. Cantieri, A. Alexandre, G. M. Vassallo, et al. 2010. PEA (Normast) in chronic neuropathic pain caused by compression lumbosciatalgia: a multicentric clinical trial. DOLOR 25:35–42.

Impellizzeri, D., G. Bruschetta, M. Cordaro, R. Crupi, R. Siracusa, E. Esposito, et al. 2014. Micronized/ultramicronized palmitoylethanolamide displays superior oral efficacy compared to nonmicronized palmitoylethanolamide in a rat model of inflammatory pain. J. Neuroinflammation 11:136.

Indraccolo, U., and F. Barbieri. 2010. Effect of palmitoylethanolamide-polydatin combination on chronic pelvic pain associated with endometriosis: preliminary observations. Eur. J. Obstet. Gynecol. Reprod. Biol. 150:76–79.

Intox. 2015a. Micronized palmitoylethanolamide (particle size 0.5-10 um): *Salmonella typhimurium*, reverse mutation assay (Ames test). Report No. R/14812/AMES/15, July 16, 2015, 54 pp.

Intox. 2015b. Micronized palmitoylethanolamide (particle size 0.5-10 um): in vitro micronucleus test in cultured human lymphocytes. Report No. R/14813/in vitro MNT/15, December 31, 2015, 55 pp.

Intox. 2015c. Micronized palmitoylethanoalmide (particle size 0.5-10 um): acute oral toxicity study in rat. Report No. R/14809/AOR-15, December 31, 2015, 31 pp.

Intox. 2015d. Micronized palmitoylethanoalmide (particle size 0.5-10 um): repeated dose (14-Day) oral toxicity study in rat. Report No. R/14810/SOR-14-DRF/15, December 31, 2015, 81 pp.

Intox. 2015e. Micronized palmitoylethanoalmide (particle size 0.5-10 um): validation of analytical method, and assessment of stability and homogeneity in dosing formulations to be used for non-clinical toxicity studies (Guideline: SANCO/030/99 rev. 4). Report No. R/AUT1731/AMV-SHA/15, December 31, 2015, 75 pp.

Intox. 2016. Micronized palmitoylethanolamide (particle size 0.5-10 um): repeated dose 90-Day oral toxicity study in rat. Report No. R/14811/SOR-90/15, 2016, 235 pp.

Kahlich, R., J. Klima, F. Cihla, and V. Frankova. 1979. Studies on prophylactic efficacy of N-2-hydroxyethyl palmitamide (Impulsin) in acute respiratory infections. Serologically controlled field trials. J. Hyg. Epidemiol. Microbiol. Immunol. 23:11–24.

Kuehl, F. A., T. A. Jr Jacob, O. H. Ganley, R. E. Ormond, and M. A. P. Meisinger. 1957. The identification of N-(2-hydroxyethyl)-palmitamide as a naturally occurring anti-inflammatory agent. J. Am. Oil Chem. Soc. 79:5577–5578.

Marini, I., M. L. Bartolucci, F. Bortolotti, M. R. Gatto, and G. A. Bonetti. 2012. Palmitoylethanolamide versus a nonsteroidal anti-inflammatory drug in the treatment of temporomandibular joint inflammatory pain. J. Orofac. Pain 26:99–104.

Maron, D. M., and B. N. Ames. 1983. Revised methods for the Salmonella mutagenicity test. Mutat. Res. 113:173–215.

Masek, K. 1980. PEA, N-(2-hydroxyethyl)-palmitamide. Results, reports, papers and documents (1966–1980; unpublished English summary).

Masek, K., and H. Raskova. 1967. Pharmacology of palmitoylethanolamide. Pp. 199–209 *in* A. Leonardi and J. Walsh, eds. Drugs of animal origin. Ferro Edizioni, Milano.

Masek, K., F. Perlik, J. Klima, and R. Kahlich. 1974. Prophylactic efficacy of N-2-hydroxyethyl palmitamide (Impulsin®) in acute respiratory tract infections. Eur. J. Clin. Pharmacol. 7:415–419.

OECD. 1997. OECD No. 471, Bacterial reverse mutation test, the organization for economic co-operation and development (OECD) Guidelines for the testing of chemicals, adopted by the council on 21 July, 1997.

OECD. 1998. OECD No. 408, Repeated dose 90-day oral toxicity study in rodents, the Organization for economic co-operation and development (OECD) guidelines for the testing of chemicals, section 4, OECD Publishing, Paris, adopted by the Council on 21 September, 1998.

OECD. 2008a. *Test No. 425: Acute oral toxicity: up-and-down procedure*, OECD guidelines for the testing of chemicals, section 4, OECD Publishing, Paris, adopted by the council on 3 October, 2008.

OECD. 2008b. OECD No. 407, Repeated dose 28-Day oral toxicity study in rodents, the organization for economic co-operation and development (OECD) Guidelines for the testing of chemicals, section 4, OECD publishing, Paris, adopted by the council on 3 October, 2008.

OECD. 2014. OECD No. 487, In vitro mammalian cell micronucleus test, the organization for economic co-operation and development (OECD) Guidelines for the testing of chemicals, adopted by the council on 26 September, 2014.

Paladini, A., M. Fusco, T. Cenacchi, C. Schievano, A. Piroli, and G. Varrassi. 2016. Palmitoylethanolamide, a special food for medical purposes, in the treatment of chronic pain: a pooled data meta-analysis. Pain Physician 19:11–24.

Pescosolido, N., A. Librando, M. Puzzono, and M. Nebbioso. 2011. PEA effects on intraocular pressure after Nd:YAG laser iridotomy: an experimental clinical study. J. Ocul. Pharmacol. Ther. 27:629–635.

Schifilliti, C., L. Cucinotta, V. Fedele, C. Ingegnosi, S. Luca, and C. Leotta. 2014. Micronized palmitoylethanolamide reduces the symptoms of neuropathic pain in diabetic patients. Pain Res. Treat. 2014. doi:10.1155/2014/849623.

Skaper, S. D., L. Facci, and P. Giusti. 2013. Glia and mast cells as targets for palmitoylethanolamide, an anti-inflammatory and neuroprotective lipid mediator. Mol. Neurobiol. 48:340–352.

Skaper, S. D., L. Facci, M. Fusco, M. F. Della Valle, M. Zusso, B. Costa, et al. 2014. Palmitoylethanolamide, a naturally occurring disease-modifying agent in neuropathic pain. Inflammopharmacology 22:79–94.

Truini, A., A. Biasiotta, G. Di Stefano, S. La Cesa, C. Leone, C. Cartoni, et al. 2011. PEA restores myelinated-fibre function in patients with chemotherapy-induced painful neuropathy. CNS Neurol. Disord. Drug Targets 10:916–920.

9

Development of a nutrient-dense complementary food using amaranth-sorghum grains

Judith Kanensi Okoth[1], Sophie Atieno Ochola[2], Nicholas K. Gikonyo[3] & Anselimo Makokha[1]

[1]Department of Food Science and Technology, Jomo Kenyatta University of Agriculture and Technology, P.O. Box 62000-00200, Nairobi, Kenya
[2]Department of Foods, Nutrition and Dietetics, Kenyatta University, P.O. Box 43844-00100, Nairobi, Kenya
[3]Department of Pharmacy and Complementary/Alternative Medicine, Kenyatta University, P.O. Box 43844-00100, Nairobi, Kenya

Keywords
Antinutrients, grain amaranth, nutrients, processing, stunting

Correspondence
Judith Kanensi Okoth, Department of Food Science and Technology, Jomo Kenyatta University of Agriculture and Technology, P.O. Box 62000-00200 Nairobi, Kenya.
E-mail: kanensi@gmail.com

Funding Information
This work was supported by Jomo Kenyatta University of Agriculture and Technology and Kenya Agricultural Productivity Project, Project number KAPP06/PRC-SECBCCI-06FP2006023.

Abstract

Thin porridge from cereals and starchy tubers is a common complementary food in Sub Saharan Africa. It may be high in antinutrients, low in energy, and nutrient density hence inadequate in providing infants' high energy and nutrients requirements per unit body weight. Consequently, undernourishment levels among children under 5 years are high. Therefore, there is need to avail nutrient-dense complementary foods especially for children in low-resource settings. The study was aimed at developing a nutrient-dense complementary food from amaranth and sorghum grains. Amaranth grain, a pseudocereal, though rarely used as a complementary food in Kenya has a higher nutritional quality than other staples. Plant-based foods are known to have high levels of antinutrients. Steeping and germination were used to reduce the levels of antinutrients and enhance the bioavailability of minerals in the grains. Various steeped and germinated amaranth and sorghum grains formulations were made to find the ratio with the highest nutrient content and lowest antinutrient levels. The 90% amaranth-sorghum grains formulation had significantly ($F = 32.133$, $P < 0.05$) higher energy (5 kcal per g on dry weight basis) than the other formulations and a protein content of 14.4%. This is higher than the estimated protein needs from complementary foods even for a 12–23 months child of low breast milk intake (9.1 g/d). Antinutrients could not be detected which could imply enhanced nutrient bioavailability. Therefore, a nutrient-dense complementary food product was developed from steeped and germinated amaranth and sorghum grains with 90% amaranth grain. In ready to eat form, it would give an energy content of 1.7 kcal per g (dilution of 1:2 amaranth-sorghum flour to water) and 1.2 kcal per g (dilution of 1:4 amaranth-sorghum flour to water). It can be used as a nutrient-dense complementary food and for other vulnerable groups.

Introduction

According to Kenya Demographic Health Survey 2014 (KNBS and ICF Macro 2015), the proportion of stunted and wasted children in Kenya was 26% and 4%, respectively. Children aged 6–11 months had the highest wasting rates of 7%. These children fail to attain their full potential of growth and development, suffer long-term deprivation of energy, nutrients, and consequently chronic protein energy malnutrition (PEM), often accompanied by micronutrient deficiencies. The period 6–24 months of age is one of the most critical periods in the growth of the infant. At this age, their demand for nutrients relative to their body size is high. However, there are limitations in the quality and quantity of available complementary foods (Dewey and Adu-Afarwuah 2008; Owino et al. 2008; Imdad et al. 2011).

Some of the challenges during this period include the use of plant-based complementary foods that are too bulky for the weanling with a tiny stomach to eat the necessary quantities that provide adequate nutrients and energy to meet their requirements. Besides plant-based foods notably

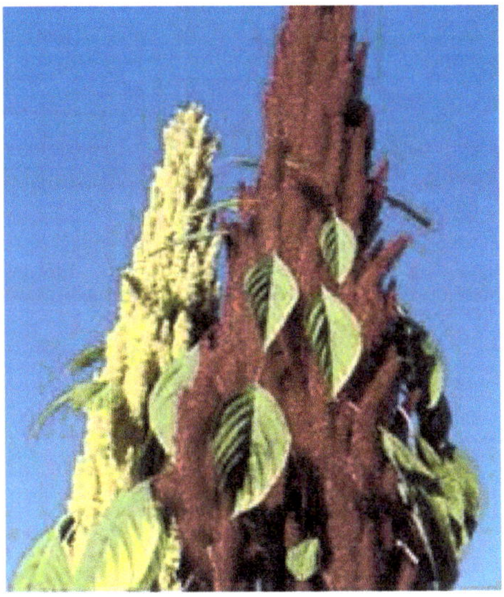

Figure 1. Amaranth grain.

unrefined cereals, legumes, and nuts contain high levels of phytates and at times polyphenols (Gibson and Ferguson 2008). These components vary in the degree to which they inhibit iron and zinc absorption (Gibson and Ferguson 2008; WHO/FAO 2004). Therefore, the children who mainly rely on these unprocessed foods may develop PEM and micronutrient deficiencies. Hence, there is a need to develop nutrient-dense complementary foods for such children.

There is currently, a lot of interest in the nutritional value of amaranth plant, whose leaves are eaten as a vegetable in many parts of Kenya (Mlakar et al. 2010). Amaranth seeds (Fig. 1) contain more protein than most grains such as wheat, maize, rice, and sorghum (Mlakar et al. 2010; Mburu et al. 2012). Further, they contain relatively high levels of micronutrients especially iron, phosphorus, magnesium, vitamin A and E (Kauffman and Weber 1990; Alemu 2008). Besides, amaranth grain is recommended for infants because of its high protein digestibility, absorption, and retention by the baby's body system (Kauffman and Weber 1990). In addition, amaranth has satisfactory lysine and tryptophan contents by FAO/WHO standards. This makes it a valuable complement to staples like maize or sorghum which are limited in amino acid lysine and tryptophan, respectively. Amaranth seed is, however, deficient in the amino acid leucine. Kauffman and Weber (1990) reported threonine as the limiting amino acid in amaranth seeds. However, amaranth grain is not commonly consumed in Kenya, though it could give a nutrient-dense complementary food. In this study, sorghum grain was used to complement amaranth grain because it is a drought-tolerant traditional staple cereal that is widely utilized in Kenya.

A number of traditional food processing technologies such as germination and lactic acid fermentation have been proposed as ways to improve nutrient density of complementary foods and reduce antinutrients (Gibson and Hotz 2007). This study, therefore, aimed at developing a nutrient-dense high-quality complementary food from amaranth and sorghum grains through processing (steeping and germination).

Methodology

Amaranth-sorghum grains product development (processing)

The ingredients were processed to optimize the nutrient density while reducing the antinutrient content. Then product formulation was done followed by nutrient and antinutrient content determination.

Preparation of raw materials

One batch, each of amaranth and sorghum grains were prepared as shown in Figure 2. The grains were sorted, washed, steeped, and germinated at room temperature. They were then dried in an oven at 60°C for 48 h and the rootlets were removed. The grains were then boiled until soft for (30 min), dried, and ground into flour. A second batch of amaranth grain was roasted immediately after germination to find out if the nutrient content would be better than when it was only boiled after germination. The flours were stored in sealed cellophane bags in a cold room at 10°C.

Formulation of the complementary food from amaranth-sorghum flours

Amaranth grains that were steeped for 5 h and germinated for 24 h as well as sorghum grains steeped for 24 h and germinated for 72 h, were ground into flour, and then mixed in various ratios as shown in Table 1 (Okoth et al. 2011). The product formulation was aimed at providing adequate energy and protein content while minimizing antinutrients content. The formulations were then stored in cellophane bags at 0°C prior to laboratory analyses.

Determination of energy and protein content of the formulations

The gross energy content was determined using a bomb calorimeter (C400) (Gallenkamp, Loughbrough, UK) while the protein content was determined using the semi-micro kjeldahl method (AOAC 1995; Method 20.87-32.1.22).

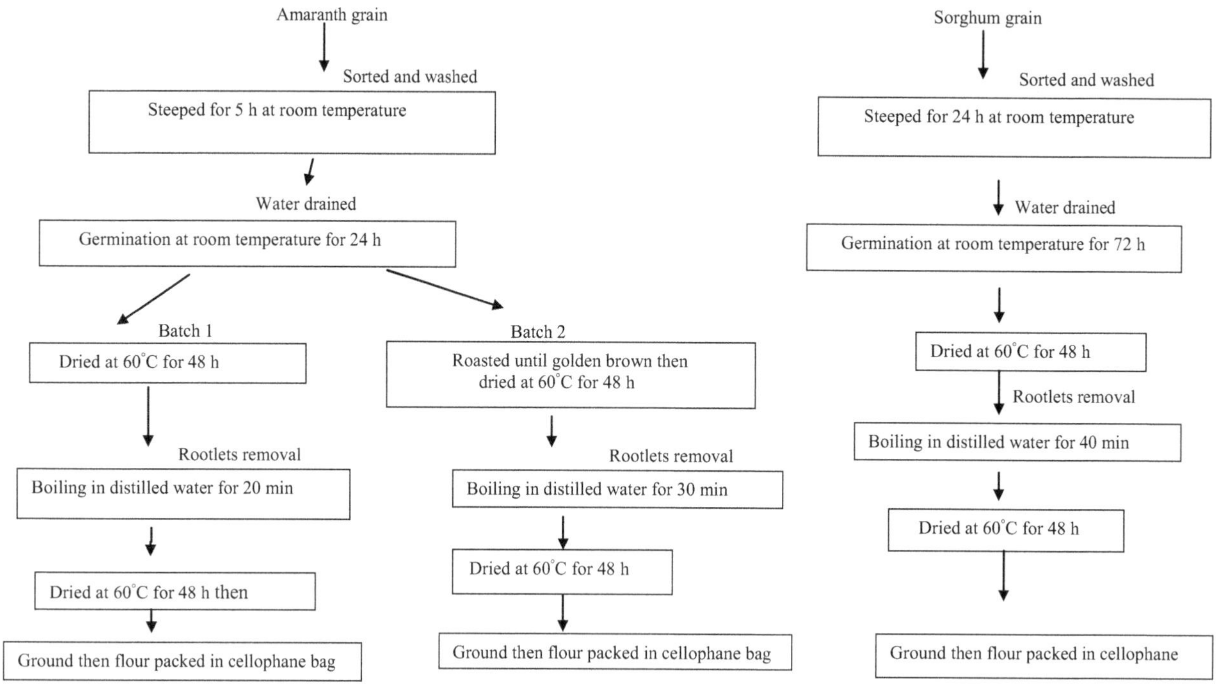

Figure 2. Processing of amaranth and sorghum grains for product development.

Table 1. Formulation of nutrient-dense complementary food.

Formulations of the grains	Amaranth:sorghum ratios
Amaranth boiled + sorghum boiled	90:10
Amaranth boiled + sorghum boiled	80:20
Amaranth boiled + sorghum boiled	70:30
Amaranth boiled + sorghum boiled	60:40
Amaranth roasted, boiled + sorghum boiled	90:10
Amaranth roasted, boiled + sorghum boiled	80:20
Amaranth roasted, boiled + sorghum boiled	70:30
Amaranth roasted, boiled + sorghum boiled	60:40

Determination of the nutritional profile of the developed amaranth and sorghum grains product

Moisture and fat contents were determined by hot air drying (AOAC 1995, Method 925. 10-32.1.03) and Soxhlet extraction (AOAC 1995; Method 920.85-32.1.13) methods, respectively. Fatty acids were converted to methyl esters using 5% HCl in methanol (w/v), followed by extraction with hexane (Ichihara and Fukubayashi 2009). The methyl esters were then separated and quantified by gas chromatography and flame ionization detection (Ciftci et al. 2009). Crude Fiber content was quantified using the Henneberg–Stohmann method (AOAC 1995; Method 920.86-32.1.15). Total mineral content was determined by dry ashing method (AOAC 1995; Method 923.03-32.1.05). The total iron and zinc contents were determined by wet digestion and with an atomic absorption spectrophotometer (AAS) (AOAC 1995; Method 970.12). Product carbohydrate content was calculated by difference method as described by FAO (2010), Shahnawaz et al. (2009) and James (1995) given below:

$$\text{Total carbohydrate in 100 g of food} = 100 - \text{weight in g of (Protein + Water + Ash + Fat)}$$

where g = grams.

The HCl extractable iron and zinc in the product were determined as described by Mbithi-Mwikya et al. (2000). Iron and zinc availability in the product was determined by the method described by Svanberg et al. (1993) and modified by Matuschek et al. (2001). Sugars were separated and quantified using AOAC (1995), method 980.13. β-carotene was determined using UV-visible spectrophotometric method as described by Srivastava and Sanjeev (1998).

Determination of the antinutrient content of the amaranth-sorghum product

The tannin content of the amaranth-sorghum product was determined using the modified vanillin–HCl method (Makokha et al. 2002 adapted from Price et al. 1978 and Burns 1963). The phytate content was determined by the Camire and Clydesdale (1982) method. In vitro-protein digestibility was determined by the Mertz et al. (1984) method.

Table 2. The mean of moisture, energy, and protein content of the formulations (dwb).

Nutrients	Formulation amaranth:sorghum ratio	Moisture content (%)	Energy (kcal per g dwb)	Protein content (% dwb)
ABSI	90:10	4.8 ± 0.3	5.0 ± 0.2[1]	14.4 ± 0.6
ABS2	80:20	4.8 ± 0.3	4.7 ± 0.1[1]	14.9 ± 0.7
ABS3	70:30	5.2 ± 0.0	4.5 ± 0.2[1]	14.2 ± 0.3
ABS4	60:40	4.4 ± 0.0	3.5 ± 0.2	14.0 ± 0.1
ARBS1	90:10	2.7 ± 0.3	4.8 ± 0.1[1]	17.4 ± 0.0
ARBS2	80:20	2.9 ± 0.1	4.7 ± 0.2[1]	15.0 ± 0.2
ARBS3	70:30	3.2 ± 0.7	4.6 ± 0.1[1]	14.1 ± 0.0
ARBS4	60:40	3.8 ± 0.4	4.4 ± 0.1	12.9 ± 0.0

$N = 3$. Values are means ± standard deviation of triplicate analysis. dwb, dry weight basis. Key: ABS1, Amaranth boiled + Sorghum, steeped, germinated, boiled; ABS2, Amaranth boiled + Sorghum, steeped, germinated, boiled; ABS3, Amaranth boiled + Sorghum, steeped, germinated, boiled; ABS4, Amaranth boiled + Sorghum, steeped, germinated, boiled; ARBS1, Amaranth roasted, boiled + sorghum steeped, germinated, boiled; ARBS2, Amaranth roasted, boiled + sorghum steeped, germinated, boiled; ARBS3, Amaranth roasted, boiled + sorghum steeped, germinated, boiled; ARBS4, Amaranth roasted, boiled + sorghum steeped, germinated, boiled. Significantly different $P < 0.05$.
The energy content of the formulation with 90% amaranth grain was significantly higher than that of the other formulations (F=32.133, $P < 0.05$).

Results and Discussion

Formulation of the amaranth-sorghum (complementary) food product

The various formulations that were made, their moisture, energy, and protein content are given in Table 2. The mean energy content of the formulations was 4.5 kcal with, a minimum of 3.5 kcal and a maximum of 5 kcal. The mean protein content of the formulations was 14.7% with a minimum of 12.9% and a maximum of 17.4%. The formulation with germinated and boiled amaranth grain and germinated and boiled sorghum grain in the ratio of 90:10 had the highest energy (5.0 ± 0.2 kcal per g). This is higher as compared to energy obtained from 1 g of both carbohydrate (4 kcal) and protein (4 kcal). The energy content of the formulation with 90% amaranth grain was significantly higher than that of the other formulations ($F = 32.133$, $P < 0.05$). However, there were no significant difference between the protein content of the 90% amaranth formulation and the other formulations ($F = 2.319$, $P = 0.127$). On the basis of energy content, the 90:10 amaranth to sorghum content formulation was chosen as the best for the complementary food. The moisture content was used to express the results on dry weight basis (dwb).

"Energy value should be viewed in light of its density in the ready to eat form of a complementary food because of differences in the viscosity in foods leading to bulk densities" (Mbithi-Mwikya et al. 2000). According to Wardlaw and Kessel (2002), a child at 6 months requires 700 kcal of energy per day. To meet this need, a 6-month-old child will need to take two cups (350 mL each) of the complementary food in a day with the assumption that 1 mL/g of the food provides about 1 kcal. A child between 1 and 3 years requires 1022 kcal of energy per day (Burgess, A., and P, Glasauer. 2004). Therefore, they would need to take two cups of 300 mL of the amaranth-sorghum food in a day with a dilution of 1:2 (Amaranth-sorghum product to water).

The formulation with a ratio of 90 (steeped, germinated, roasted, and boiled amaranth grain):10 (germinated and boiled sorghum grain) had the highest protein content. However, the differences in protein content among the different formulations were not significant. The formulation chosen for the product had a protein content of 14.4%. This is higher than the estimated protein needs from complementary foods even for a 12–23-month-old child of low breast milk intake (9.1 g/d). The formulation chosen contains 28.8 g protein per 1000 kcal. This is considerably higher than that in the World Health Organization/Food and Agriculture Organization (WHO/FAO) report on protein requirements (WHO 2007), which recommended a minimum of 6.9% energy contributed by protein.

Nutritional properties of developed amaranth-sorghum product and the effect of processing on the nutrients

The proximate composition of the product is given in Table 3. The carbohydrate content was 71.4%. It provides

Table 3. Nutritional profile of the developed complementary food on dwb.

Nutrient	Quantity
Moisture %	5.2 ± 0.0
Energy kcal per g	5.0 ± 0.2
Protein %	14.4 ± 0.3
Fat %	6.8 ± 0.4
Ash %	2.2 ± 0.1
Crude fiber %	3.0 ± 0.1

Values are means ± standard deviation of triplicate analysis. dwb, dry weight basis.

Table 4. Nutritional value of commonly used food aid commodities.

	Energy (kcal per 100 g)	Fat (MJ/100 g)	Fat (E %)	Protein (g per 100 g)	Protein (E %)
Corn Soy blend	3.8	1.6	14.2	18.0	18.9
Wheat Soy blend	3.7	1.55	14.6	20.0	21.1
Corn Soy milk	3.8	1.6	14.2	20.0	21.1

Source: WFP (2000); Michaelsen et al. (2008).

an energy content of 1.2 kcal per 1 g wet weight basis. The product provides 28.8 g protein per 1000 kcal of energy. It had a glucose content of 14.8 g per 100 g, fructose 9.3 g per 100 g, and sucrose content of 12.3 g per 100 g. Michaelsen et al. (2008) reported that the most important dietary mono- and disaccharides are glucose, fructose, lactose, and sucrose (sugar). These sugars are good sources of energy and will typically increase the energy density of a diet (Michaelsen et al. 2008).

The proximate composition of fortified blended foods (FBF) commonly used by World Food Programme (WFP) to rehabilitate moderately malnourished children is given in Table 4. The FBF nutritional value was compared with that of the developed food product (Table 3). The developed complementary food has a higher energy content compared to the FBF. The developed amaranth-sorghum product protein (14.4%) provides 28.8 g protein per 1000 kcal of energy. This is higher than the protein per kcal in FBF (Table 4). Further, there was no indigestible protein detected in the product. The inability to detect indigestible protein in the product can be attributed to the decrease in the level of antinutrients (Singh et al. 1982; Kataria et al. 1989; Mbithi-Mwikya et al. 2000).

In the study, no fat was added to the product, as is usually done in commercially blended foods. Usually in FBFs, the oil is added at the time of distribution to minimize use of oil for other purposes. Fat tends to reduce the shelf life of food. The energy content supplied by fat in the amaranth-sorghum product was 12.2% of the total energy in the product. Linoleic acid (LA) was the highest in amount compared with the other fatty acids in the product as given in Table 5 while lauric acid (0.34 mg/100 g) was the least. The essential fatty acids in the product provided 7.4% energy (E %) of the total energy on dwb. The n-3 polyunsaturated fatty acids (PUFA) provided by the developed product was 1.8 E %.

There are two types of essential fatty acids, the n-6 and the n-3 PUFA, which in most diets are provided by vegetable oils in the form of LA (25 C18:2n-6) and α-linolenic acid (ALA, C18:3n-3), respectively. According to Wulf et al. (2008) and Michaelsen et al. (2009), the fat intake of young children (1–2 years) should have a quality that provides 5–10 E % as essential fatty acids

Table 5. Essential fatty acids and fatty acid profile of the complementary food.

Fatty acid composition	Abbreviation	Quantity (mg per 100 g dwb)
Caprylic acid	C8:0	0.68
Lauric acid	C12:0	0.034
Myristic acid	C14:0	47.6
Palmitic acid	C16:0	115.6
Oleic	C18:1	176.8
Linoleic acid	C18:2	231
Linolenic acid	C18:3	10.2
Stearic acid	C18:0	11.6

Values are means ± standard deviation of triplicate analysis. dwb, dry weight basis.

including at least 1 E % of n-3 PUFA and have a ratio of n-6 to n-3 PUFA between 3 and 9. For complementary feeding of children who are well nourished, a level of 30–45 fat E % was recommended, including the fat from breast milk (Dewey and Brown 2003). Several authors have recommended that fat should supply 30–45% of energy intake for children less than 2 years of age (Michaelsen and Jorgensen 1995; Mbithi-Mwikya et al. 2000; Wardlaw and Kessel 2002).

The crude fiber was less than 5%. It is recommended that insoluble fibers should be present in low amounts in the diet because they increase bulk and reduce gastrointestinal transit time (Michaelsen et al. 2009). Dietary fibers may reduce energy intake through a suppressing effect on appetite and they may increase fecal losses of energy due to reduced absorption of fat and carbohydrate (Aggett et al. 2003; Michaelsen 2009). The amaranth-sorghum product had a total iron content of 6 mg/100 g, a value slightly lower than that of raw amaranth grains (6.6 mg per 100 g) (Fig. 3). It had a higher HCl extractability of iron than its ingredients (93.3%) and its bioavailable iron was 5.5 mg per 100 g (dwb) (11.2 mg per 1000 kcal).

The amaranth-sorghum product had a total zinc content of 3.2 mg per 100 g as given in Figure 4. The HCl extractable zinc in the food product was 84% which was higher than both its ingredients. Also, it had 2.8 mg per 100 g (dwb) (5.6 mg per 1000 kcal) bioavailable zinc.

The developed amaranth-sorghum food product had a higher availability of iron and zinc compared to raw amaranth and sorghum grains. For a food-based approach and for most formulated diets, it is important that the basic ingredients be such that the iron is more available (Golden 2009). According to Wardlaw and Kessel (2002), the recommended daily intake of iron and zinc for children 7–12 months is 11 mg per day (mg/d) while those 1–3 years it is 7 mg/d. HCl extractability of minerals and trace elements under simulated gastric conditions is an

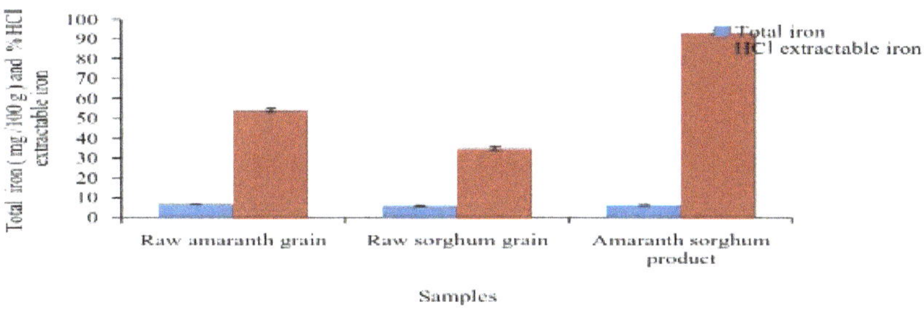

Figure 3. Total iron and HCl extractable iron content of the product and its ingredients (dry weight basis).

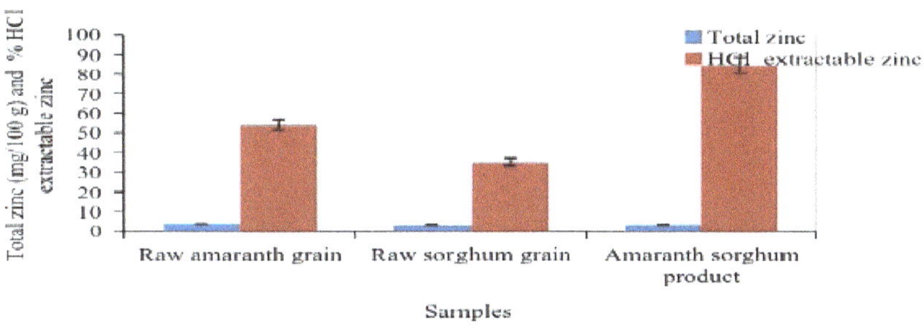

Figure 4. The total and HCl extractable zinc content in the product and its ingredients.

indicator of bioavailability in foods (Antony and Chandra 1998). The improvement in in vitro iron and zinc bioavailability observed in this study could be attributed to a decrease in phytic acid among other antinutrients.

The complementary food contained 4.2 μg per 100 g of β-carotene (7.1 I.U of vitamin A; 0.35 retinol activity equivalents per 100 g) on dwb. It also provided 0.7 retinol activity equivalents/1000 kcal. The recommended daily allowance of vitamin A is 400, 500, and 300 retinol equivalents for children 0–6 months, 7–12 months, and 1–3 years, respectively. The complementary food, therefore, will not supply the estimated needs of vitamin A for children below 23 months.

Antinutritional components of the amaranth-sorghum product (dwb)

Raw amaranth grain had a tannin content of 0.8% CE while sorghum had a tannin content of 24.9% CE. No tannins could be detected in the product. Phytates levels (inositol hexaphosphate) were 7.9 and 252 mg per 100 g in raw amaranth and sorghum grains, respectively. No phytates were detected in the developed complementary food. The most important antinutritional food constituent in diets in low-income countries in terms of negative nutritional impact is phytate, primarily contributed by cereal staples and secondarily by legumes and other plant foods (Michaelsen et al. 2009). Phytate forms insoluble complexes with a range of nutrients and thereby inhibits the absorption of protein and minerals in particular iron, zinc, and calcium. One of the most widespread groups of polyphenols with antinutritional properties is soluble tannins (Michaelsen et al. 2009). The antinutritional effect of polyphenols is complex formation with iron and other minerals, and precipitation of protein, which reduces absorbability. The fact that the antinutrients in the product could not be detected in the steeped and germinated grain implies that minerals and nutrients usually bound by them could be more bioavailable.

Conclusion

A complementary food from amaranth and sorghum grains with an energy density of 5 kcal per g sufficient to meet the recommendations for children 6–23 months of age at 2–3 servings per day was developed. The food product was also low in antinutrients and therefore of correspondingly high nutrient availability and digestibility.

Acknowledgments

We express special thanks to Jomo Kenyatta University of Agriculture and Technology for the study leave and financial support during the research. We acknowledge the Kenya Agricultural Productivity Project, Project number KAPP06/PRC-SECBCCI-06FP2006023 under N. K. Gikonyo, the Principal Investigator for the financial support too.

Conflict of Interest

None declared.

References

Aggett, P. J., C. Agostoni, I. Axelsson, C. A. Edwards, O. Goulet, O. Hernell, et al. 2003. Non digestible carbohydrates in the diets of infants and young children. J. Pediatr. Gastroenterol. Nutr. 36:329–337.

Alemu, J. 2008. The African executive development. Artsvisval. Available at: www.africanexecutive.com/modules/ma (accessed 28 April 2008).

Antony, U., and T. S. Chandra. 1998. Antinutrient reduction and enhancement in protein, starch and mineral availability in fermented flour of finger millet (*Eleusine corocan*). J. Agric. Food Chem. 46:2578–2582.

AOAC. 1995. Official methods of analysis. 16th ed. Association of Official Analytical Chemists, Washington, DC.

Burgess, A., and P. Glasauer. 2004. Family nutrition guide. Food and Agriculture Organization of the United Nations, Rome.

Burns, R. E. 1963. Methods of tannin analysis for forage crop evaluation. Georgia Agric. Exp. Stn. Tech. Bull. 32:1–14.

Camire, A. L., and F. M. Clydesdale. 1982. Analysis of phytic acid in foods by HPLC. J. Food Sci. 47:575–578.

Ciftci, H., A. Ozkaya, and E. Kariptas. 2009. Determination of fatty acids, vitamins and trace elements in *Pistacia terebinthus* coffee. J. Food Agric. Environ. 7:72–74.

Dewey, K. G., and S. Adu-Afarwuah. 2008. Systematic review of the efficacy and effectiveness of complementary feeding interventions in developing countries. Matern. Child Nutr. 4(Suppl. 1):24–85.

Dewey, K. G., and K. H. Brown. 2003. Update on technical issues concerning complementary feeding of young children in developing countries and implications for intervention programs. Food Nutr. Bull. 24:5–28.

FAO. 2010. Food and Agriculture Organization of the United Nations. Available at: http://faostat.fao.org/site/567/defult.aspx//ancor (accessed 1 July 2009).

Gibson, R. S., and C. Hotz. 2007. Traditional food-processing and preparation practices to enhance the bioavailability of micronutrients in plant-based diets. Symposium: Food-Based Approaches to Combating Micronutrient Deficiencies in Children of Developing Countries. J. Nutr. 137:1097–1100. (accessed 26 July 2009).

Gibson, F. S., and E. L. Ferguson. 2008. An interactive 24-hour recall for assessing the adequacy of iron and zinc intakes in developing countries. HarvestPlus technical monograph 8. International Food Policy Research Institute (IFPRI) and International Center for Tropical Agriculture (CIAT), Washington, DC and Cali, Available at: www.harvestplus.org/sites/default/files/tech08.pdf (Accessed on 28 April 2011)

Golden, M. 2009. Nutrient requirements of moderately malnourished populations of children. Food Nutr Bul. 30:S267–343.

Ichihara, K., and Y. Fukubayashi. 2009. Preparation of fatty acid methyl esters for gas-liquid chromatography. J. Lipid Res. 51:635–640. doi:10.1194/jlr.D001065. Available at: www.ncbi.nlm.nih.gov/pubmed/19759389 (accessed 23 July 2010).

Imdad, A., Y. Y. Mohammad, and A. B. Zulfiqar. 2011. Impact of maternal education about complementary feeding and provision of complementary foods on child growth in developing countries. BMC Public Health 11(Suppl. 3):S25. Available at: http://www.biomedcentral.com/1471-2458/11/S3/S25 (accessed 20 January, 2014).

James, C. S. 1995. Analytical chemistry of food. Seale Hayne Faculty of Agriculture, Food and Land use. Department of Agriculture and Food studies. University of Polymouth, UK. 1:96-97.

Kataria, A., B. M. Chauhan, and S. Gandhi. 1989. Antinutrients and protein digestibility (in vitro) of mungbean as affected by domestic processing and cooking. Food Chem. 32:9–17.

Kauffman, S. C., and E. L. Weber. 1990. Grain amaranth. Available at: www.hort.purdue.du/newcrop/proceed (accessed 28 April 2008).

Kenya National Bureau of Statistics (KNBS) and ICF Macro. 2015. Kenya Demographic and Health Survey 2014. KNBS and ICF Macro, Calverton, Maryland.

Makokha, O. M., K. R. Oniango, and M. S. Njoroge. 2002. Malting characteristics of some sorghum (*Sorghum bicolor*) and finger millet (*Eleusine coracona*) grain varieties grown in Kenya. Ph.D. thesis.

Matuschek, E., E. Towo, and U. Svanberg. 2001. Oxidation of polyphenols in phytate-reduced high-tannin cereals: effect on different phenolic groups and in-vitro accessible iron. Food Chem. 49:5630–5638.

Mbithi-Mwikya, S., J. V. Camp, and A. Huyghebaert. 2000. Development of a fingermillet based complementary food for children. Ph.D. thesis, 198.

Mburu, M. W., N. K. Gikonyo, G. M. Kenji, and A. M. Mwasaru. 2012. Properties of a complementary food based on amaranth grain (*Amaranthus cruentus*) grown in Kenya. J. Agric. Food Technol. 1:153–178.

Mertz, E. T., M. M. Hassen, C. Cairns-Wittern, A. W. Kirleis, L. Tu, and J. D. Axtell. 1984. Pepsin digestibility of sorghum and other major cereals. Proc. Natl. Acad. Sci. USA 81:1–2.

Michaelsen, K. F., and M. H. Jorgensen. 1995. Dietary fat content and energy density during infancy and childhood; the effect on energy intake and growth. Eur. J. Clin. Nutr. 49:467–483.

Michaelsen, F. K., C. Hoppe, S. G. Andersen, S. Jacobsen, C. Mølgaard, H. Friis, and T. P. Sangild. 2008. The Use of Whey or Skimmed Milk Powder in Fortified Blended Foods for Vulnerable Groups. J. Nutr. 138:145S–161S.

Michaelsen, K. F., C. Hoppe, N. Roos, P. Kaestel, M. Stougaard, L. Lauritzen, et al. 2009. Choice of foods and ingredients for moderately malnourished children 6 months to 5 years of age. Food Nutr. Bull. 30(3 Suppl.):S343.

Mlakar, G. S., M. Turinek, M. Jakop, M. Bavec, and F. Bavec. 2010. Grain amaranth as an alternative and perspective crop in temperate climate. J. Geogr. 5:135–145.

Okoth, J. K., S. Ochola, N. K. Gikonyo, and A. Makokha. 2011. Optimization of the period of steeping and germination for amaranth grain. J. Agric. Food Technol. 1:101–105.

Owino, V., B. Amadi, M. Sinkala, S. Filteau, and A. Tomkins. 2008. Complementary feeding practices and nutrient intake from habitual complementary foods of infants and children aged 6-18 months old in Lusaka, Zambia. Afr. J. Food Agric. Nutr. Dev. 26 July 2009.

Price, M. L., S. W. Van Scoyoc, and L. G. Butler. 1978. A critical evaluation of the vanillin reactions as an assay for tannins in sorghum grain. J. Agric. Food Chem. 26:1214–1218.

Shahnawaz, M., A. S. Sheikh, and S. M. Nizamani. 2009. Determination of nutritive values of Jamun fruit *(Eugenia jambolana)* products. Pak. J. Nutr. 8:1275–1280. ISSN 1680-5194.

Singh, U., M. S. Kherdekhar, and R. Jambunathan. 1982. Studies on desi and kabuli chickpea (Cicer arietinum L.) cultivars, the levels of amylase inhibitors, levels of oligosaccharides and in vitro starch digestibility. J. Food Sci. 47:510–512.

Srivastava, R. P., and K. Sanjeev. 1998. Pp. 360–361 *in* Fruit and vegetable preservation: principles and practices. International Book Distributing Co. (Publishing Division), Lucknow.

Svanberg, U., W. Lorri, and A. S. Sandberg. 1993. Lactic fermentation of non-tannin and high-tannin cereals: effects on in vitro estimation of iron availability and phytate hydrolysis. J. Food Sci. 58:408–412.

Wardlaw, G. M., and M. Kessel. 2002. Perspectives in nutrition. McGraw Hill Publishers. 5th ed. Pp 673.

WHO. 2007. Protein and amino acid requirements in human nutrition. Report of a Joint WHO/FAO/UNU Expert Consultation. WHO Technical Report Series 935. WHO, Geneva. Available at: http://www.who.int/nutrition/publications/nutrientrequirements/WHO_TRS_935/en/ (accessed 30 May 2009).

WHO/FAO (World Health Organization/Food and Agriculture Organization). 2004. Vitamin and mineral requirements in human nutrition. 2nd ed. WHO, Geneva. 232–233, 250–254. Available at: www.who.int/nutrition/publications/nutrient requirements (accessed 10 June 2009).

World Food Programme (WFP). 2000. Handbook for Food and Nutrition. WFP. Page 114. Available at repository.forcedmigration.org/show_metadata (accessed 26 July 2009).

Wulf, B., L. Niels, N. Agnes, N. A. Pedersen, A. Antti, F. A. Mikael, P. Inga, et al. 2008. Nordic nutrition recommendations 2004 – integrating nutrition and physical activity. Scand. J. Nutr. 48:178–187. Available at http://www.jchimp.net/index.php/fnr/article/download/1633/1504 Accessed on 20 July 2009

10

BioActivities of *Coturnix japonica* (quail) egg yolk and albumen against physiological stress

Gideon O. Oladipo & Emmanuel O. Ibukun

Department of Biochemistry, Federal University of Technology Akure, Akure, Ondo State, Nigeria

Keywords
Antistress, cold-restraint stress, hepatopathy, immobilization stress, quail egg yolk and albumen

Correspondence
Emmanuel O. Ibukun, Department of Biochemistry, Federal University of Technology Akure, Ondo State, Nigeria.
E-mail: oladipo402@yahoo.com

Funding Information
No funding information provided.

Abstract

Cold and immobilization stressors can generate oxidative stress as well as skeletal muscle fatigue. Free radicals cause oxidative degradation of lipids, proteins, nucleic acids, and carbohydrates molecules thereby compromising cell integrity and function. *Coturnix japonica* (quail) egg had been described as being very functional biochemically, due to the essential biomolecules it contains in very regulated quantity. This study was designed to evaluate the in vitro antioxidant activity of extracts of quail egg yolk and the albumen. The assessment of the antioxidant potentials was typified using the total antioxidant capacity, and ABTS, DPPH (1-diphenyl-2-picrylhydrazyl) and hydroxyl radicals scavenging activities. Others are reducing power, metal chelating and lipid peroxidation inhibition activities. The antistress activities of quail egg yolk and albumen were evaluated on hepatopathic enzymes as well as endogenous antioxidant enzymes. The total antioxidant activities of the yolk extract (YE) and the albumen extracts (AE) were, respectively, 186.57 ± 6.441 mg/g and 172 ± 10.690 mg/g AAE (Ascorbic Acid Equivalent). The YE exhibited significant, potent and appreciable antioxidant activities than AE in a concentration-dependent manner. The study confirmed that quail egg yolk contained highly antioxidative bioactive compounds not present in albumen, contributing to its (yolk) overall antioxidant and anti-inflammatory (antistress) properties, thus necessitating their (albumen and yolk) beneficial effects in the management of oxidative and inflammatory conditions.

Introduction

A vast amount of research has been conducted to understand the intricate cascade of events that occur once the brain detects a disruption in homeostasis (a stressor) and the hormonal responses driven by these systems (Thomas and Lena 2010; Kyrou and Tsigos 2009; Charmandari and Tsigos 2005). The key components of the "stress system" are the hypothalamic-pituitary-adrenal (HPA) axis and the sympathetic nervous system (SNS). When the hypothalamus is triggered by a stressor, corticotropin-releasing hormone (CRH or CRF, corticotropin-releasing factor), and arginine vasopressin (AVP) are secreted, eliciting both the production of adrenocorticotropin hormone (ACTH) from the posterior pituitary and the activation of the noradrenergic neurons of the locus caeruleas/norepinepherine (LC/NE) system in the brain. The LC/NE system is primarily responsible for the immediate "fight or flight" response driven by epinephrine and norepinephrine, whereas ACTH drives the production of cortisol from the adrenal cortex. Under normal conditions, the production of CRH and ACTH fluctuate in a predictable circadian cycle and are inhibited by high levels of blood cortisol via a well-described negative feedback loop Experimental and clinical evaluations are specific for a wide range of body changes also called adaptation syndrome, which are predictable rhythm and responses of the HPA axis (Thomas and Lena 2010).

Cold and immobilization stressors can generate oxidative stress as well as skeletal muscle fatigue. Cold immobilization stress also called immobilization stress and cold-restraint stress had been described by Popovic et al. (2009) as experimental induction of very extreme condition which cannot be carried out on human, but believed to have same effect on human as it revealed in animal models. Free radicals cause oxidative degradation of lipids, proteins, nucleic acids, and carbohydrates molecules thereby compromising cell integrity and function. The large generation of free radicals, particularly reactive oxygen species and their high activity play important roles in the progression of a great number of pathological disorders like inflammation, atherosclerosis, stroke, heart disease, diabetes mellitus, multiple sclerosis, cancer, Parkinson's, and Alzheimer's diseases (Aina and Oyedapo 2013; Ozgen et al. 2006; Mensor et al. 2001).

Several studies had predicted quail egg as medically relevant in elevating antioxidant status of experimental rats. However, this study was aimed to evaluate the antistress properties of quail egg yolk and albumen on hepatic function as well as modulation of the antioxidant status of the animals, the toxicological evaluation of diazepam used as standard antistress drug on antioxidant modulation was established.

Methodology

Reagents and Chemicals used in this experiment were obtained from different sources such as British Drug House (BDH) and Sigma Aldrich limited and were all of good analytical grades. All the solutions, buffers, and reagents were prepared using glass distilled water. Diazepam was used in this experiment as standard antistress drug (reference drug) was obtained from Martadol pharmaceutical shop, Akure, Ondo State. Nigeria and was NAFDAC registered.

Extraction of bioactive components involved (Jianping et al.2011); approximately 100 g of freeze-dried egg yolk was extracted with 500 mL of 80% methanol (80:20, vol/vol) adjusted to pH 1.5 with 1 mol/L HCl. Albumen extraction was done by enzymatic hydrolysis using pepsin (Davalos et al. 2004). The samples were then mixed thoroughly using a vortex mixer for 2 min and centrifuged at 6000g for 10 min at 4°C. The supernatant was collected, freeze-dried, and reconstituted to 40 mL.

In Vitro antioxidant assays

Since the determination of antioxidant activities is a quantitative analysis, all assays were performed in triplicate. For each test performed, various concentrations (1–5 mg/mL) of the extract and standards were prepared.

Assay for total antioxidant activity

To the reagent solution; sulfuric acid (0.6 mol/L), sodium phosphate (28 mmol/L), and ammonium molybdate (4 mmol/L); 0.3 mL of sample was added and incubated at 95°C in a water bath for 90 min. After cooling to room temperature absorbance was recorded at 765 nm against reagent blank. The absorbance of the sample was extrapolated on the ascorbic acid standard curve to obtain concentration of the sample in mg/ml then the total antioxidant activity (mg/g ascorbic acid equivalence) was calculated.

Assay of reducing power activity

The reducing power of the extracts was determined according to the method of Oyaizu (1986). Extract (0.5 mL) was mixed with 1.25 mL each of phosphate buffer and potassium ferricyanide ($C_6N_6FeK_3$). The mixture was incubated at 50°C for 20 min. Trichloroacetic acid (1.25 mL) was then added and the mixture centrifuged at 3000 g for 10 min. Thereafter, 1.25 mL of the upper layer of the solution was mixed with 1.25 mL of distilled water and 0.25 mL of $FeCl_3$. The absorbance was read at 700 nm. Higher absorbance of the reaction mixture indicates greater reductive potential.

Assay of DPPH radical scavenging (1, 1-diphenyl-2-picrylhydrazyl) activity

The DPPH radical scavenging activity of the extracts was evaluated according to the method described by Leong and Shui (2002). Exactly 1 mL of 0.3 mmol/L DPPH prepared in methanol was added to 1 mL of extract of various concentrations (1–5 mg/mL) and allowed to react at room temperature for 30 min. The reaction mixture was vortexed thoroughly and left in the dark at room temperature for 30 min. The absorbance of the mixture was measured spectrophotometrically at 517 nm and the percentage scavenging activity was calculated using the formula below.

$$\%\ \text{scavenging activity} = ((Ac - As)/Ac) \times 100$$

where Ac is the absorbance of control and As the absorbance of the extract.

Assay of 2,2'-azino-bis-(3-ethylbenzothiazoline-6-sulfonic acid) (ABTS) radical scavenging activity

ABTS radical scavenging activity of the plant extract was determined according to the method of Re et al. (1999). The stock solutions were of 7 mmol/L $ABTS^+$ and 2.4 mmol/L potassium persulfate. The working solution was then prepared by mixing the two stock solutions in equal quantities and allowing them to react for 16 h at room temperature in the dark. The solution was diluted by mixing 5 mL $ABTS^+$ solution with 145 mL of distilled water to obtain an absorbance of 0.076 ± 0.001 units at 734 nm. Extracts (1 mL) at various concentrations (1–5 mg/mL) were allowed to react with 1 mL of $ABTS^+$ solution, and the absorbance was measured at 734 nm after 30 min using a spectrophotometer and the percentage scavenging activity was calculated using the formula below.

% scavenging activity = ((Ac–As)/Ac) × 100

where Ac is the absorbance of control and As the absorbance of the extract.

Assay of metal chelating activity

The metal chelating activity was determined according to the method of Haro-Vicente et al. (2006). Extract (1 mL) was added to 100 μL of 1 mmol/L $FeSO_4.7H_2O$. The reaction mixture was left at room temperature for 2 min. After which 0.5 mL of 0.5 mmol/L 1, 10-phenanthroline was added and the mixture was incubated for 10 min at room temperature. The absorbance was read at 510 nm. The Fe^{2+} chelating capacity was calculated thus:

Fe^{2+} chelating activity (%) = ((Ac–As)/Ac) × 100

Assay of hydroxyl radical scavenging activity

The hydroxyl radical scavenging activity was measured by studying the competition between deoxyribose and the extracts for hydroxyl radicals generated from the Fe^{2+} / ascorbate/EDTA/H_2O_2 system according to the method of Halliwell et al. (1987). The reaction mixture contained 1 mL (3.0 mmol/L deoxyribose, 0.1 mmol/L EDTA, 2 mmol/L H_2O_2, 0.1 mmol/L L-Ascorbic acid, 0.1 mmol/L $FeCl_3.6H_2O$ in 10 mmol/L phosphate buffer, pH 7.4) and various concentrations of the extracts (1–5 mg/mL). The reaction mixtures were incubated at 37°C for 1 h, followed by the addition of 1 mL of 1 % (w/v) TBA (in 0.25 N HCl) and 1.0 mL 10 % (w/v) TCA. The reaction mixtures were heated in boiling water bath at 100°C for 20 min and the pink chromogen (malondialdehyde-(TBA) adduct) was extracted into 1.0 mL of butan-1-ol and the absorbance was read at 532 nm against reagent blank. The hydroxyl radical scavenging activity calculated thus: Hydroxyl radical (OH^-)

scavenging activity (%) = ((Ac–As)/Ac) × 100.

Assay of lipid peroxidation inhibition activity

The inhibition of lipid peroxidation was ascertained according to the method of Ohkawa et al. (1979). Albino rats were killed by cervical dislocation. The liver was carefully excised and washed in ice cold 1.15% potassium chloride solution, blotted with filter paper and weighed. The liver homogenized in four volumes phosphate buffer (pH 7.4) using a Teflon homogenizer. The resulting homogenate was centrifuged at 3000 rpm for 10 min to obtain the supernatant. A 200 μL aliquot of each of the supernatant was mixed with 60 μL 0.1 mol/L Tris HCl buffer (pH 7.4) and extracts of various concentrations (1–5 mg/mL) followed by the addition of 50 mmol/L $FeSO_4$ and 240 μL of distilled water. The resultant mixture were incubated at 37°C for 1 h. 600 μL of 8.1% SDS was added followed by the addition of 1200 μL of 1.3 mol/L Acetic acid buffer (pH 3.4) and 1200 μL 0.8 % TBA. The mixture was heated at 100°C for 1 h to complete the reaction. Then the samples were cooled, centrifuged at 3000 rpm for 10 min. The intensity of pink colored complex was measured at 532 nm and the inhibition of lipid peroxidation was calculated thus:

Inhibition (%) = ((Ac–As)/Ac) × 100

Experimental Design

Immobilization Stress combined with cold-restraint stress

Male albino rats were used according to the standard guidelines of the Care and Use of Experimental Animal Resources. 40 male albino rats weighing 200 ± 10 g were used to evaluate the ability of the quail egg yolk and albumen extracts to combat stress and were obtained from standard animal house. The rats were housed 5 per cage under constant environmental conditions (20–24°C; 12 h light/dark cycle), and were given ad libitum access to standard pelleted food and water. After the administration of quail egg yolk and albumen extracts for 21 days, combined IS and cold-restraint stress (CRS) test was performed by immobilizing animals in the cold chamber at 4 ± 0.3°C; the plexiglass cage volume was adjusted to the size of the animal, to restrain completely their movements (Popovic et al. 2009) for 2 h, except group 1. Group 2 animals were treated after stress with diazepam (5 and 10 mg/mL BW). Immobilization was done in a plastic container with the aid of paper glue.

Group 1: Untreated, unstressed group-Negative control group (C–).

Group 2: Untreated, stressed group-Positive control group (C+).

Group 3: Diazepam treated (5.0 mg/mL/BW/0.2 mL ip), stressed group (D1).

Group 4: Diazepam treated (2.5 mg/mL/BW/0.2 mL ip), stressed group (D2).

Group 5: Treated (albumen 5 mg/mL/BW/0.5 mL orally), stressed group (A1).

Group 6: Treated (albumen10 mg/mL/BW/0.5 mL orally), stressed group (A2).

Group 7: Treated (yolk 5 mg/mL/BW/0.5 mL orally), stressed group (Y1).

Group 8: Treated (yolk 10 mg/mL/BW/0.5 mL orally), stressed group (Y2).

Preparation of serum and tissue homogenates

Blood samples were collected by ocular punctures into plain bottles. Serum was prepared by aspiration of the clear liquid after clotting and centrifuged for 10 min at 3000 g in a bench centrifuge. Rats were anaesthetized by cervical dislocation and killed loss of consciousness. The liver and kidneys were excised, washed in ice cold 1.15% potassium chloride solution, blotted with filter paper and weighed, and were homogenized in ice cold 5 % w/v sodium phosphate buffer (pH 7.4) using a Teflon homogenizer. The resulting homogenates were stored at 4°C and then used for biochemical analysis.

In vivo Biochemical Estimation

Liver function evaluations

Assay of determination of TP in liver tissues

This was carried out using the manufacturer protocol of Randox laboratory limited, United Kingdom. Total Protein Kit based on Weichselbaumin, Randox laboratory limited, United Kingdom (1995). 1 mL of reagent R1(Sodium hydroxide (100 mmol/L), sodium-potassium tartrate (16 mmol/L), potassium iodide (15 mmol/L), and copper II sulfate [6 mmol/L]) was added to 0.02 mL of the test sample, the mixture was incubated at 25°C and the absorbance was then measured against the reagent blank at a wavelength of 546 nm.

Total Protein Concentration = ((Abs Sample/ Abs Standard) x standard concentration.

Assay of aspartate amino transferase activity in serum

Activity of AST was evaluated using manufacturer protocol of Randox AST Kit based on the principle of Reitman and Frankel (1957). Diluted sample (0.1 mL) was mixed with 0.5 mL of R1 (phosphate buffer (100 mmol/L, pH 7.4), L-aspartate (100 mmol/L), and α-oxoglutarate [2 mmol/L]) and the mixture incubated for 30 min at 37°C after which 0.5 mL of R2 (2, 4-dinitrophenylhydrazine (2 mmol/L]) was added to the reaction mixture and allowed to stand for another 20 min at 25 ^{0} C. Then, 5.0 mL of NaOH (0.4 mol/L) was added and the absorbance was read against the reagent blank after 5 min at 546 nm. The activity of AST in homogenate was obtained following the extrapolation of absorbance value on AST standard curve.

Assay of alanine amino transferase activity in serum

Assay of alanine amino transferase (ALT) activity was carried out using the manufacturer protocol of Randox ALT Kit based on the principle described by Reitman and Frankel (1957). Reagent1 (0.5 mL) containing Phosphate buffer (100 mmol/L, pH 7.4), L-alanine [200 mmol/L), and α-oxoglutarate (2.0 mol/L) was added to a test tube already containing 0.1 mL of serum sample and the mixture was incubated at 37°C for 30 min. Then, 0.5 mL of R2 containing 2, 4-dinitrophenylhydrazine (2.0 mmol/L) was added and the mixture incubated again at 20°C for 20 min. Finally, 5 mL of NaOH was added. The mixture was allowed to stand for 5 min at room temperature and the absorbance was read at 546 nm. The activity of ALT in the homogenate was obtained from a standard curve.

Assay of alkaline phosphatase activity in serum

Assay of alkaline phosphatase (ALP) activity was carried out according to the procedure provided by Randox Kit Manufacturer which is based on the method of Englehardt (1970). ALP activity was measured by monitoring the concentration of p-nitrophenol formed when ALP reacted with p-nitrophenyl phosphate. Exactly 1.0 mL of the reagent (1 mol/L, pH 9.8 Diethanolamine buffer, 0.5 mmol/L $MgCl_2$; substrate: 10 mmol/L p-nitrophenolphosphate) was added to 0.02 mL of sample and then mixed. The absorbance was read for 3 min at intervals of 1 min at a wavelength of 405 nm.

Calculation

ALP activity was determined using the formula:

U/l = 2760 × A405 nm/min.

Assay of determination of bilirubin concentration in serum

The colorimetric method based on that described in Randox kit protocol. Total bilirubin is determined in the presence of caffeine, which releases albumin bound bilirubin, by the reaction with diazotized sulfanilic acid, absorbance was read at 578 nm.

Evaluation of GGT activity in serum

The assay was conducted using a Randox kit protocol. Using a water-bathe set at 37°C for the incubation of the reaction, the reaction is constituted of 100 μL of the sample extract 1000 μL of the reagent at a pH of 8.25 using tris-buffer of 100 mmol/L concentration. The reagent contains glycylglycine (100 mmol/L) and L-γ-glutamyl-3-carboxy-4-nitroanilide (2.9 mmol/L). The absorbance of the mixture was read at 405 nm.

Calculation

To calculate the GGT activity use the following formula.

U/L = 1158 × A 405 nm/min.

Evaluation of endogenous antioxidant enzyme in serum

Superoxide dismutase activity

SOD activity was assayed by the method of Kakkar et al. (1984). Reaction mixture contained 1.2 mL of sodium pyrophosphate buffer (0.052 mmol/L, pH 7.0), 0.1 mL of phenazine methosulfate (PMS) (186 μmol/L), 0.3 mL of nitro blue tetrazolium (NBT) (300 μmol/L). 0.2 mL of the supernatant obtained after centrifugation (1500g, 10 min followed by 10,000g, 15 min) of 10% kidney homogenate was added to reaction mixture. Enzyme reaction was initiated by adding 0.2 mL of NADH (780 μmol/L) and stopped precisely after 1 min by adding 1 mL of glacial acetic acid. Amount of chromogen formed was measured by recording color intensity at 560 nm. Results are expressed as units/mg protein.

Glutathione peroxidase activity (GSH-Px)

Glutathione peroxidase (GSH-Px) activity was measured by NADPH oxidation, using a coupled reaction system consisting of glutathione, glutathione reductase, and cumene hydroperoxide (Tappel 1978). 100 μL of enzyme sample was incubated for 5 min with 1.55 mL stock solution (prepared in 50 mmol/L Tris buffer, pH 7.6 with 0.1 mmol/L EDTA) containing 0.25 mmol/L GSH, 0.12 mmol/L NADPH, and 1 unit glutathione reductase. The reaction was initiated by adding 50 μL of cumene hydroperoxide (1 mg/mL), and the rate of disappearance of NADPH with time was determined by monitoring absorbance at 340 nm. One unit of enzyme activity is defined as the amount of enzyme that transforms 1 μmol of NADPH to NADP per min. Results are expressed as units/mg protein.

Catalase activity

The activity of Catalase activity (CAT) was measured using its perioxidatic function according to the method of Johansson and Borg (1988). 50 μL potassium phosphate buffer (250 mmol/L, pH 7.0) was incubated with 50 μL methanol and 10 μL hydrogen peroxide (0.27%). The reaction was initiated by addition of 100 μL of enzyme sample with continuous shaking at room temperature (20°C). After 20 min, reaction was terminated by addition of 50 μL of 7.8 mol/L potassium hydroxide. 100 μL of purpald (4-Amino-3-hydrazino-5-mercapto-1,2,4-triazole, 34.2 mmol/L in 480 mmol/L HCl) was immediately added, and the mixture was again incubated for 10 min at 20°C with continuous shaking. Potassium peroxidate (50 μL 65.2 mmol/L) was added to obtain a colored compound. The absorbance was read at 550 nm in a spectrophotometer. Results are expressed as micromoles of formaldehyde produced/mg protein.

Reduced glutathione (GSH)

Reduced glutathione (GSH) level in the liver was assayed following the method of Ellman (1959), modified by Hissin and Hilf (1973). The homogenate (720 μL) was double diluted and 5% TCA was added to it to precipitate the protein content of the homogenate. After centrifugation (10,000g for 5 min) at 4°C the supernatant was taken, 5,5'-dithiolbis-2-nitrobenzoic acid (DTNB) solution (Ellmam's reagent) was added to it and the absorbance was measured at 412 nm on a spectrophotometer. A standard graph was drawn using different concentrations of standard GSH solution (1 mg/mL). With the help of the standard graph, GSH contents in the homogenates of the experimental animals were calculated.

Glutathione-S-transferase

Glutathione-S-transferase (GST) catalyzes the conjugation reaction with glutathione in the first step of mercapturic acid synthesis. GST activity was measured by the method of Habig and Jakoby (1974). The reaction mixture contained suitable amount of the enzyme (25 μg of protein in homogenates), 1 mL of KH_2PO_4 buffer, 0.2 mL of EDTA, 0.1 mL of 1-chloro-2,4-dinitrobenzene (CDNB), and GSH. The reaction was carried out at 37°C and monitored spectrophotometrically by the increase in absorbance of the conjugate of GSH and CDNB at 340 nm. A blank was run in the absence of the enzyme. One unit of GST activity is 1 μmol product formation per minute.

All values are expressed as mean ± standard deviation. Statistical evaluation was done using One Way Analysis of Variance (ANOVA) followed by Duncan's Multiple Range Test (DMRT). The significance level was set at $P < 0.05$.

Result and Discussion

The total antioxidant capacities of the extracts of the quail egg yolk and albumen (Table 1) were 186.57 ± 6.441 and

Table 1. Total antioxidant (mg/g AAE).

Extracts	Total antioxidant (mg/g AAE)
Yolk	186.57 ± 6.441[a]
Albumen	172.04 ± 10.690[a]

Values are expressed as mean ± standard deviation (n = 3). Values with different superscript are significantly different ($P < 0.05$). AAE, Ascorbic Acid Equivalent.

172.04 ± 10.690 mg/g Ascorbic acid equivalent (AAE), respectively, these results revealed that the yolk extract (YE) had higher antioxidant activity than albumen extract (AE).

Table 2 shows the iron reducing activities of extracts of quail egg yolk and albumen increasing in a concentration-dependent manner. It was observed that, the iron reducing potential of YE and AE were significantly lower ($P < 0.05$) than ascorbic acid at all working concentrations (1–5 mg/mL) ($P < 0.05$). However, YE gave significantly higher ferric reducing activity than AE at all concentration ($P < 0.05$).

DPPH radical scavenging activity (Table 3) showed the proton-donating property of the extracts at all concentrations. At 5 mg/mL the variation was significantly different; ascorbic acid (93.02 ± 0.59%) exhibited a higher radical scavenging activity than albumen (50.33 ± 2.30%) but a significantly lower activity than yolk extracts (95.61 ± 0.14%). This radical protonating activities of ascorbic acid and YE did not replicate their ferric reducing properties, however, contradicted it.

Table 2. Reducing power activities of extracts of yolk and albumen.

CONC (mg/ml)	Ascorbic acid	Yolk	Albumen
1	1.37 ± 0.025[g]	0.48 ± 0.032[c]	0.2 ± 0.002[c]
2	1.85 ± 0.013[i]	0.65 ± 0.02[d]	0.21 ± 0.009[c]
3	2.31 ± 0.011[j]	0.78 ± 0.018[e]	0.20 ± 0.008[c]
4	2.38 ± 0.032[k]	0.92 ± 0.026[f]	0.36 ± 0.002[b]
5	3.26 ± 0.03[l]	1.44 ± 0.111[h]	0.39 ± 0.035[b]

Values are expressed as mean ± standard deviation (n = 3). Values with different superscript are significantly different ($P < 0.05$).

Table 3. DPPH radical scavenging activities of extracts of yolk and albumen.

CONC (mg/ml)	Ascorbic acid	Yolk	Albumen
1	83.55 ± 1.09[e]	88.86 ± 0.27[g]	22.25 ± 0.1[a]
2	87.57 ± 1.18[f]	89.61 ± 0.23[gh]	26.27 ± 0.58[b]
3	90.63 ± 0.27[hi]	89.74 ± 0.079[gh]	36.39 ± 0.86[c]
4	91.92 ± 0.99[ij]	94.43 ± 0.08[kl]	51.19 ± 1.06[d]
5	93.02 ± 0.59[jk]	95.61 ± 0.14[l]	50.33 ± 2.3[d]

Values are expressed as mean ± standard deviation (n = 3). Values with different superscript are significantly different ($P < 0.05$).

Table 4. 2,2'-azino-bis-(3-ethylbenzothiazoline-6-sulfonic acid (ABTS) radical scavenging activities of extracts of yolk and albumen.

CONC (mg/ml)	Trolox	Yolk	Albumen
1	48.33 ± 0.13[a]	75.81 ± 0.43[e]	67.96 ± 0.34[b]
2	74.69 ± 0.41[d]	79.11 ± 0.87[g]	73.15 ± 0.90[c]
3	79.08 ± 0.35[g]	85.32 ± 0.95[j]	77.26 ± 0.35[f]
4	86.43 ± 0.11[k]	92.89 ± 0.47[m]	82.15 ± 0.64[h]
5	89.31 ± 0.08[l]	97.15 ± 0.44[n]	84.15 ± 0.66[i]

Values are expressed as mean ± standard deviation (n = 3). Values with different superscript are significantly different ($P < 0.05$).

The YE and AE of quail egg were fast and effective scavengers of the ABTS radical and this activity was comparable to that of trolox (Table 4). Efficiency in quenching free radicals in the system is dependent on the concentration of YE and AE, and result of Table 4 presented YE (97.15 ± 0.440%) to have significant activity than trolox (89.31 ± 0.079%) and AE (84.15 ± 0.66%) at 500 μg/mL ($P < 0.05$). ABTS radical scavenging activities were concentration dependent ($P < 0.05$).

The metal (iron) chelating activities of the extracts at different concentrations were represented in Table 5. The chelating abilities of YE and AE were found to be comparable to the reference compound (EDTA) at all working concentrations and exhibited high chelating ability which were significantly different. At 5 mg/mL concentration, YE had a lower activity (77.47 ± 0.25%) which is significantly different ($P < 0.05$) from EDTA (95.62 ± 0.16%). The albumen (35.75 ± 0.08%) had much lower activities at 5 mg/mL concentrations; inferring that its potency to chelate metals and inhibit the Fenton chemistry was lowest significantly compared to EDTA and YE.

The hydroxyl radical scavenging activity (Table 6) represents the percentage hydroxyl ion scavenging activities of the YE and AE at varying concentrations (1–5 mg/mL). It was revealed that the concentration of the reference compound-mannitol tested (at 5 mg/mL), significantly scavenged hydroxyl radical more than AE (91.86 ± 0.77%), no significant difference existed between

Table 5. Metal chelating activities of extracts of yolk and albumen.

CONC (mg/mL)	EDTA	Yolk	Albumen
1	67.25 ± 0.04[h]	35.52 ± 0.22[d]	22.91 ± 0.06[a]
2	75.5 ± 0.12[i]	47.52 ± 0.26[e]	25.81 ± 0.05[b]
3	79.67 ± 0.11[k]	56.21 ± 0.11[f]	26.07 ± 0.12[b]
4	84.35 ± 0.17[l]	64.51 ± 0.23[g]	26.56 ± 0.19[c]
5	95.62 ± 0.16[m]	77.47 ± 0.25[j]	35.75 ± 0.08[d]

Values are expressed as mean ± standard deviation (n = 3). Values with different superscript are significantly different ($P < 0.05$).

Table 6. Hydroxyl radical scavenging activities of extracts of yolk and albumen.

CONC (mg/ml)	Mannitol	Yolk	Albumen
1	68.22 ± 0.08^{d}	53.21 ± 0.02^{c}	32.57 ± 0.18^{a}
2	76.37 ± 0.06^{f}	74.69 ± 0.07^{e}	46.46 ± 0.36^{b}
3	92.26 ± 0.12^{h}	94.32 ± 0.2^{i}	87.68 ± 0.06^{g}
4	95.54 ± 0.09^{j}	96.51 ± 0.07^{k}	94.86 ± 1.39^{ij}
5	97.51 ± 0.15^{l}	97.81 ± 0.06^{l}	91.86 ± 0.77^{h}

Values are expressed as mean ± standard deviation ($n = 3$). Values with different superscript are significantly different ($P < 0.05$).

the activity of the YE (97.81 ± 0.06) and mannitol (97.51 ± 0.154) ($P < 0.05$).

The lipid peroxidation inhibition activity (Table 7) was peculiar with the YE and AE. YE and AE had lipid peroxidation inhibition activities that were significantly lower compared to quercetin, at all concentrations ($P < 0.05$).

Biochemical estimations

The profile of biochemical indices such as, alanine aminotransferase (ALT), aspartate aminotransferase (AST), alkaline phosphatase (ALP), Gamma-glutamyl transferase (GGT), catalase activities, SOD, Glutathione peroxidase (GSH-Px) activities, and reduced glutathione (GSH) level total bilirubin and total protein concentration, were used in assessing the antistress properties of the YE and AE.

Exposure to immobilization stress may lead to increment of free radical generation which may have changed liver enzyme activities, and lipid peroxidation elevation in plasma of rats. Cold restraint and immobilization stressors in rats are known to produce oxidative stress and skeletal muscle fatigue.

Acute emotional stress (immobilization or restraint, alone or in combination with cold exposure) is one form of emotional stress, that has been widely used as a technique for and physiological changes coping ability of animals in response to stress (Pearl et al.1966). It had been reported that rats with restraint stress demonstrated elevation in the plasma levels of ACTH and corticosterone which occur during stress response via activation of the hypothalamic-pituitary-adrenal (HPA) axis (Lou et al. 2008). In response to stress, ACTH is released, which acts on the adrenal cortex to stimulate the synthesis and release of cortisol (Sadock and Sadock 2003). Increased plasma cortisol influences the mobilization of stored fat and carbohydrate reserves which in turn increases blood glucose level. The increased cortisol levels are reversed by antistress agents. Previous reports had also established that chronic vitamin E administration reduces an increase in plasma corticosterone level in rats with cold stress or immobilization stress (Lu et al. 2003).

Liver damage or hepatopathy could be confirmed by elevated activities of AST, ALP, and ALT. Chida et al. (2006) reported that although all the interactions between stress and the liver are not completely understood, there appears to be a negative association between stress on liver disease progression (Chida et al. 2006). The result of this study is in agreement with Chida et al. (2006) and some previous report on the effect of stress on liver enzymes.

Table 8 revealed the effect of quail egg yolk and albumen on physiological stress on liver enzyme markers in the serum; the alterations in the activities of ALT, AST, and ALP. Pretreatment with doses of yolk (5 and 10 mg/mL/BW) and albumen (5 and 10 mg/mL/BW), and the standard drug (diazepam) (5.0 and 2.5 mg/mL/BW) in the stressed groups, significantly ($P < 0.05$) reduced the elevated liver ALP, AST, and ALT levels, which could be due to inhibition of stimulation of sympathetic nervous system by the polyphenolic and/or other antioxidants compounds. The ability of quail egg yolk and albumen to significantly ameliorate hepatopathy by reducing the activities of ALP, AST, and ALT due to the induced stress indicated anti-stress activity which may also be due to their membrane stabilizing ability. The slight increase (though not/slightly significant) in liver ALP, AST, and ALT levels observed in the treated stressed group with 5.0 mg/mL/BW of diazepam may be due to slight toxicity to the liver of the dose of the standard drug used.

Gamma glutamyl transferase activity was evaluated in the serum. The untreated but stressed group (C+) revealed higher activity for GGT, confirming the denaturing effect of stress. All the treated groups demonstrated ameliorative indices, however, administration of yolk extract of 10 mg/mL/BW demonstrated more ameliorative activity than albumen and leading to the reduced production of this enzyme by hepatic cells. Elevated serum GGT can be found in patients with hepatitis, biliary, and pancreas related disorders. The primary role of cellular GGT is to

Table 7. Lipid peroxidation inhibition activities of extracts of yolk and albumen.

CONC (mg/ml)	Quercetin	Yolk	Albumen
1	64.75 ± 0.53^{d}	57.52 ± 0.51^{c}	34.89 ± 0.48^{a}
2	73.48 ± 0.29^{g}	65.97 ± 0.67^{e}	46.19 ± 0.29^{b}
3	81.59 ± 0.14^{i}	73.73 ± 0.42^{g}	56.97 ± 0.55^{c}
4	87.32 ± 0.38^{j}	78.93 ± 0.52^{h}	66.59 ± 0.27^{e}
5	92.25 ± 0.12^{l}	88.69 ± 0.33^{k}	68.86 ± 0.28^{f}

Values are expressed as mean ± standard deviation ($n = 3$). Values with different superscript are significantly different ($P < 0.05$).

Table 8. Results of biochemical effects of yolk and albumen on serum.

GRPS	GSH (mg/g tissue)	ALT (U/L)	TOTAL BILIRUBIN (mg/dl)	AST (U/L)	ALP (U/L)	TOTAL PROTEIN (mg/dl)	SOD (μmol/min/g tissue)	GSH-Px (μmol/min/g tissue)	CATALASE (μmol/min/g tissue)	GGT (U/L)	GST (μmol/min/g tissue)
C-	51.19 ± 4.01^{e}	18.26 ± 4.55^{a}	1.15 ± 0.08^{ab}	36.37 ± 3.71^{a}	34.28 ± 0.93^{a}	17.05 ± 0.81^{e}	149.89 ±4.34^{g}	44.59 ± 2.92^{e}	90.46 ± 1.83^{e}	12.61 ± 0.42^{a}	5.42 ± 0.79^{d}
C+	12.846 ± 0.65^{a}	30.25 ± 1.09^{d}	3.38 ± 0.12^{e}	55.97 ± 5.89^{e}	68.80 ± 0.94^{d}	3.31 ± 0.89^{a}	38.6 ± 4.47^{a}	12.00 ± 1.12^{a}	26.83 ± 1.42^{a}	44.83 ± 0.02^{f}	0.45 ± 0.13^{a}
D1	20.182 ± 1.20^{b}	24.22 ± 4.26^{bc}	1.36 ± 0.15^{bc}	44.28 ± 1.74^{cd}	36.02 ± 2.14^{ab}	12.83 ± 0.30^{d}	76.154 ± 5.48^{c}	20.19 ± 2.52^{c}	37.5 ± 3.09^{b}	21.52 ± 0.82^{d}	1.40 ± 0.27^{b}
D2	31.124 ± 0.76^{d}	21.67 ± 1.81^{ab}	1.03 ± 0.19^{a}	40.43 ± 1.50^{abc}	35.73 ± 0.84^{ab}	12.9 ± 0.33^{d}	109.89 ± 8.34^{f}	26.68 ± 1.52^{d}	78.33 ± 1.54^{d}	14.98 ± 0.62^{b}	2.78 ± 0.45^{c}
A1	18.11 ± 2.41^{b}	26.77 ± 2.64^{cd}	1.02 ± 0.05^{a}	45.47 ± 3.81^{d}	40.12 ± 0.93^{c}	5.49 ± 0.21^{b}	57.622 ± 5.27^{b}	14.86 ± 1.92b	29.15 ± 1.81^{a}	27.37 ± 0.82^{e}	1.63 ± 0.47^{a}
A2	24.702 ± 1.15^{c}	24.81 ± 1.86^{bc}	1.36 ± 0.03^{bc}	42.32 ± 2.16^{bcd}	37.8 ± 1.78^{b}	8.36 ± 0.66^{c}	84.686 ± 6.01^{d}	19.35 ± 1.22^{c}	47.09 ± 1.35^{c}	21.17 ± 0.12^{d}	1.63 ± 0.49^{b}
Y1	23.02 ± 2.25^{c}	20.93 ± 2.56^{ab}	1.65 ± 0.24^{d}	39.30 ± 2.03^{ab}	40.35 ± 1.22^{c}	4.94 ± 0.67^{b}	88.634 ± 2.91^{d}	20.89 ± 1.72^{c}	45.29 ± 6.94^{c}	20.28 ± 0.52^{c}	1.67 ± 0.26^{b}
Y2	28.996 ± 2.36^{d}	18.95 ± 1.84^{a}	1.53 ± 0.26^{cd}	37.96 ± 3.18^{ab}	37.16 ± 2.92^{b}	8.66 ± 0.55^{c}	96.694 ± 4.17^{e}	24.75 ± 2.42^{d}	74.48 ± 7.79^{d}	14.30 ± 0.82^{b}	2.74 ± 0.10^{c}

Values are expressed as mean ± standard deviation (n = 5). Values with different superscript are significantly different ($P < 0.05$) for each assay.
ALP, Assay of alkaline phosphatase; ALT, Assay of alanine amino transferase; AST, Assay of aspartate amino transferase; GGT, gamma-glutamyl transferase; GSH; Reduced glutathione; GST, Glutathione-S-transferase; SOD, Superoxide dismutase.

metabolize extracellular reduced glutathione (GSH), allowing for precursor amino acids to be assimilated and reutilize for intracellular GSH synthesis (Lee et al. 2004). The frequent denaturation of protein in the extracellular environment by activities of free radicals promote the activities of the GGT as more amino acids are made available for transmembrane mobility leading to the generation of glutathione necessary for the endogenous antioxidant activities against the radicals. However, Lee et al. (2004) reported that the increased in the activity GGT in the presence of iron and other transition metals would lead to the generation of free radicals through the reducing ability of cysteinylglycine which reduces F^{3+} to Fe^{2+} which is one of the deleterious radical of protein, lipid, and nucleic acids. We can therefore infer that the increase in GGT ectoactivity is a compromising factor leading to the cell proliferation.

Bilirubin is a natural product of heme catabolism by heme oxygenase in the liver when worn out red blood cell is broken down often due to oxidative proliferation. Serum bilirubin is considered as one of the true test of liver function since it reflects the liver ability to take up bilirubin and metabolize it to bile. Elevated levels of total bilirubin as a result of the unconjugated form indicate the severity of the acute hepatopathy resulting from physiological stress. The serum levels of the total bilirubin by antistress effect of the extracts were shown in Table 8. From the result, all the extracts have ameliorating properties. The stressed but untreated (C+) group had higher total bilirubin which was significantly different from the unstressed and untreated group (C−). The result also expressed toxic effect of posttreatment with 5 mg/mL/BW diazepam, whereas the 2.5 mg/mL/BW had a reduced total bilirubin which is significantly different from 5 mg/mL/BW. This suggested 2.5 mg/mL/BW diazepam as better antistress dose over 5 mg/mL/BW. Yolk administered group showed higher total bilirubin than albumen and diazepam. This was due to the conjugated bilirubin which on aggregate contributed to the total bilirubin concentration. The relationship between total bilirubin and stress could be traced to be oxidative proliferation of the erythrocyte membrane leading to denaturation of hemoglobin, this further led to cascade of reaction that generated total bilirubin. Moreover, hepatopathy would cause defect in the conjugation of bilirubin, leading to increased release of unconjugated bilirubin into the blood, justifying the hepatoprotective properties of the quail egg yolk and albumen.

The contributions of the bioactive compounds in the yolk and albumen to the inhibition of denaturation could not be simplified. We assume that the antidenaturation effects of the quail egg yolk and albumen revealed their relevance as possessing the ability to prevent the proliferation of the proteins by scavenging-free radicals generated by physiological stress. The result of the liver tissue total protein evaluation revealed that there was no significant difference between the two diazepam concentrations administered, however, they showed considerable ameliorating effects but were not able to nullify the effect of the cold immobilization stress. Yolk (10 mg/mL/BW) and albumen (10 mg/mL/BW) ameliorated stressed condition but without significant difference ($P < 0.05$).

The modulation of endogenous antioxidant biomolecules in the blood revealed that the yolk and albumen facilitated the hepatic antioxidant system from the damage induced by the stress. Cells have cooperative defense systems for the reduction in oxidizing agents. The defense systems contain numerous enzymatic and nonenzymatic antioxidants, including SOD, catalase (CAT), glutathione peroxidase (GPx), reduced glutathione (GSH), and glutathione S-transferase (GST). However, when there is an over-flux of free radical, protective systems are overwhelmed. Catalase catalyzes the breakdown of hydrogen peroxide which is a reactive oxygen species to water and molecular oxygen, thus minimizing the proliferation of cells. SOD is one important enzyme involved in the dismutation of superoxide radical. SOD protects against free radical injury by converting superoxide radical to hydrogen peroxide and prevents the formation of hydroxyl radical. In the stressed and untreated group (C+) there was significant decrease in the activities of SOD and catalase. During the advent of free radicals, the antioxidant system of the body is compromise. Initially, there will be increase in the activities of the enzymes. However, prolong assault will result in proliferation of the hepatocytes as well as other sites of synthesis of these enzymes, thus leading to reduction in their activities. The result revealed endogenous-enzymes-activity promoting ability of yolk and albumen which increased as the dose increased. Yolk demonstrated significantly higher ameliorative property than albumen. Excess free radicals have been shown to react with several amino acid residues *in vitro*, making active enzymes denatured (Stadtman and Berlett 1998). Thus, treatment with yolk and albumen had a significant reduction in free radicals influence. The bioactive compounds of the extracts act as ligands that promote the genetic transcriptional and translational production of these endogenous antioxidant enzymes increasing the antioxidant status of the experimental animals.

Conclusion

This study revealed that the extracts of egg yolk and albumen have antioxidant activities. The yolk demonstrated higher antistress and antioxidant modulating activity than higher concentrations of diazepam and albumen. The activity of 5 mg/mL/kg BW diazepam was revealed as toxic dose. The albumen antistress property could be as a result of the free R-group of the peptides which had been described to be responsible for the biological roles of the amino acids. This study thus established that the increased consumption of *Coturnix japonica* (quail) egg could curtail physiological stress.

Conflict of Interest

The authors declare no conflict of interest.

References

Aina, O. I., and O. O. Oyedapo. 2013. In vitro investigations into the antioxidant and anti-Inflammatory potentials of the fractions and ethanolic extract of *Cyclosorus afer* (christ.) Ching, stalks. Life J. Sci. 15:235–249.

Charmandari, E., and C. Tsigos. 2005. Endocrinology of the stress response. Annu. Rev. Physiol. 67:259–284.

Chida, Y., N. Sudo, and C. Kubo. 2006. Does Stress Exacerbate Liver Disease? J. Gastroenterol. Hepatol. 20:202–208.

Davalos, A., M. Miguel, B. Bartolome, and R. Lopez-Fandino. 2004. Antioxidant activity of peptides derived from egg white proteins by enzymatic hydrolysis. J. Food Prot. 9:1939–1944.

Ellman, G. L. 1959. Tissue sulfhydryl group. Arch. Biochem. Biophys. 82:70–77.

Englehardt, A. 1970. Measurement of alkaline phosphatase. Aerztl Labor 16:42–43.

Habig, W. H., and W. B. Jakoby. 1974. Glutathione Stransferases. The first enzymatic step in mercapturic acid formation. J. Biol. Chem. 249:7130–7139.

Halliwell, B., J. M. C. Gutteridge, and O. I. Aruoma. 1987. The deoxyribose method: a simple 'test tube' assay for determination of rate constants for reactions of hydroxyl radicals. Anal. Biochem. 165:215–219.

Haro-Vicente, J. F., C. Martinez-Gracia, and G. Ros. 2006. Optimisation of invitro measurement of available iron from different fortification in citric fruit juices. J. Food Chem. 98:639–648.

Hissin, P. J., and R. Hilf. 1973. A fluorometric method for the determination of oxidized and reduced glutathione in tissue. Anal. Biochem. 74:214–226.

Jianping, W., L. Daise, S. Andreas, and N. Chamila. 2011. Free aromatic amino acids in egg yolk show antioxidant properties. Food Chem. 129:155–161.

Johansson, L. H., and L. A. Borg. 1988. A spectrophotometric method for determination of catalase activity in small tissue samples. Anal. Biochem. 174:331–336.

Kakkar, P., B. Das, and P. N. Viswanathan. 1984. A modified spectrophotometeric assay of superoxide dismutase. Ind. Biochem. Biophys. 21:130–132.

Kyrou, I., and C. Tsigos. 2009. Stress hormones: physiological stress and regulation of metabolism. Curr. Opin. Pharmacol. 9:787–793.

Lee, D., R. Blomhoff, and D. R. Jacobs. 2004. Is serum gamma-glutamyltransferase a marker of oxidative stress? Free Radical Res. 38:535–539.

Leong, L. P., and G. Shui. 2002. An investigation of antioxidant capacity of fruits in Singapore markets. Food Chem. 76:65–75.

Lou, L. X., B. Geng, J. B. Du, and X. C. Tang. 2008. Hydrogen sulfide-induced hypothermia attenuates stress-induced ulceration in rats. J. Exp. Pharmacol. Physiol. 35:223–228.

Lu, P., N. Yaras, A. Agar, S. Gümüslü, S. Bilmen, and G. Özkaya. 2003. The effect of vitamin E on stress-induced changes in visual evoked potentials (VEPs) in rats exposed to different experimental stress models. Acta Ophthalmol. Scand. 81:181–187.

Mensor, L. L., F. S. Menezes, G. G. Leitao, A. S. Reis, T. C. Dos-Santos, C. S. Coube, et al. 2001. Screening of Brazilian plant extracts for antioxidant activity by the use of DPPH free radical method. Phytother. Res. 15:127–130.

Ohkawa, H., N. Ohishi, and K. Yagi. 1979. Assay for lipid peroxides in animal tissues by thiobarbituric acid reaction. Anal. Biochem. 95:351–358.

Oyaizu, M. 1986. Studies on products of browning reactions: antioxidant activities of products of browning reaction prepared from glucose amine. Jpn. J. Nutr. 44:307–315.

Ozgen, M., R. N. Reese, A. Z. Tulio, J. C. Scheerens, and A. R. Miller. 2006. Modified 2, 2- azino-bis-3-ethylbenzothiazoline-6-sulfonic acid (ABTS) method to measure antioxidant capacity of selected small fruits and comparison to ferric reducing antioxidant power (FRAP) and 2, 2'- diphenyl-1-picrylhydrazyl (DPPH) methods. J. Agri. Food Chem. 54:1151–1157.

Pearl, W., T. Balazs, and D. A. Buyske. 1966. The effect of stress on serum transaminase activity in the rat. Life Sci. 5:67–74.

Popovic, M., S. J. Hudomal, B. Kaurinovic, J. Rasic, S. Trivic, and M. Vojnović. 2009. Antioxidant effects of some drugs on immobilization stress combined with cold restraint stress. Molecules 14:4505–4516. doi:10.3390/14114505.

Re, R., N. Pellegrini, A. Proteggente, A. Pannala, M. Yang, and C. Rice-Evans. 1999. Antioxidant activity applying an improved ABTS radical cation decolorization assay. Free Rad. Biol. Med. 26:1231–1237.

Reitman, S., and S. A. Frankel. 1957. Colorimetric method for the determination of serum level of glutamate-oxaloacetate and pyruvate transaminases. Am. J. Clin. Pathol. 28:56–63.

Sadock, B., and V. Sadock. 2003. Synopsis of psychiatry. 9thed. Williams and Wilkins, PA philadelphia.

Stadtman, E. R., and B. S. Berlett. 1998. Reactive oxygenmediated oxidation in aging and disease. Drug Metab. Rev. 30:225–243.

Tappel, A. L. 1978. Glutathione peroxidase and hydroperoxides. Methods Enzymol. 52:506–513.

Thomas, G. G., and E. Lena. 2010. Chronic stress and the HPA axis: clinical assessment and therapeutic considerations. A review of natural and nutraceutical therapies for clinical practice. 9; Article 2. Available at: www.pointinstitute.org/wp-content/uploads/2012/10/standard_v_9.2_hpa_axis.pdf

Weichselbaumin, T. E. 1995. An accurate and rapid method for the determination of protein in small amount of blood serum. Am. J. Clin. Pathol. 16:40.

11

Nutritional, antioxidative, and antimicrobial analysis of the Mediterranean hackberry (*Celtis australis* L.)

Ajda Ota[1], Ana Miklavčič Višnjevec[2], Rajko Vidrih[1], Željko Prgomet[3], Marijan Nečemer[4], Janez Hribar[1], Nina Gunde Cimerman[1,5], Sonja Smole Možina[1], Milena Bučar-Miklavčič[2] & Nataša Poklar Ulrih[1,5]

[1]Biotechnical Faculty, University of Ljubljana, Jamnikarjeva 101, Ljubljana SI-1000, Slovenia
[2]Science and Research Centre of Koper, University of Primorska, Zelena ulica 8, Izola SI-6310, Slovenia
[3]Agricultural Department in Poreč, University of Rijeka, Carla Huguesa 6, Poreč, Croatia
[4]Institute Jožef Stefan, Jamova cesta 39, Ljubljana SI-1000, Slovenia
[5]Centre of Excellence for Integrated Approaches in Chemistry and Biology of Proteins (CIPKeBiP), Jamova cesta 39, Ljubljana SI-1000, Slovenia

Keywords
Antimicrobial activity, *Celtis australis*, nutritional analysis, phenols, triple-quadrupole tandem mass spectrometry, ultrahigh-pressure liquid chromatography

Correspondence
Nataša Poklar Ulrih, Department of Food Science and Technology,Biotechnical Faculty, University of Ljubljana, Jamnikarjeva 101, SI-1000 Ljubljana, Slovenia.
E-mail: natasa.poklar@bf.uni-lj.si

Funding Information
This study was founded by European Regional Development Funds (Rast Istre, SI-HR-3-2-001), the Slovenian Research Agency, and the Slovenian Government Office for Development and European Cohesion Policy.

Abstract

Celtis australis is a deciduous tree commonly known as Mediterranean hackberry or the European nettle tree. The fruit of hackberry are seldom used for nutritional purposes. The nutritional and physicochemical properties of ripe hackberry fruit from Istria (Marasi village near Vrsar, Croatia) were determined, including water, total fiber, protein, vitamin, mineral, and phenolic contents. This analysis demonstrates that the hackberry fruit is a valuable source of dietary fiber, protein, and vitamins, and of pigments such as lutein, β-carotene, zeaxanthin, and tocopherols. The seasonal differences associated with the different growth stages for the element composition, total phenolic content, and phenolic profile were also determined for hackberry mesocarp and leaves. Water and ethanol extracts were prepared from mesocarp and leaves harvested at different growth stages and their phenolic profiles and antioxidant and antimicrobial activities were investigated. This study demonstrates that water and ethanol extracts of hackberry fruit and leaves collected at different growth stages contain epicatechin, gallic acid, vanillic acid, 3,4-dihydroxybenzaldehyde, delphinidin-3,5-di-O-glucoside, cyanidin-3,5-di-O-glucoside, and pelargonidin-3,5-di-O-glucoside. They also show some antimicrobial and antifungal activities. Further studies are needed to identify and define the active ingredients of these hackberry leaf ethanol extracts.

Introduction

Celtis australis L. is known as the Mediterranean hackberry, European nettle tree, or the lote tree, and it grows wild in mild Mediterranean regions (e.g., southern Europe, northern Africa) and in southeast Asia (Baytop 1994). It was initially placed into the *Ulmaceae* family, but was later re-classified into the *Cannabaceae* family (Sytsma et al. 2002). The genus *Celtis* comprises about 70 species that are valued mainly for their wood (Bean 1981); (Chiej 1984); (Facciola 1990). In eastern North America, the hackberry *Celtis occidentalis* prevails, while the more humid soils in central North America are dominated by the shorter sugarberry tree, *Celtis laevigata* (Demır et al. 2002). Although the Mediterranean hackberry grows better in deep moist soils, it can often be found in poor soils among dry rock (Costa et al. 1998).

The fruit of the Mediterranean hackberry ripen in autumn as spherical drupes of 9–12 mm in diameter. These fruits are astringent in taste and contain a single seed that comprises approximately 38% of the fruit dry mass. The fruit has a high sugar content, which has been reported as up to 81.5% (Herrera 1987) and they are considered to be very effective medicinally due to their lenitive and stomachic properties (Chiej 1984; Chevallier 1996). Leaf and fruit preparations have preventive effects in the treatment of amenorrhea, colic, diarrhea, dysentery, peptic ulcers, and menstrual bleeding (Chevallier 1996; Chopra et al. 1986). The leaves of *Celtis australis* contain rare flavonoid C-glycosides, such as acacetin 7-O-glucoside, isovitexin, and cytisoside (Spitaler et al. 2009; Zehrmann et al. 2010; Sommavilla et al. 2012).

A study into the nutritional and physical properties of hackberry fruit was carried out by Demır et al. (2002), who analyzed hackberry fruit for their crude oil, protein, crude fiber, and ash and mineral contents. The aim of this study was to initially determine the crude-fiber, protein and fatty-acid content in hackberry seeds, along with the sugar, vitamin (i.e., carotenes, tocopherols), and total phenol and mineral contents in the mesocarp and leaves of ripe hackberry fruit from Istria (Marasi village near Vrsar, Croatia). Total phenols were determined in water and ethanol extracts of these hackberry fruit. In addition, several phenolic compounds were identified using ultrahigh-pressure liquid chromatography (UHPLC) linked to triple-quadrupole tandem mass spectrometry (QqQ-MS/MS). Also, as plant extracts are considered to be valuable sources of biologically active compounds that have antimicrobial activities, the antibacterial and antifungal activities against selected bacteria and fungi were determined for extracts from hackberry fruit mesocarp and leaves harvested at the different growth stages. To the best of our knowledge, this is the first study that includes determination of the nutritional and physicochemical properties along with the antibacterial and antifungal activities associated with the Mediterranean hackberry.

Materials and Methods

Materials

Chemicals and reagents

Folin-Ciocalteu reagent, 2,2-diphenyl-1-picrylhydrazyl (DPPH), RPMI medium, 2-p-iodophenyl-3-p-nitrophenyl-5-phenyl tetrazolium chloride, gallic acid, lutein, α-carotene, β-carotene, and tocopherol were from Sigma, Germany. Mueller–Hinton broth and Mueller–Hinton Agar were from Oxoid, (Hampshire, UK), and zeaxanthin was from Applichem. Total Dietary Fibre kits (Merck, Darmstadt, Germany) were used for fiber determination. Standard methanol solutions of gallic acid (Sigma), vanillic acid (Fluka Chemika, Buchs, Switzerland), 3,4-dihydroxybenzaldehyde (3,4-dihydroxybenzaldehyde (DHA); Acros Organics), epicatechin (Sigma), delphinin-3,5-di-*O*-glucoside, cyanidin-3,5-di-*O*-glucoside, and pelargonidin-3,5-di-*O*-glucoside (Extrasythese, France) were used for determination of the phenolic compounds All other solvents, buffers, and reagents were analytically pure.

Plant material and extraction procedure

Unripe and ripe mature hackberry fruit and leaves were collected at different growth stages (i.e., end of June, end of October) in Istria (Marasi village near Vrsar, Croatia) and transported on the same day to the laboratory at the Biotechnical Faculty, University of Ljubljana, Slovenia. The fruit was deseeded and samples of mesocarp and seeds were lyophilized. Water and ethanol extracts from mesocarp and dry leaves of hackberry fruit were prepared by extraction of 5 g lyophilised powdered mesocarp and leaves in water and in 70% aqueous ethanol for 4 h. The extracts were centrifuged, dried by rotary evaporation, lyophilized, and kept at −20°C until use.

Methods

Nutritional properties

Nutritional properties of the hackberry fruit mesocarp and seeds were determined according to the AOAC International reference methods (AOAC Official Method, 1997). Soluble solids were measured using a hand refractometer (Atago, Tokyo, Japan). The reducing sugars were determined using the Luff-Schoorl method (Alexander et al. 1985). Total, soluble, and insoluble fibers were determined according to the modified enzymatic–gravimetric method of Prosky, using Total Dietary Fiber kit (Merck, Germany). The analysis was performed according to the manufacturer's instructions. The soluble and insoluble dietary fiber residues minus the ash and crude protein in the residues were taken as the respective dietary fiber fraction. The total dietary fiber was calculated as the sum of the soluble and insoluble dietary fiber.

Mineral element composition

The mineral element compositions of the ripe mesocarp and leaves were analyzed using energy dispersive X-ray fluorescence spectrometry. From 0.5 g to 1.0 g of powdered samples were used to prepare pellets, using a pellet die and a hydraulic press. The disc radioisotope excitation sources of ^{55}Fe (25 mCi) and ^{109}Cd (20 mCi) (Eckert & Ziegler, Berlin, Germany) were used as the primary excitation sources. The emitted fluorescence radiation was measured using an energy dispersive X-ray spectrometer composed of a Si(Li) detector (Canberra), a spectroscopy amplifier (Canberra M2024), an analog-to-digital converter (Canberra M8075), and PC-based multichannel analyzer (S-100, Canberra). The spectrometer was equipped with a vacuum chamber. The energy resolution of the spectrometer was 175 eV at 5.9 keV.

Analysis of the complex X-ray spectra was performed using the AXIL spectral analysis program (Nečemer et al. 2008, 2011);. The evaluated uncertainty of this procedure included the statistical uncertainty of the measured intensities and the uncertainty of the mathematical fitting procedure. The overall uncertainties of the spectral measurements and the analyses were in most cases better than 1%. Quantification was then performed using the quantitative analysis of environmental samples software that was developed in our laboratory (Nečemer et al. 2008, 2011). The estimated uncertainty of the analysis was 5–10%. This relatively high total estimated uncertainty is mainly due to the contributions of the matrix correction and geometry calibration procedures, which included errors in the tabulated fundamental parameters, and also error contributions from the spectrum acquisition and analysis.

Lutein and β-carotene contents

The lutein and β-carotene contents of the ripe hackberry fruit mesocarp were determined according to the method described by (Sircelj and Batic 2007). Here, about 0.1 g lyophilized sample was mixed with 5 mL cold acetone. This mixture was homogenized using an Ultra-Turrax (Janke & Kunkel GmBH & Co., Staufen, Germany) at 20,000 rpm for 20 sec, and centrifuged at 2300 g for 5 min. The supernatant was then filtered through a 0.45 μm filter, and the tocopherol content was determined using high-performance liquid chromatography (HPLC; Spectra-Physics, Santa Clara, CA, USA), with a P4000 pump (SpectraSYSTEM), an AS1000 autosampler (SpectraSYSTEM) and a UV-Vis detector. The samples were injected into a precolumn (Spherisorb ODS2 5U; 5 μm, 50 × 4.6 mm), from where they passed into the main column (Spherisorb ODS2 5U; 5 μm, 250 × 4.6 mm). The injection volume was 20 μL. The mobile phase comprised acetonitrile/ H_2O/ methanol (A; 100:10:5, v/v/v) and acetone/ ethylacetate (B; 2:1, v/v) with a gradient of B in A of 10–75% in 18 min, 75–70% in 7 min, and 70–100% in 5 min. The flow rate was 1 mL/min. The column temperature was 5°C (Mistral tip 880, Spark Holland) and the autosampler temperature was 4°C. The detection wavelength was 440 nm, and the time of the analyses was 30 min. Lutein and β-carotene were identified by comparison of their retention times with those of authentic standards (Sigma). Quantification was based on the external standard method.

Tocopherols contents

The extraction procedure for the tocopherols was the same as that described for lutein and β-carotene, and the tocopherols contents were determined according to the method described by Wildi and Lutz (1996), using fluorescence detection after chromatography. The same HPLC system was used as that for the determination of lutein and β-carotene (i.e., Spectra-Physics HPLC system), and the parameters used were the same, except that the mobile phase was methanol, the column temperature was 20°C, and the detection used an excitation wavelength of 295 nm and an emission wavelength of 325 nm. The tocopherols were identified by comparisons of their retention times with those of authentic standards (Sigma). The quantification was based on the external standard method.

Fatty-acid composition

The fatty acids were determined as their methyl esters after transesterification, according to AOAC Official Method, (1997), using gas chromatography (HP 5890, series II; Hewlett Packard Corp., Palo Alto) equipped with a fused-silica capillary column (SP2380; Supelco; 30 m × 0.25 mm; film thickness, 0.20 μm). The stationary phase was poly(biscyanopropyl/ cyanopropylphenyl siloxane) (9:1, v/v). The carrier gas was helium, at a flow rate of 1 cm^3/min. The internal standard was heptadecanoic acid. The column temperature was set for 150–210°C at 5°C/min. The injector and flame-ionization detector temperatures were set at 220°C and 250°C, respectively. The injection volume was 1 μL. Identification was achieved by comparison of the retention times for the fatty acid methyl esters (FAMEs) of the investigated oil samples with the retention times of FAME standards (FAME Mix rapeseed oil). The data are given as weight percentages of the total fatty acids. The analyses were carried out in duplicate. The standard errors of determination were between 0.01% and 0.25%.

Total phenolics

The total content of phenolic compounds in the mesocarp and leaf extracts of *C. australis* were determined spectrophotometrically (Waterman and Mole 1994). An appropriately diluted extract or gallic acid (as the calibration standard) was mixed with freshly prepared Folin-Ciocalteau reagent, sodium carbonate solution (20%, w/v), and Milli-Q water. After 40 min, the total phenolic compounds in the extracts of the mesocarp and leaves were determined at 765 nm. The total amounts of phenolic compounds are expressed per gram gallic acid. The analyses were conducted in triplicate, with the data given as means ± SEM.

Identification of phenolics by *UHPLC–QqQ-MS/MS*

For the identification of the phenolic compounds, the freeze dried extracts were reconstituted with ultrapure water (Milli-Q) and ethanol. The phenolic compounds were identified and determined, using UHPLC interfaced to QqQ-MS/MS, on an HPLC system (Agilent 1260) equipped with a degasser (model G4225A), a binary gradient pump (model G1312A,) a thermoautosampler (model G1329B), a column oven (model G1316A), a diode array detection system (model G4212B), and a Poroshell 120 column (EC-C18; 2.7 μm; 3.0 × 50 mm). Elution was with a gradient of water/ formic acid (99.5:0.5; v/v) (A) and acetonitryl /methanol (50:50; v/v) (B) as follows: 0 min, 96% A/ 4% B; 3.96 min, 50% A/ 50% B; 4.45 min, 40% A/ 60% B; 5.94 min, 0% A/ 100% B, which was held until completion at 7.13 min. In addition, a further HPLC column was used (Ascentis; 2.7 μm; 15 cm × 4.6 mm) with a gradient of water/ formic acid (99.5:0.5; v/v) (A) and acetonitryl/ methanol (50:50; v/v) (B) that was adjusted properly according to the retention time. The flow was 0.2 mL/min, and the sample injection volume was 1 μL. The HPLC system was connected in series with a triple quadrupole mass spectrometer (6420; Agilent Technology, Santa Clara, CA, USA). The standard phenolic compounds were dissolved in methanol and infused, to optimize the acquisition parameters. The MS and MS/MS spectra of the compounds under investigation were acquired using the following optimized conditions: fragmentor voltage, 80–220 V; collision energy, 15–45 eV; capillary voltage, 4.0 kV; cell acceleration voltage, 7 V; sheath gas temperature, 400°C; cone gas flow, 10 L/min; desolvation gas flow, 12 L/min; and collision gas, nitrogen. For multiple reactions, monitoring (MRM) of the individual compounds, the positive ion (anthocyanins, system I) and negative ion (nonanthocyanin phenolic compounds, system II) modes were selected for the first quadrupole, and the collision energies were adjusted to optimize the signal for the most abundant product ions. The limit of detection (LOD) of the method was 0.04 μg/100 g sample for epicatechin, 0.002 μg/100 g sample for gallic acid, 0.001 μg/100 g sample for vanillic acid, 0.04 μg/100 g sample for 3,4-DHA, and 2 μg/100 g sample for delphinidin-3,5-di-O-glucoside, cyanidin-3,5-di-O-glucoside, and pelargonidin-3,5-di-O-glucoside. The determined levels of delphinidin-3,5-di-O-glucoside, cyanidin-3,5-di-O-glucoside and pelargonidin-3,5-di-O-glucoside were calculated on the basis of calibration curves constructed using their respective chlorides.

Antioxidant activity

The antioxidant activities of the ethanol and water extracts of the hackberry mesocarp and leaves from different growth stages were determined spectrophotometrically, using the DPPH reagent, 2,2-diphenyl-1-picryl-hydrazyl (Brand-Williams et al. 1995). The analyses were performed in triplicate for each extract.

Antibacterial activity

The antibacterial activities of the ethanol and water extracts of the hackberry mesocarp and leaves from different growth stages were tested against a panel of pathogenic microorganisms, including Gram-positive *Staphylococcus aureus* ATCC 25923 and *Listeria monocytogenes* ŽMJ58a, and Gram-negative *Escherichia coli* O157:H7 ŽMJ370 and *Pseudomonas aeruginosa* ŽMJ87 (all clinical isolates). The cultivation/ assay media were Mueller–Hinton broth or Mueller–Hinton agar (Oxoid, Hampshire, UK). The minimum inhibitory concentrations (MICs) for the extracts were determined using the broth microdilution method, as previously described (Klančnik et al. 2010). Briefly, 50 μL of each bacterial suspension in suitable growth medium was added to the wells of a sterile 96-well microtiter plate that already contained 50 μL of twofold serially diluted plant extracts in the relevant growth medium. The final volume in each well was 100 μL. Control wells were prepared with culture medium, bacterial suspension only, plant extracts only, and ethanol at the concentration corresponding to the highest concentration present. The MICs were the lowest concentrations where no viability was observed after 24 h on the basis of the metabolic activity. To indicate respiratory activity, the presence of color was determined after addition of 10 μL/well 2 mg/mL 2-p-iodophenyl-3-p-nitrophenyl-5-phenyl tetrazolium chloride (Sigma) dissolved in water, and an incubation under the appropriate cultivation conditions for 30 min in the dark (Klančnik et al. 2010). All of the measurements of the MICs were carried out in duplicate.

Antifungal activity

The antifungal activities of only the ethanol extracts of the hackberry mesocarp and leaves were tested against eight ubiquitous opportunistic pathogenic fungi: *Saprochaaete clavata* EX 5631, *Candida albicans* EX 9382, *Candida papapsilosis* EX 9370, *Aureobasidium pullulans* EX 3105, *Aspergillus fumigatus* EX 8280, *Fusarium dimerum* EX 9214, *Exophiala dermatitidis* EX 5586, and *Rhodotorula mucilaginosa* EX 9762, as the most frequent fungal colonizers of dishwashers (Zalar et al. 2011; (Gümral et al. 2015) and washing machines (Babič et al. 2015) around the world. All of the fungal cultures are deposited in the Ex Culture Collection of Extremophilic Fungi, as part of the Infrastructural Centre Mycosmo (MRICUL) at the Department of Biology, Biotechnical Faculty, University of Ljubljana, Slovenia. The tests were carried out according to the M27-A3 and M38-A2 reference methods for broth dilution antifungal susceptibility testing of yeast (CLSI 2008a) and filamentous fungi (CLSI 2008b), respectively. For the broth microdilution test, 50 μL of each inoculum suspension with final cell counts of approximately 10^4 cells/mL in RPMI medium was added to the wells of a sterile 96-well microtiter plate that already contained 50 μL twofold serially diluted plant extracts in the relevant growth medium. The final volume in each well was 100 μL. The MICs were determined after 48 h incubation at 30°C. The MICs of the antifungal agents are defined as the lowest concentrations that inhibited visible fungal growth. All of the measurements of the MICs were carried out in duplicate.

Results and Discussion

Nutritional properties of hackberry fruit

The nutritional properties of hackberry fruit are given in Tables 1 and 2. The data for water, soluble solids, and reducing sugars in the air-driedmesocarp, and for total fat in the air-dried seeds are given in Table 1. The mesocarp of the ripe hackberries contained 30.0% water, while that of the seeds was 18.1% in the air-dried samples (Table 1). The fruit contained 3.4 g/100 g protein and 10.2% total dietary fiber, 8.2% insoluble fiber, and 2.0% soluble fiber. According to Demır et al. (2002), the mesocarp contains 90.2% dry matter, which is higher than that determined in the present study. The difference in the water contents is probably due to loss of water prior to harvest.

Table 1. Water, soluble solids, and reducing sugars in air-dried mesocarp and total fat in air-dried seeds.

Analysis	Mesocarp	Seeds
Water (%)	30.0 ± 1.2	18.1 ± 0.98
Soluble solids (%Brix)	53.4 ± 0.1	–[1]
Reducing sugars (g/100 g fw)	50.9 ± 0.19	–
Total fat (g/ 100 g dw)	–	8.1 ± 1.0

Data are means ± SD.
fw, fresh weight, dw, dry weight.
[1]not measured.

Table 2. Mineral content in hackberry fruit mesocarp and leaves.

	Mesocarp (mg/100 g dw)	Leaves (mg/100 g dw)	
Element	October	June	October
Si	ND	1280 ± 135	2570 ± 162
P	143 ± 2	141 ± 1	131 ± 18
S	20.8 ± 3.2	102 ± 17	84 ± 8
Cl	71 ± 4.9	240 ± 24	343 ± 21
K	1060 ± 64	834 ± 75	975 ± 59
Ca	269 ± 16	5970 ± 537	5590 ± 339
Mn	1.2 ± 0.01	6.0 ± 0.54	11.8 ± 3.0
Fe	5.1 ± 0.4	11.4 ± 0.6	17.8 ± 2.6
Ni	0.25 ± 0.09	0.24 ± 0.09	1.72 ± 0.75
Cu	0.45 ± 0.06	1.09 ± 0.09	2.01 ± 0.47
Zn	0.35 ± 0.07	0.79 ± 0.08	1.03 ± 0.01
Se	0.09 ± 0.01	0.08 ± 0.01	0.34 ± 0.01
Pb	0.07 ± 0.03	0.16 ± 0.03	0.70 ± 0.25
Br	0.69 ± 0.04	0.96 ± 0.05	2.01 ± 0.18
Rb	1.04 ± 0.09	0.32 ± 0.04	0.56 ± 0.18
Sr	0.50 ± 0.03	6.00 ± 0.26	5.92 ± 0.30
Mo	0.04 ± 0.01	0.04 ± 0.01	0.17 ± 0.01

Data are means (n = 2) ± SD.
ND, not detected.

Table 2 gives the mineral contents in the mesocarp of ripe hackberry and the leaves collected during the different growth stages (i.e., end of June, end of October), expressed per 100 g dry weight. Among the minerals, K was at the highest concentration in mesocarp, followed by Ca and P. In the leaves collected at the same time, the Ca content (5.59 g/100 g) reached more than fivefold that of K. The major difference between the leaves collected at the different growth stages at the end of June and the end of October was seen for Si, the content of which increased twofold over this 4-month period.

For the microelements in mesocarp, Fe was the major microelement at 5.05 mg/100 g, followed by Mn (1.20 mg/100 g) and Rb (1.04 mg/100 g), and slightly lower concentrations for Br (0.69 mg/100 g), Cu (0.45 mg/100 g) and Zn (0.35 mg/100 g) (Table 2). Only one literature source was found regarding mineral contents (Demır et al. 2002). These samples of Demır et al.(2002) contained threefold more K, slightly more P, and one-sixteenth of the Ca levels. With regard to the microelements also determined by Demır et al. (2002); our samples contained similar amounts of Zn, slightly more Pb, Cu, and Ni, and twice as much Fe and Mn. The mineral contents of fruit depend on genetic factors and pedoclimatic conditions. The hackberry trees from which the fruit was harvested in the present study were growing wild, with no agricultural practices applied. We hypothesize that the main reason for the differences observed between this study and the study of Demır et al. (2002) lies in the different pedoclimatic conditions, although no mineral analyses of the soils were carried out in either case. The reason for the much higher content of Na in the fruit in this study might be the proximity of the sea. In comparison to mesocarp, leaves contained more than 20-fold more Ca (5.97 g/100 g), with this as the predominant element, followed by Si, which was not detected in the mesocarp, and K. The element compositions of leaves changed depending on the growth stage. The major difference that was observed was the increase in Si levels from 1.28 g/100 g to 2.57 g/100 g from the end of June to the end of October.

Regarding the pigments and tocopherols in the mesocarp of the ripe hackberry fruit, among the carotenoids, β-carotene was the most abundant (5.58 μg/g), followed by lutein (1.41 μg/g) and zeaxanthin (0.74 μg/g). The mesocarp of hackberry fruit also contained α-, γ- and δ-tocopherols. Here, α-tocopherol was the most abundant among the tocopherols, at 150.13 μg/g dry matter (dm), while γ-tocopherol and δ-tocopherol were at 4.9 μg/g dm and 2.8 μg/g dm, respectively. For the pigments, hackberry contained 3.7 μg/g dm chlorophyll a. In the literature, there appears to be the single report for carotenoids of 7.5 μg/g in hackberry fruit (Boudraa et al. 2010), which is higher in comparison to values for β-carotene determined in the present study.

Regarding the fatty acid composition, the seeds of these hackberry fruit contained mainly linoleic acid, at 5.109 g/100 g seeds, which represented 76.25% of all of the fatty acids. The remaining main fatty acids were oleic acid (0.951 g/100 g seeds; 14.18%), palmitic acid (0.452 g/100 g seeds; 6.72%), and stearic acid (0.188 g/100 g seeds; 2.81%). No data for the fatty acid composition of hackberry seeds were found in the literature.

The visual and textural appearance of the hackberry mesocarp resembles that of dried dates and dried figs. When the chemical composition of hackberry fruit determined here was compared to a previous study on fig, these hackberries contained similar amounts of total fibre and protein, but fivefold greater amont of β-carotene (Saxholt et al. 2008);. Hackberry also contained a similar mineral chemical composition to figs, in particular with respect to K, Ca, and P (Saxholt et al. 2008).

Total phenolic compounds

When the water extracts were examined, for the ripe mesocarp they contained 0.27 g/100 g total phenols (as gallic acid equivalents), and for unripe mesocarp they contained 0.05 g/100 g total phenols. The total phenols determined in the ethanol extract of ripe mesocarp gave 0.24 g/100 g total phenols, while that for the unripe mesocarp contained 0.10 g/100 g total phenols. Compared to dates (*Phoenix dacttyfera* L.), the present analyses of ripe hackberry mesocarp showed comparable total phenols (Saafi et al. 2009).

Contrary to literature data (Sommavilla et al. 2012), seasonal differences were observed for total phenolics content between leaves harvested at the different growth stages at the end of June and at the end of October. Water extracts contained higher amounts of total phenols in the ripe mesocarp (i.e., end of October; 0.27 g/100 g), while this was lower in the unripe mesocarp (i.e., end of June; 0.05 g/100 g). The water extracts of leaves collected at the end of October also contained more than twofold higher concentrations of phenols (0.17 g/100 g) than leaves harvested at the end of June (0.08 g/100 g). The total phenols content in the water extract of leaves was comparable to that reported for *Ficus carica* leaves (Konyalıoğlu et al. 2005. The total amount of phenols determined in the ethanol extract of leaves collected at the end of June was 0.07 g/100 g total phenols, while their concentration increased 10-fold (to 0.89 g/100 g) by the end of October.

In addition to their function as antioxidants, the phenolic compounds act as screening agents against effects of UV-B radiation and water deficit, which potentially explains the increased phenolics contents in mesocarp and leaves harvested at the end of October (Grace 2005; Petridis et al. 2012).

The individual phenolic compounds identified in the water and ethanol extracts obtained from mesocarp and leaves (Fig. 1) harvested at different growth stages are presented in Table 3. The levels of these phenolic compounds were generally lower in the water extracts compared to the ethanol extracts. The predominant phenolic compound in the present study was in the ethanol extracts of mesocarp of both unripe and ripe hackberry fruit, which was cyanidin-3,5-di-O-glucoside; this was followed by pelargonidin-3,5-di-O-glucoside and 3,5 DHA, with a ripe mesocarp containing at least 10-fold more than the unripe mesocarp. Pelargonidin-3,5-di-O-glucoside, cyanidin-3,5-di-O-glucoside, 3,5 DHA, vanillic acid, and epicatechin were detected in the ethanol extract of leaves harvested in June. Over the next 4 months to the October sampling, the levels of epicatechin increased 100-fold, while those of cyanidin-3,5-di-O-glucoside and vanillic acid almost doubled. However, more data need to be collected to confirm these seasonal variations in the phenolic compounds determined here. Previously acacetin 7-O-glucoside, isovitexin, and cytisoside were isolated from leaves of hackberry (Spitaler et al. 2009) although there are no data available for seasonal variations of pelargonidin-3,5-di-O-glucoside, cyanidin-3,5-di-O-glucoside, 3,5 DHA, vanillic acid, and epicatechin. The overall increases in the phenols during this 4-month period will contribute to the protective effects of certain phenolic compounds against damage from UV-B radiation and water deficit (Grace 2005; Petridis et al. 2012). Nevertheless, it should be noted that we have here defined only a few of the phenolic compounds that are present in the Mediterranean hackberry. Therefore, more phenolic compounds need to be identified and their levels determined.

Antioxidative potential

As seen from Figure 2, the highest antioxidative potential (given as gallic acid equivalents) of mesocarp was in the water extract, followed by the ethanol extract, as also observed by Zehrmann et al. (2010). For the leaves, the

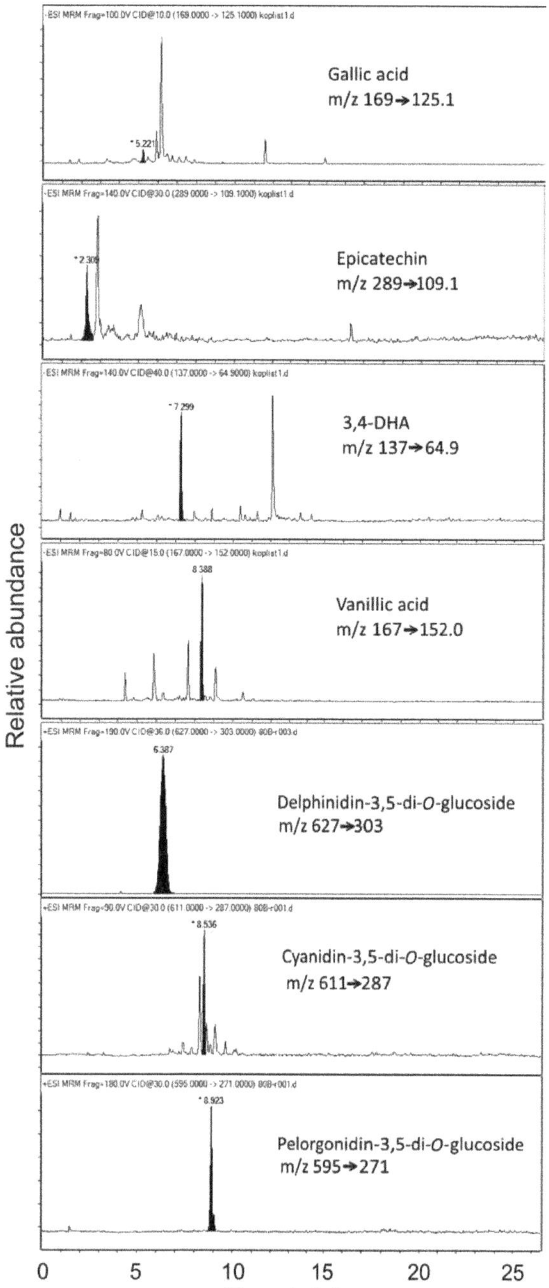

Figure 1. Representative chromatograms (as indicated) from combined ultrahigh-pressure liquid chromatography and triple-quadrupole tandem mass spectrometry of phenols in *Celtis australis*.

ethanol extract harvested at the end of October contained 50-fold the level of antioxidants than the leaves harvested at the end of June. This is consistent with the significantly increased levels of epicatechin (100-fold), which shows a positive and high correlation with antioxidant capacity (Othman et al. 2010), and the doubled levels of cyanidin-3,5-di-O-glucoside and vanillic acid found.

Antibacterial activity

Antibacterial activity tests were performed with the water and ethanol extracts of hackberry mesocarp and leaves collected at the different growth stages. The antimicrobial activities were measured against two Gram-positive bacteria, *Staphylococcus aureus* and *Listeria monocytogenes*, and two Gram-negative bacteria, *Pseudomonas aeruginosa* and *Escherichia coli* O157:H7. These data are given in Table 4.

The extracts prepared from the hackberry mesocarp and leaves harvested at the end of October showed low antibacterial activities, while those harvested earlier (i.e., in June) showed weaker, or in the case of the hackberry mesocarp, no antibacterial activity against these bacterial species. As previously described bySowkat et al. (2012), the water extract from leaves had a higher antibacterial activity against *S. aureus*, compared to *P. aeruginosa*. This was confirmed also in the present study with leaves collected in October; in addition, comparable activities were also found for the fruit mesocarp (Table 4). Badoni et al. (2010) also studied the antimicrobial activities of crude extracts from hackberry fruit and reported antibacterial activities against *S. aureus*, *B. subtilis*, *P. aeruginosa*, and *E. coli*. Although different extraction solvents were used and lower MICs were determined, the growth of *S. aureus* was again inhibited at lower concentrations than for *P. aeruginosa*. Indeed, the different methods of extraction and solvents used will be one of the reasons for the differences in these MICs. These data are comparable to the antibacterial activities of *Ficus carica* leaves, where weak antibacterial activity was shown against *E. coli* and *S. aureus* (*Jeong* et al. 2009).

Antifungal activity

The most frequent fungal colonizers of both dishwashers and washing machines were selected to determine the antifungal activities of the ethanol extracts of mesocarp and leaves. These were *Saprochaaete clavata* EX 5631, *Candida albicans* EX 9382, *Candida papapsilosis* EX 9370, *Aureobasidium pullulans* EX 3105, *Aspergillus fumigatus* EX 8280, *Fusarium dimerum* EX 9214, *Exophiala dermatitidis* EX 5586, and *Rhodotorula mucilaginosa* EX 9762.

While the mesocarp ethanol extract showed no antifungal activities, extracts prepared from leaves harvested at the end of October inhibited the growth of *C. albicans*, *C. parapsilosis* (MICs, 0.156 mg/mL), and *R. mucilaginosa* (MIC, 0.313 mg/mL), although the growth of other tested fungi was not inhibited. These data can be explained by the significantly higher (i.e., 10-fold) amounts of phenols in the ethanol extract of leaves. This is of particular importance as over the last 30 years the fungi in indoor environments have increasingly been recognized as a potential

Table 3. Total and individual phenolic compounds in the water and ethanol extracts from mesocarp and leaves harvested at the different growth stages.

Extract	Compound	Mesocarp (mg/100 g fw)		Leaves (mg/100 g fw)	
		June	October	June	October
Water	Epicatechin	<LOD	<LOD	<LOD	<LOD
	Gallic acid	<LOD	0.114 ± 0.020	0.013 ± 0.003	<LOD
	Vanillic acid	<LOD	<LOD	<LOD	<LOD
	3,5-Dihydroxybenzaldehyde	<LOD	<LOD	<LOD	<LOD
	Delphinidin-3,5-di-O-glucoside	<LOD	0.016 ± 0.001	<LOD	0.004 ± 0.000
	Cyanidin-3,5-di-O-glucoside	<LOD	<LOD	<LOD	0.003 ± 0.001
	Pelargonidin-3,5-di-O-glucoside	<LOD	0.018 ± 0.001	<LOD	0.007 ± 0.001
	Total phenolics	53.3 ± 0.4	274.4 ± 9.2	76.1 ± 0.9	168.3 ± 1.4
Ethanol	Epicatechin	<LOD	<LOD	0.133 ± 0.014	13.522 ± 0.655
	Gallic acid	<LOD	<LOD	<LOD	<LOD
	Vanillic acid	<LOD	<LOD	0.463 ± <LOD	0.784 ± 0.008
	3,5-Dihydroxybenzaldehyde	0.373 ± 0.023	3.480 ± 0.030	1.183 ± 0. 024	1.011 ± 0.062
	Delphinidin-3,5-di-O-glucoside	<LOD	<LOD	<LOD	<LOD
	Cyanidin-3,5-di-O-glucoside	0.004 ± 0.001	0.051 ± 0.001	0.005 ± 0.001	0.011 ± 0.0010
	Pelargonidin-3,5-di-O-glucoside	0.002 ± 0.001	0.033 ± 0.001	0.007 ± 0.001	0.007 ± 0.001
	Total phenolics	101.6 ± 1.4	239.1 ± 3.2	74.1 ± 1.9	894.2 ± 21.2

Data are means ± SD.
fw, fresh weight; LOD, limit of detection.

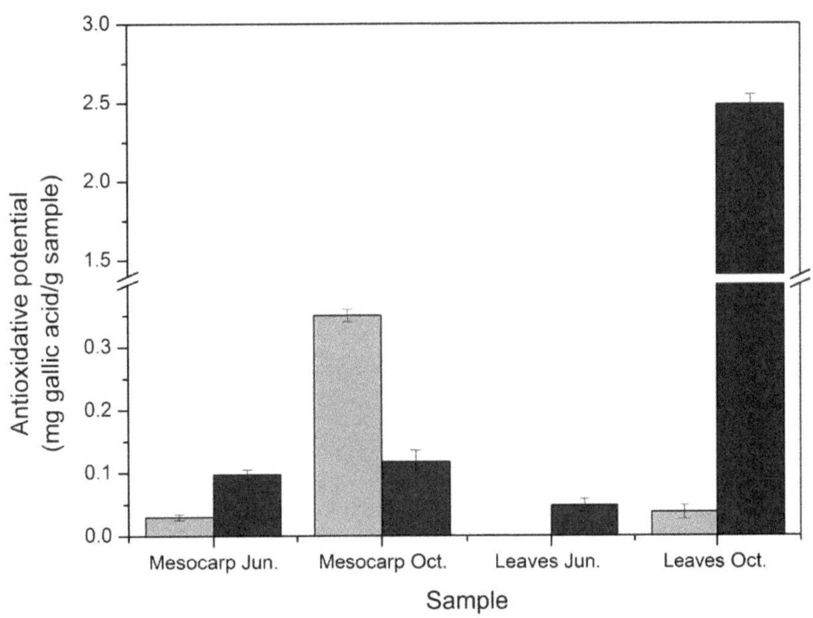

Figure 2. Influence of water (light gray) and 70% ethanol (dark gray) as the extraction medium on the antioxidative potential of hackberry mesocarp and leaves extracts collected at different growth stages.

health problem, which is linked to the growingly immunocompromised population (de Vos et al. 2009; (Neofytos et al. 2007). Conditions inside household appliances were originally considered to be prohibitive for fungal growth; however, novel energy-saving trends have led to the use of these appliances at lower temperatures and with biodegradable detergents. These conditions have thus become selective for thermo tolerant, oxidative stress resistant, and generally stress-tolerant fungi, many of which are opportunistic human pathogens (Gostinčar et al. 2011). In the light of the small number of appropriate antifungal agents, and as both *R. mucilaginosa* and *C. parapsilosis* have been reported to be new emerging pathogens that can cause primarily catheter-related infections and opportunistic

Table 4. Antibacterial activities of water and ethanol extracts of hackeberry mesocarp and leaves collected at the different growth stages.

	Minimum inhibitory concentrations (mg/mL)							
	Water extract				Ethanol extract			
	Mesocarp		Leaves		Mesocarp		Leaves	
Bacterium	June	October	June	October	June	October	June	October
Escherichia coli	>10	5	5	2.5	>10	5	2.5	5
Listeria monocytogenes	>10	>10	>10	10	>10	5	>10	5
Pseudomonas aeruginosa	>10	>10	>10	>10	>10	2.5	>10	>10
Staphylococcus aureus	>10	5	>10	5	>10	1.25	>10	1.25

nosocomial fungemia in immunocompromised patients (Neofytos et al. 2007; Pfaller et al. 2007; van Asbeck et al. 2009; Miceli et al. 2011), these data show promise for the development of new types of biodegradable detergents based on plant extracts.

Conclusions

Celtis australis L. has to date been valued mainly for its wood. Hackberry fruit are thus small, and they have a relatively large stone, with the consequent low yield of mesocarp. These fruits are seldom consumed fresh, although sometimes they are used to produce liqueurs by mixing them with fruit brandy. Sensory properties and mineral composition of hackberry fruits are also similar to that of figs.

Our data show that these fruits are interesting from the nutritional point of view, as they contain dietary fiber, phenols, vitamins (tocopherols, carotenoids), and minerals. The amounts of total fiber and protein are comparable to those observed for figs.

The antioxidant activities of the water and ethanol extracts studied here increased with the amounts of total phenols that they contained. This study revealed the presence of epicatechin, gallic acid, vanillic acid, 3,5 DHA, delphinin-3,5-di-*O*-glucoside, cyanidin-3,5-di-*O*-glucoside, and pelargonidin-3,5-di-*O*-glucoside in these extracts. As the concentrations of these phenols varied according to the growth stage, the knowledge gained here can be applied to determine the optimal harvest time to maximize the yields of such bio-active phenolics. Additionally, these fruits are a rich source of water-soluble polyphenolic compounds, which are here identified, and some publications have indicated that leaves of *C. australis* contain the rare flavonoid C-glycosides, such as acacetin 7-O-glucoside, isovitexin, and cytisoside.

Antimicrobial and, in particular, antifungal activities were also detected for the ethanol extracts prepared here from hackberry leaves, against the most important fungal opportunistic pathogen *C. albicans*, and against two emerging opportunistic pathogenic yeast *C. parapsilosis* and *R. mucilaginosa*. Further studies are thus needed to identify and define the active ingredients of these hackberry leaf ethanol extracts.

Acknowledgments

This study was founded by European Regional Development Funds (Rast Istre, SI-HR-3-2-001), the Slovenian Research Agency, and the Slovenian Government Office for Development and European Cohesion Policy.

Conflict of Interest

The authors declare that they have no conflicts of interest.

References

Alexander, R. R., J. Griffiths, and M. Wilkinson. 1985. Basic Biochemical methods. John Wiley & Sons, New York.

AOAC Official Method. 1997. Official methods of analysis. 16th ed. AOAC International, Gaithersburg.

van Asbeck, E. C., K. V. Clemons, and D. A. Stevens. 2009. *Candida parapsilosis*: a review of its epidemiology, pathogenesis, clinical aspects, typing and antimicrobial susceptibility. Crit. Rev. Microbiol. 35:283–309.

Babič, M. N., P. Zalar, B. Ženko, H.-J. Schroers, S. Džeroski, and N. Gunde-Cimerman. 2015. *Candida* and *Fusarium* species known as opportunistic human pathogens from customer-accessible parts of residential washing machines. Fungal Biol. 119:95–113.

Badoni, R., D. K. Semwal, and U. Rawat. 2010. Fatty acid composition and antimicrobial activity of *Celtis australis* L Fruits. J Sci Res 2:397–402.

Baytop, T. 1994. Türkçe Bitki Adlari Sözlügü [A Dictionary of Vernacular Names of Wild Plants of Turkey], No. 578. The Turkish Language Society, Ankara.

Bean, W. 1981. Trees and shrubs hardy in the British Isles. Vol. 1. A-C. John Murray, London.

Boudraa, S., L. Hambaba, S. Zidani, and H. Boudraa. 2010. Composition minérale et vitaminique des fruits de cinq espèces sous exploitées en Algérie: *Celtis australis* L., *Crataegus azarolus* L., *Crataegus monogyna* Jacq., *Elaeagnus angustifolia* L. et *Zizyphus lotus* L. Fruits 65:75–84.

Brand-Williams, W., M. E. Cuvelier, and C. Berset. 1995. Use of a free radical method to evaluate antioxidant activity. LWT - Food Sci. Technol. 28:25–30.

Chevallier, A. 1996. The encyclopedia of medicinal plants: a practical reference guide to over 550 key herbs and their medicinal uses. Dorling Kindersley, London.

Chiej, R. 1984. Encyclopaedia of medicinal plants (Macdonald encyclopedias). Brown, Little, Edinburgh.

Chopra, R. N., S. L. Nayar, and I. C. Chopra. 1986. Glossary of Indian medicinal plants. Council of Scientific and Industrial Research, New Delhi.

CLSI. 2008a. CLSI reference method for broth dilution antifungal susceptibility testing of yeasts approved standard CLSI document M27-A3. 3rd ed. Clinical and Laboratory Standards Institute, Wayne, PA.

CLSI. 2008b. CLSI Reference method for broth dilution antifungal susceptibility testing of filamentous fungi approved standard CLSI document M38-A2. 2nd ed. Clinical and Laboratory Standards Institute, Wayne, PA.

Costa, M., C. Morla, and H. Sainz, eds. 1998. Los bosques Ibéricos. Editorial Planeta, Barcelona.

Demır, F., H. Doğan, M. Özcan, and H. Haciseferoğullari. 2002. Nutritional and physical properties of hackberry (*Celtis australis* L.). J. Food Eng. 54:241–247.

Facciola, S. 1990. Cornucopia: a source book of edible plants. Kampong Publications, Vista.

Gostinčar, C., M. Grube, and N. Gunde-Cimerman. 2011. Evolution of fungal pathogens in domestic environments? Fungal Biol. 115:1008–1018.

Grace, S. C. 2005. Phenolics as Antioxidants. Pp. 141–168 *in* N. Smirnoff, ed. Antioxidants and reactive oxygen species in plants. Oxford, Blackwell Publishing Ltd.

Gümral, R., B. Özhak-Baysan, A. Tümgör, et al. 2015. Dishwashers provide a selective extreme environment for human-opportunistic yeast-like fungi. Fungal Divers. 76:1–9. doi:10.1007/s13225-015-0327-8.

Herrera, C. M. 1987. Vertebrate-dispersed plants of the Iberian Peninsula: a study of fruit characteristics. Ecol. Monogr. 57:305. doi:10.2307/2937089.

Jeong, M. R., H. Y. Kim, and J. D. Cha. 2009. Antimicrobial activity of methanol extract from *Ficus carica* leaves against oral bacteria. J. Bacteriol. Virol. 39:97–102.

Klančnik, A., S. Piskernik, B. Jeršek, and S. S. Možina. 2010. Evaluation of diffusion and dilution methods to determine the antibacterial activity of plant extracts. J. Microbiol. Methods 81:121–126.

Konyalıoğlu, S., H. Sağlam, and B. Kıvçak. 2005. α-Tocopherol, flavonoid, and phenol contents and antioxidant activity of *Ficus carica* leaves. Pharm. Biol. 43:683–686.

Miceli, M. H., J. A. Díaz, and S. A. Lee. 2011. Emerging opportunistic yeast infections. Lancet Infect. Dis. 11:142–151.

Nečemer, M., P. Kump, J. Ščančar, et al. 2008. Application of X-ray fluorescence analytical techniques in phytoremediation and plant biology studies. Spectrochim. Acta Part B At. Spectrosc. 63:1240–1247.

Nečemer, M., P. Kump, and K. Vogel-Mikuš. 2011. Use of X-ray fluorescence-based analytical techniques in phytoremediation. Pp. 331–358 *in* I. A. Golubev, ed. Handbook of phytoremediation. New York, Nova Science Publishers Inc.

Neofytos, D., D. Horn, and J. A. De Simone Jr. 2007. *Rhodotorula mucilaginosa* catheter-related fungemia in a patient with sickle cell disease: case presentation and literature review. South. Med. J. 100:198–200.

Othman, A., A. M. M. Jalil, K. K. Weng, A. Ismail, N. Abd Ghani, and I. Adenan. 2010. Epicatechin content and antioxidant capacity of cocoa beans from four different countries. Afr. J. Biotechnol. 9:1052–1059.

Petridis, A., I. Therios, G. Samouris, et al. 2012. Effect of water deficit on leaf phenolic composition, gas exchange, oxidative damage and antioxidant activity of four Greek olive (*Olea europaea* L.) cultivars. Plant Physiol. Biochem. 60:1–11.

Pfaller, M. A., D. J. Diekema, D. L. Gibbs, et al. 2007. Results from the ARTEMIS disk global antifungal surveillance Study, 1997 to 2005: an 8.5-year analysis of susceptibilities of Candida species and other yeast species to *Fluconazole* and *Voriconazole* determined by CLSI standardized disk diffusion testing. J. Clin. Microbiol. 45:1735–1745.

Saafi, E. B., Arem A. El, M. Issaoui, M. Hammami, and L. Achour. 2009. Phenolic content and antioxidant activity of four date palm (*Phoenix dactylifera* L.) fruit varieties grown in Tunisia. Int. J. Food Sci. Technol. 44:2314–2319.

Saxholt, E., A. T. Christensen, A. Møller, H. B. Hartkopp, K. Hess Ygil, and O Hels. 2008. Danish food composition databank, revision 7. Technical University of Denmark, National Food Institute.

Sircelj, H., and F. Batic.2007. Evaluation of selected nutritional factors in *Aposeris foetida* (L.) Less. during the harvesting period. J. Appl. Bot. Food Qual. 81:121–125.

Sommavilla, V., D. Haidacher-Gasser, M. Sgarbossa, and C. Zidorn. 2012. Seasonal variation in phenolics in leaves of *Celtis australis* (Cannabaceae). Biochem. Syst. Ecol. 41:110–114.

Sowkat, A., S. Rejendra, M. Surabhi, and G. Ankur. 2012. Antibacterial activity of *Celtis australis* by in vitro study. Int. J. Pharm. Sci. 4:629–631.

Spitaler, R., S. Gurschler, E. Ellmerer, B. Schubert, M. Sgarbossa, and C. Zidorn. 2009. Flavonoids from *Celtis australis* (Cannabaceae). Biochem. Syst. Ecol. 37:120–121.

Sytsma, K. J., J. Morawetz, J. C. Pires, M. Nepokroeff, E. Conti, M. Zjhra, et al. 2002. Urticalean rosids: circumscription, rosid ancestry, and phylogenetics based on rbcL, trnL-F, and ndhF sequences. Am. J. Bot. 89:1531–1546.

de Vos, P., M. Bucko, P. Gemeiner, et al. 2009. Multiscale requirements for bioencapsulation in medicine and biotechnology. Biomaterials 30:2559–2570.

Waterman, P. G., and S. Mole. 1994. Analysis of phenolic plant metabolites. Blackwell Scientific Publications, Oxford.

Wildi, B., and C. Lutz. 1996. Antioxidant composition of selected high alpine plant species from different altitudes. Plant, Cell Environ. 19:138–146.

Zalar, P., M. Novak, G. S. de Hoog, and N. Gunde-Cimerman. 2011. Dishwashers-a man-made ecological niche accommodating human opportunistic fungal pathogens. Fungal Biol. 115:997–1007.

Zehrmann, N., C. Zidorn, and M. Ganzera. 2010. Analysis of rare flavonoid C-glycosides in *Celtis australis* L. by micellar electrokinetic chromatography. J. Pharm. Biomed. Anal. 51:1165–1168.

12

Prevention of microbial hazard on fresh-cut lettuce through adoption of food safety and hygienic practices by lettuce farmers

Lateefah A. Oyinlola[1], Adewale O. Obadina[1], Adebukunola M. Omemu[2] & Olusola B. Oyewole[1]

[1]Department of Food Science and Technology, Federal University of Agriculture, Abeokuta, Nigeria
[2]Department of Hospitality and Tourism Management, Federal University of Agriculture, Abeokuta, Nigeria

Keywords
Food safety, hygiene, lettuce, microbial contamination, pathogens

Correspondence
Adewale Olusegun Obadina, Department of Food Science and Technology, Federal University of Agriculture, Abeokuta, Nigeria.
E-mail: obadinaw@gmail.com

Funding Information
This work was supported by the My Community, Our Earth (MyCOE) project sponsored by AAG, USAID, and SERVIR (Grant/Award Number: "Effect of climate variability on fresh cut vegetable")

Abstract

Lettuce is consumed raw in salads and is susceptible to microbial contamination through environment, agricultural practices, and its morphology, thus, a potential vehicle for food-borne illness. This study investigated the effect of adoption of food safety and hygienic practices by lettuce farmers on the microbial safety of field sourced lettuce in Lagos State, Nigeria. Ten structured questionnaires were administered randomly to 10 lettuce farmers to assess food safety and hygienic practices (FSH). Two farmers who practice FSH and two farmers who do not practice NFSH were finally used for this study. Samples of ready-to-harvest lettuce, manure applied, and irrigation water were obtained for a period of five months (August – December 2013) and analyzed for total plate count (TPC), total coliform count (TCC), *Escherichia coli, Listeria spp., Salmonella spp.,* and *Shigella spp.* counts. Result of microbial analyses of lettuce samples was compared with international microbiological specification for ready-to-eat foods. Results showed that the range of TPC on lettuce was 6.00 to 8.11 LogCFU/g from FSH farms and TPC of lettuce samples from NFSH farms ranged from 6.66 to 13.64 LogCFU/g. 1.49 to 4.85LogCFU/g were TCC ranges from lettuce samples obtained from FSH farms while NFSH farms had TCC ranging between 3.95 and 10.86 LogCFU/g, respectively. The range of isolated pathogen count on lettuce from FSH and NFSH farms exceeded the international safety standard; there was a significant difference in the microbial count of lettuce from FSH farms and NFSH farms. This study concludes that the lettuce samples obtained did not pass the international microbial safety standards. FSH compliance is a major determinant of the microbial safety of lettuce. Hence, the institution of FSH on farm to improve microbial safety of lettuce produced for public consumption is emphasized.

Introduction

Lettuce (*Lactuca sativa*) is a temperate annual or biennial plant of the daisy family Asteraceae (ITIS, 2010). It is often grown as a leafy vegetable eaten raw notably in salads, sandwiches, and hamburgers. Lettuce is healthy to eat because it is low in calories and contain essential nutrients (Gueye and Diouf 2007). Depending on the variety, lettuce is a good source of vitamin A, vitamin K, and Potassium with higher concentrations of vitamin A found in darker green lettuces. It also provides some dietary fiber (concentrated in the spine and ribs), carbohydrates, protein, and a small amount of fat with the exception of the iceberg type. Lettuce provides some vitamin C, calcium, iron, and copper, with vitamins and minerals largely found in the leaf (Katz and Weaver 2003). Lettuce is one of the vegetables that have attracted high consumption and have high economic importance throughout the world (FAOSTAT, 2010). It is a cool-season crop that grows easily in a well-drained, good soil rich in organic fertilizers with adequate supply of water. Water is the most dominant limiting factor for lettuce production (Coelho et al. 2005).

Human and animal enteric pathogens except soil-borne spore formers such as *Clostridium perfringens* and *Bacillus cereus* are usually absent from fresh vegetables at harvest, unless they have been fertilized with human or animal wastes or irrigated with water containing such wastes (Generld et al. 2006). Raw vegetables and fruits may introduce pathogens into processing plants and kitchen environments, thus, contaminate other foods (Generld et al. 2006). Viruses, including hepatitis A, calicivirus, and Norwalk-like strain have been found in lettuce (USFDA, 2012).

At production areas, irrigation and rinse waters have received attention, as they might be some of the major sources of microbial contamination. Irrigation and rinse waters might contain pathogenic bacteria such as *Salmonella* spp. and *Escherichia coli* O157:H7 (Generld et al. 2006). Usually, irrigation and rinse waters are used without any previous treatment when obtained from rivers, streams, lakes, or wells adjacent to the cropping areas (Pacheco et al. 2002; Abreu et al. 2010; Salem et al. 2011; Ilic et al. 2012; Olaimat and Holley 2012).

Food safety practices (FSH) are Good Agricultural Practices with bias for food safety on the farm. The concept of FSH evolved recently as a result of the big concern about food safety and quality, and the environmental sustainability of agriculture. FSH offers benefits to the farmers and consumers to meet specific objectives of food security, food quality, production efficiency, livelihood, and environmental protection. In a broad sense, FSH applies available knowledge in addressing environmental, economic, and social sustainability for on-farm production and postproduction processing, resulting in a safe and healthy food and non-food agricultural products.

A better understanding of the interaction between human pathogens and produce interaction is needed in the development of intervention strategies to increase the safety of lettuce supply. Thus, investigation on the microbial ecology of human pathogens, and factors affecting survival and growth of human pathogens in an agricultural/farm environment, including water and soil amendments, is essential to developing and implementation of the intervention to reduce the risk of contaminating fresh produce from the agricultural production environment.

Materials and Methods

Administration of questionnaires

Questionnaires were administered to 10 lettuce farmers within Badagry, Amuwo-Odofin, and Ikorodu local governments of Lagos State, South Western Nigeria. The questionnaires were drafted to assess the food safety hygiene (FSH) practices of the farmers. Two farmers who practice (FSH) and two farmers who do not practice (NFSH) gave their consent to participate fully in the research work and thus used for this study. The different samples used for the analysis were collected from these farmers.

Sample collection

Samples collected from the farms included lettuce, irrigation water, and Manure/soil samples.

Sampling period

Sampling was done monthly between August and December 2013, which incorporated the weak rainy season and a weak dry season experienced which is an optimum period for lettuce growing in Lagos state. Sampling of lettuce, irrigation water, and soil around each sampled lettuce was done five times during the study period.

Lettuce sampling

The lettuce plants were cut just above the ground with a knife previously disinfected with 70% ethyl alcohol. The samples were placed directly into sterile plastic bags. Samples were collected in replicate randomly from the farms during each visit.

Irrigation water sampling

For the sampling of the irrigation water sources at each farm, 5 mL sample was collected in a sterilized plastic bottle. The sampling bottles were filled while turned sideways and upwards in order to avoid superficial contamination.

Manure/soil sampling

Soil/manure samples were collected from a 10 cm^2 area around each sampled lettuce plant. Soil samples were collected during every visit to the growers. At each production area, three soil samples were taken and pooled to produce one single soil sample for every grower on every visit. The samples were placed in plastic bags and transported to the laboratory for subsequent microbiological analyses.

Microbiological analysis

All the samples (lettuce, irrigation water, manure/soil) were taken to the laboratory in an ice packed container for analysis. Nutrient agar (Macconkey agar, Salmonella–Shigella agar, Eosin ethylene blue agar and Brilliance Listeria agar) were used for total plate count (TPC), total coliform count (TCC), *Salmonella spp.*, *Shigella spp.* *E. coli*, and *Listeria spp.*, counts, respectively, using standard bacteriological techniques as described by Eni et al. (2010). Isolates were identified using cultural, morphological, and biochemical characteristics. All media used were sourced from Oxoid, UK and prepared according to manufacturer's instructions. Microbial load on lettuce samples were compared with specification of "Guidelines for Assessing the Microbiological Safety of Ready-to-eat foods placed in Market" by "Health Protection Agency (2009)" and "Centre for Food Safety (2007)", while irrigation water samples result was compared with the World Health Organization standards for irrigating fresh produce. (WHO, 1989, 2006)

Data analysis

All procedures were carried out in triplicates and data collected from the study were subjected to analysis of variance (ANOVA). Differences among means were separated using Duncan's multiple range test and significances were accepted at 5% level ($P < 0.05$) (Duncan, 1955) Pearson correlation coefficient between the relative humidity, temperature, and rainfall of the sampling period as well as pathogenic load of manure, irrigation water, and lettuce samples was calculated. Statistical Package for Social Sciences 16.0 version was used for statistical.

Results and discussion

The use of food safety and hygienic (FSH) practices among lettuce farmers was compared and summarized in Table 1. The farms visited received technical support, related to organic production practices, that was provided by extension services of the Lagos state ministry of agriculture, but the focus was mainly on the control of chemical hazards, example of which is pesticide residue, as this was derived from the interviews with the farmers. The workers were very compliant, responsive to changes, and concerned with possible quality improvements.

The majority of lettuce farmers (53%) applied raw poultry droppings to their lettuce plant, 70% applied raw cow dung, and none of the respondent made use of human waste. All (100%) the respondent agreed that they make use of composted or aged manure on lettuce farm. All the respondents had no control in place on the lettuce

Table 1. Food safety hygiene (FSH) compliance by farmers. ($n = 10$).

		Response (%)	
Question on hygiene and food safety practices		Yes	No
1	Do you apply raw poultry droppings?	80	20
2	Do you apply raw cow dung?	70	30
3	Do you use human waste?	0	100
4	Is composted or aged animal manure used to supplement the soil?	100	0
5	If composted manure is used, are there records to show that animal manures are properly composted such as certifications or Standard Operating Procedures for composting?	0	100
6	Are there controls in place to prevent indirect contamination of raw animal manure from adjacent properties?	0	100
7	Do you keep untreated animal dungs with harvested vegetables?	0	100
8	Is the quality of water source assessed?	0	100
9	Do you use surface water for irrigation?	60	40
10	Do you use well water for irrigation?	40	60
11	Do you use pipe borne water for irrigation?	0	100
12	Do animals have access to irrigation water?	60	40
13	Do you store manure near source of irrigation?	30	70
14	Do you wash your hands before harvesting lettuce?	20	80
15	Do you wash lettuce vegetables after they are harvested?	0	100
16	Do you clean container for harvest before reusing them?	0	100
17	Do you use disinfectants to clean your harvest containers?	0	100
18	Do you have daily contact with animals (Poultry, Dogs, Goats, and Sheep)?	30	70
19	Do you wash your hands after touching animals?	0	100
20	Do birds or wildlife enter your vegetable farm?	60	40
21	Do you wash your hands after toilet use?	90	10
22	Do you wash your hands before eating?	80	20
23	Are you aware of anyone getting diarrhea from eating lettuce?	0	100
24	Is there a management program to identify potential contamination risks during the growing and harvesting of lettuce?	0	100

farms visited to prevent indirect contamination of raw animal manure from adjacent properties, while none of the respondents kept untreated animal dungs with harvested lettuce vegetables. The survey questionnaire result demonstrated that most of the lettuce farms operated in a high microbial risk context with respect to lettuce production, harvest, and packaging. Result also show that none (0%) of the respondents assessed the quality of the water, only 60% of the respondent uses surface water for irrigation, while 40% of the respondent used well water for irrigation and none (0%) of the respondent have access to tap water for irrigation purposes. Sixty percent (60%) of the respondent have birds or wildlife entering their farms and as such agreed that animals do have access to their source of irrigation water and majority (70%) of the respondent store their manure near source of irrigation water. Most (80%) of the respondent practice the hygiene of washing hands before harvesting lettuce vegetables, 90% claimed to wash their hands after using the toilet, 80% wash their hands before eating, and none of the respondents wash lettuce vegetables after they are harvested. None of the respondent uses disinfectant to clean harvest containers nor do they clean their containers before reusing them. Few (30%) of the respondents have daily contact with animals but none of the respondents washes their hand after touching animals.

Heaton and Jones (2008) reported that its a known and acceptable fact that fruit and vegetable consumption is a risk factor for infection of enteric pathogens, unfortunately, lettuce farmers interviewed lacked knowledge of lettuce contamination with food-borne pathogens, and human illness. None of the respondents have been informed of anyone getting diarrheal infection from eating lettuce grown on their farm. Also, none (0%) of the respondents have a management program to identify potential contamination risk during the growing and harvesting of lettuce.

The farms visited received technical support, related to organic production practices, that was provided by extension services of the Lagos state ministry of agriculture, but the focus was mainly on the control of chemical hazards, example of which is the pesticide residue, as this was derived from the interviews with the farmers. The workers were very compliant, responsive to changes, and concerned with possible quality improvements.

On the average, TPC values from lettuce samples obtained from FSH 2 farm is the lowest, while TPC values from lettuce obtained from NFSH2 farm is the highest. A maximum acceptable concentration of 5.0 LogCFU/g of aerobic mesophylls on fresh-cut vegetables is suggested by literature (Mossel 1982; Solberg et al. 1990) but TPC values obtained from this study ranged from 6.00 logCFU/g to 13.64 LogCFU/g. Munuera et al. (1994) also had lettuce samples with TPC values higher than 5.0 LogCFU/g in 61.5% of lettuce from different markets and street stands TPC values of 5.7, 7.8, 5.2, and 6.1 LogCFU/g were also reported for lettuce from salad bar, retail outlets, packaged vegetables, and grocery stores, respectively (Ercolani 1976; Garg et al. 1990; King et al. 1991; Albrecht et al. 1995).

The total coliform count (TCC) of lettuce samples obtained from FSH1 farm ranged from 4.77 LogCFU/g in November to 1.49 LogCFU/g in October, while FSH 2 farm had TCC values that ranged from 4.85 LogCFU/g in November to 3.78 LogCFU/g in December. TCC values of NFSH 1 farm ranged from 8.62 LogCFU/g in October to 3.95 LogCFU/g in December and TCC from NFSH 2 farm ranged from 10.86 LogCFU/g in November to 4.24 LogCFU/g in September. The mean TCC of lettuce samples obtained in each month of sampling were not significantly different from one another at $P < 0.05$, while the mean TCC values from different farms were significantly different $P < 0.05$ from one another as presented in Table 2. Total coliform count TCC on lettuce samples was at maximum with lettuce samples obtained from NFSH 2 (1.49 LogCFU/g) and was at minimum in FSH 1 lettuce samples (10.86 LogCFU/g) as presented in Table 2. Rodr′iguez de lecea and Soto Esteras (1981)while reporting 3.0 LogCFU/g as the standard TCC value expected on leafy greens TCC values found values lower than 3.0 LogCFU/g from his study, while Albrecht et al. (1995); Brocklehurst et al. (1987); Ercolani (1976) and Ruiz et al. (1987) found TCC higher values than 3.0 LogCFU/g. Due to their natural characteristics and the contact with soil, irrigation water, and animal intrusion, several studies have demonstrated that leafy greens frequently present contamination by fecal coliforms (Fischer-Arndt et al. 2010; James 2006; Levantesi et al. 2012; Millner 2003; Moyne et al. 2011; Oliveira et al. 2012b; and Oliveira et al. 2012b). In this study, there is neither 95% nor 99% correlation between TCC of lettuce and TCC of manure/soil samples as shown in Table 3.

Mean *Shigella spp.* count, *E. coli* count, *Listeria spp.* count as well as *Salmonella spp.* count was at minimum from lettuce samples obtained from FSH 2 farm and peaked with lettuce samples obtained from NFSH 1 farm. *Listeria spp.* count obtained from lettuce samples throughout the research period exceeded the satisfactory limits of <1 LogCFU/g and border line of between 1 LogCFU/g and ≤2 LogCFU/g in ready-to-eat vegetables. Chukwu et al.(2006) reported that outbreak of listeriosis has not yet been reported in Nigeria and there is limited report on the occurrence of the organism, this might be due to limited attention on the existence of the organism by public health workers and/or poor knowledge of its isolation and identification procedures. *E. coli* count on lettuce

Table 2. Microbial load of lettuce samples between August and December 2013.

Months	Farm	TPC (Log CFU/g)	TCC (Log CFU/g)	*Shigella spp.* Log CFU/25 g	*Listeria spp.* (Log CFU/25 g)	*E. coli* (Log CFU/25 g)	*Salmonella spp.* (Log CFU/25 g)
August	FSH 1	$7.24 \pm 1.16_{a}$	$4.47 \pm 0.61_{a}$	$2.30 \pm 0.17_{a}$	$4.30 \pm 0.33_{a}$	$2.00 \pm 0.03_{a}$	$2.00 \pm 0.47_{a}$
	FSH 2	$7.20 \pm 0.96_{ab}$	$4.64 \pm 0.91_{ab}$	$2.00 \pm 0.55_{a}$	$4.36 \pm 0.65_{a}$	$3.86 \pm 0.67_{a}$	$2.00 \pm 0.48_{a}$
	NFSH	$8.49 \pm 1.72_{c}$	$4.58 \pm 0.25_{c}$	$4.26 \pm 0.33_{a}$	$4.34 \pm 0.97_{a}$	$4.26 \pm 0.65_{a}$	$2.90 \pm 0.53_{a}$
	NFSH 2	$8.86 \pm 1.52_{bc}$	$8.14 \pm 1.01_{bc}$	$6.05 \pm 1.16_{a}$	$6.91 \pm 1.16_{a}$	$4.49 \pm 0.81_{a}$	$6.15 \pm 0.50_{a}$
September	FSH 1	$8.70 \pm 1.20_{a}$	$4.30 \pm 0.60_{a}$	$3.00 \pm 0.27_{a}$	$3.00 \pm 0.95_{a}$	$3.00 \pm 0.30_{a}$	$3.00 \pm 0.11_{a}$
	FSH 2	$7.00 \pm 0.62_{ab}$	$4.08 \pm 0.55_{ab}$	$3.00 \pm 0.20_{a}$	$3.48 \pm 0.51_{a}$	$3.00 \pm 0.30_{a}$	$3.00 \pm 0.05_{a}$
	NFSH 1	$7.20 \pm 0.62_{c}$	$4.86 \pm 0.92_{c}$	$3.47 \pm 0.32_{a}$	$5.70 \pm 0.27_{a}$	$3.00 \pm 0.30_{a}$	$3.00 \pm 0.08_{a}$
	NFSH 2	$7.70 \pm 0.82_{bc}$	$4.24 \pm 1.23_{bc}$	$3.18 \pm 0.29_{a}$	$8.30 \pm 0.30_{a}$	$3.65 \pm 0.14_{a}$	$1.69 \pm 0.57_{a}$
October	FSH 1	$7.26 \pm 0.35_{a}$	$1.49 \pm 0.99_{a}$	$4.34 \pm 0.95_{a}$	$9.08 \pm 1.82_{a}$	$0.00 \pm 0.00_{a}$	$3.00 \pm 0.28_{a}$
	FSH 2	$8.11 \pm 1.13_{ab}$	$4.20 \pm 0.77_{ab}$	$0.00 \pm 0.00_{a}$	$8.90 \pm 1.20_{a}$	$0.00 \pm 0.00_{a}$	$3.00 \pm 0.28_{a}$
	NFSH 1	$9.18 \pm 0.79_{c}$	$8.62 \pm 1.65_{c}$	$6.46 \pm 0.82_{a}$	$6.79 \pm 1.00_{a}$	$6.30 \pm 0.91_{a}$	$3.00 \pm 0.28_{a}$
	NFSH 2	$9.60 \pm 1.69_{bc}$	$6.62 \pm 1.00_{bc}$	$0.00 \pm 0.00_{a}$	$0.00 \pm 0.00_{a}$	$6.70 \pm 0.90_{a}$	$0.00 \pm 0.00_{a}$
November	FSH1	$6.26 \pm 0.21_{a}$	$4.77 \pm 0.30_{a}$	$4.56 \pm 0.00_{a}$	$5.70 \pm 0.03_{a}$	$3.00 \pm 0.15_{a}$	$3.00 \pm 0.00_{a}$
	FSH 2	$6.64 \pm 0.32_{ab}$	$4.85 \pm 0.34_{ab}$	$0.00 \pm 0.00_{a}$	$0.00 \pm 0.00_{a}$	$0.00 \pm 0.00_{a}$	$0.00 \pm 0.00_{a}$
	NFSH 1	$6.66 \pm 0.32_{c}$	$5.86 \pm 0.78_{c}$	$4.63 \pm 0.00_{a}$	$5.95 \pm 0.02_{a}$	$3.00 \pm 0.15_{a}$	$3.00 \pm 0.00_{a}$
	NFSH 2	$13.64 \pm 0.31_{bc}$	$10.86 \pm 0.44_{bc}$	$7.18 \pm 0.00_{a}$	$7.67 \pm 0.05_{a}$	$10.37 \pm 0.30_{a}$	$6.01 \pm 0.00_{a}$
December	FSH 1	$6.00 \pm 0.22_{a}$	$3.48 \pm 0.19_{a}$	$3.30 \pm 0.05_{a}$	$4.86 \pm 0.20_{a}$	$3.00 \pm 0.06_{a}$	$3.00 \pm 0.00_{a}$
	FSH 2	$6.18 \pm 0.16_{ab}$	$3.78 \pm 0.24_{ab}$	$3.30 \pm 0.08_{a}$	$4.69 \pm 0.09_{a}$	$3.00 \pm 0.06_{a}$	$3.00 \pm 0.00_{a}$
	NFSH 1	$6.93 \pm 0.20_{c}$	$3.95 \pm 0.21_{c}$	$3.48 \pm 0.12_{a}$	$4.75 \pm 0.08_{a}$	$3.00 \pm 0.06_{a}$	$3.00 \pm 0.00_{a}$
	NFSH 2	$8.53 \pm 0.37_{bc}$	$7.27 \pm 0.32_{bc}$	$4.41 \pm 0.08_{a}$	$2.30 \pm 0.12_{a}$	$5.45 \pm 0.12_{a}$	$3.01 \pm 0.00_{a}$

Figures with the different subscript across columns shows significant difference ($P < 0.05$) in the mean of microbial result from different farms within a month, while figures with same subscripts across columns shows no significant difference (at $P < 0.05$) from different farms within a month. FSH1, food safety hygiene compliance farm 1; FSH2, food safety hygiene compliance farm 2; NFSH1, food safety hygiene noncompliance farm 1, NFSH2, food safety hygiene noncompliance farm 2; TPC, total plate count; TCC, total coliform count.

Table 3. Correlation of total coliform counts in lettuce, manure, and irrigation water over season variation.

TCC	Lettuce	Rainfall	Temperature	RH	Manure	Water
Lettuce	1.000					
Rainfall (mm)	0.180	1.000				
Temperature (°C)	−0.066	−0.207	1.000			
RH (%)	0.215	0.326	−0.458[2]	1.000		
Manure	0.349	−0.007	−0.065	0.115	1.000	
Water	0.523[1]	0.284	−0.048	0.099	−0.174	1.000

TCC, total coliform count; RH, relative humidity.
[1]Correlation is significant at the 0.01 level (two-tailed).
[2]Correlation is significant at the 0.05 level (two-tailed).

exceeded the satisfactory limit of "not detected in 25 g" reported by Health Protection Agency (2009) and Center for Food Safety (2007) throughout the research period. The presence of *E. coli* in vegetables may indicate insufficient awareness of microbial hazards during farming, inadequate sanitary conditions, and an increased probability of contamination by pathogenic bacteria associated with several food-borne illnesses (Neto et al. 2012; Soriano et al. 2000).

Shigella spp. count ranged between 8.07 LogCFU/25 g in "October" and 2.19 LogCFU/25 g in "August", which were beyond the safety limits of "not detected in 25 g" reported by Health Protection Agency (2007). It also exceeded the safety level stated by Microbiological Guidelines For Ready-to-eat Food (2007) which is <1.30 LogCFU/g as satisfactory level and 1.30103 LogCFU/g to <2 LogCFU/g being acceptable limits, *Salmonella spp.* count obtained from lettuce samples from this study exceeded the satisfactory safety limits of "not detected in 25 g" stated by Health Protection Agency (2007) and Microbiological Guidelines For Ready-to-eat Food (2007).

Irrigation water samples also did not meet minimum World Health Organization (<1 LogCFU/mL) criteria for irrigating fresh produce-like lettuce (World Health Organization 1989; WORLD HEALTH ORGANIZATION 2006) as presented in Table 4, this finding was in agreement with the previous reports (Okafo et al. 2003; Chigor et al. 2010). A significant positive correlation of coliform count of irrigation water with the coliform count of lettuce ($r = 0.523$, $P < 0.01$) presented in Table 3 as well as positive correlation between *Listeria spp.* count on irrigation water and the *Listeria spp.* count on lettuce presented on Table 5 vegetables suggests irrigation water sources being a subject to lettuce contamination in this study. FSH 1 and 2 used ground water while NFSH 1 and NFSH 2 used pond. Fong et al. (2007) and Richardson et al. (2009) identified that the ground water can be contaminated with different kinds of enteric microorganisms,

Table 4. Microbiological load of irrigation water samples (LogCFU/mL) between August and December 2013.

Months	Farms	TPC (Log CFU/g)	TCC (Log CFU/g)	*Shigella spp. (Log CFU/25 g)*	*Listeria spp. Log CFU/g*	*E. coli LogCFU/25 g*	*Salmonella spp. (LogCFU/25 g)*
August	FSH 1	$1.60 \pm 0.06_a$	$1.11 \pm 0.08_a$	$0.00 \pm 0.00_a$	$0.00 \pm 0.05_a$	$0.90 \pm 0.05_a$	$1.00 \pm 0.10_a$
	FSH 2	$1.90 \pm 0.07_b$	$1.08 \pm 0.05_b$	$0.00 \pm 0.00_b$	$0.48 \pm 0.09_b$	$1.30 \pm 0.08_b$	$1.60 \pm 0.08_a$
	NFSH 1	$2.13 \pm 0.07_c$	$1.64 \pm 0.10_b$	$0.00 \pm 0.00_b$	$0.00 \pm 0.06_b$	$1.36 \pm 0.10_c$	$3.00 \pm 0.07_b$
	NFSH 2	$2.01 \pm 0.06_d$	$1.28 \pm 0.07_c$	$0.00 \pm 0.00_c$	$0.16 \pm 0.0.08_c$	$1.67 \pm 0.14_d$	$1.16 \pm 0.12_c$
September	FSH 1	$3.30 \pm 0.13_a$	$2.45 \pm 0.08_a$	$0.85 \pm 0.19_a$	$1.53 \pm 000_a$	$2.70 \pm 0.12_a$	$4.00 \pm 0.41_a$
	FSH 2	$2.30 \pm 0.10_b$	$2.42 \pm 0.08_b$	$1.40 \pm 0.17_b$	$1.91 \pm 0.05_b$	$3.00 \pm 0.10_b$	$2.42 \pm 0.40_a$
	NFSH 1	$2.85 \pm 0.17_c$	$2.95 \pm 0.05_b$	$2.30 \pm 0.20_b$	$1.71 \pm 0.06_b$	$2.09 \pm 0.13_c$	$0.00 \pm 0.70_b$
	NFSH 2	$2.83 \pm 0.12_d$	$2.62 \pm 0.11_c$	$1.50 \pm 0.18_c$	$1.73 \pm 0.03_c$	$3.21 \pm 0.14_d$	$2.14 \pm 0.50_c$
October	FSH 1	$2.70 \pm 0.15_a$	$2.33 \pm 0.01_a$	$0.00 \pm 0.00_a$	$1.41 \pm 0.07_a$	$1.95 \pm 0.14_a$	$2.22 \pm 0.12_a$
	FSH 2	$2.10 \pm 0.12_b$	$2.30 \pm 0.09_b$	$0.66 \pm 0.19_b$	$1.79 \pm 0.05_b$	$2.53 \pm 0.16_b$	$2.82 \pm 0.27_a$
	NFSH 1	$2.70 \pm 0.20_c$	$2.85 \pm 0.10_b$	$0.78 \pm 0.12_b$	$1.96 \pm 0.08_b$	$2.60 \pm 0.15_c$	$3.91 \pm 0.23_b$
	NFSH 2	$3.30 \pm 0.13_d$	$2.49 \pm 0.11_c$	$1.28 \pm 0.24_c$	$1.71 \pm 0.08_c$	$3.08 \pm 0.11_d$	$2.30 \pm 0.37_c$
November	FSH 1	$3.52 \pm 0.16_a$	$2.48 \pm 0.05_a$	$0.00 \pm 0.00_a$	$1.61 \pm 0.18_a$	$2.18 \pm 0.11_a$	$2.30 \pm 0.12_a$
	FSH 2	$2.30 \pm 0.20_b$	$2.60 \pm 0.08_b$	$1.49 \pm 0.18_b$	$2.70 \pm 0.20_b$	$2.78 \pm 0.17_b$	$2.96 \pm 0.30_a$
	NFSH 1	$3.18 \pm 0.11_c$	$3.00 \pm 0.09_b$	$1.00 \pm 0.21_b$	$2.90 \pm 0.19_b$	$2.85 \pm 0.16_c$	$4.10 \pm 0.32_b$
	NFSH 2	$3.00 \pm 0.23_d$	$2.68 \pm 0.03_c$	$0.83 \pm 0.18_c$	$2.39 \pm 0.17_c$	$3.28 \pm 0.14_d$	$2.48 \pm 0.25_c$
December	FSH 1	$2.21 \pm 0.08_a$	$1.81 \pm 0.06_a$	$0.00 \pm 0.00_a$	$0.00 \pm 0.00_a$	$1.45 \pm 0.00_a$	$1.70 \pm 0.002_a$
	FSH 2	$2.58 \pm 0.10_b$	$1.90 \pm 0.08_b$	$0.36 \pm 0.10_b$	$0.95 \pm 0.30_b$	$2.04 \pm 0.01_b$	$1.86 \pm 0.07_a$
	NFSH 1	$2.81 \pm 0.11_c$	$2.33 \pm 0.07_b$	$0.30 \pm 0.09_b$	$0.90 \pm 0.35_b$	$2.13 \pm 0.0_c$	$2.10 \pm 0.06_b$
	NFSH 2	$2.68 \pm 0.02_d$	$2.00 \pm 0.05_c$	$0.78 \pm 0.12_c$	$1.99 \pm 0.34_c$	$2.58 \pm 0.02_d$	$1.78 \pm 0.05_c$

Figures with the different subscript across columns shows significant difference ($P < 0.05$) in the mean of microbial result from different farms within a month, while figures with same subscripts across columns shows no significant difference (at $P < 0.05$) from different farms within a month. FSH1, food safety hygiene compliance farm 1; FSH2- food safety hygiene compliance farm 2; NFSH1, food safety hygiene noncompliance farm 1; NFSH2, food safety hygiene noncompliance farm 2. TPC, total plate count; TCC, total coliform count.

Table 5. Correlation of *Listeria spp.* in lettuce, manure and irrigation water over season.

Listeria spp.	Lettuce	Rainfall	Temperature	RH	Manure	Water
Lettuce	1.000					
Rainfall (mm)	0.087	1.000				
Temperature (°C)	−0.054	−0.207	1.000			
RH (%)	0.268	0.326	−0.459[1]	1.000		
Manure	−0.200	0.266	−0.082	0.085	1.000	
Water	0.377[1]	0.241	0.185	−0.017	−0.411[1]	1.000

RH, relative humidity.
[1]Correlation is significant at the 0.05 level (two-tailed).

such as *E. coli*, *Salmonellaspp.*, and *Campylobacter*. However, Richardson et al. (2009) highlighted that the ground water is generally accepted to be of better quality because the water is protected from contamination more than pond water. Irrigation water samples, collected from both the water sources (pond water) and ground water indicated contamination by *E. coli* throughout the study period. FSH 1 and FSH 2 used ground water pumped up from a dug well for drip irrigation, meanwhile NFSH 1 and NFSH 2 farms used pond water for irrigation with bowls, buckets, and watering cans. None of the farmers had control in place to prevent indirect contamination of raw animal manure from adjacent properties; the well water can be suspected to be contaminated through adjacent properties especially when the water table is close to the ground surface. The exact cause of higher coliform contamination from NFSH lettuce samples was not determined, but low water quality, cross contamination, NFSH, and unknown factors could be contributing factors. The lack of sanitary and sewage management facilities in the study area coupled with close interactions between people, livestock, water sources, and fresh produce, could result in high concentrations of enteric organisms in the environment as well as increase the risk of producing cross contamination.

The use of raw manure in vegetables produce contamination has been reported by many authors (Kudva et al. 1998; Ingham et al. 2004; Lejeune and Christie 2004). Table 6 presented the manure contamination during the research period, although an insignificant positive correlation ($r = 0.349$) existed between the TCC of the manure and TCC on lettuce samples as shown in Table 3. Manure samples from the farms showed high contamination of *E. coli* and coliforms, suggesting that composting were not thorough if practiced at all. Storage, frequency of application, and methods of application of manure were derived from the producers' own experiences. Table 7 An insignificant correlation that existed between the pathogenic

Table 6. Microbial load of manure/soil samples between August and December 2013.

Months	Farm	TPC *(LogCFU/g)*	TCC *(LogCFU/g)*	*Shigella spp. (LogCFU/25 g)*	*Listeria spp. (LogCFU/g)*	*E. coli (LogCFU/25 g)*	*Salmonella spp. (LogCFU/25 g)*
August	FSH 1	$11.19 \pm 0.12_a$	$6.79 \pm 0.28_a$	$6.51 \pm 0.21_a$	$8.70 \pm 0.04_a$	$9.23 \pm 1.12_a$	$3.30 \pm 0.05_a$
	FSH 2	$11.47 \pm 0.08_b$	$8.15 \pm 0.30_b$	$6.86 \pm 0.17_b$	$9.23 \pm 0.10_{bc}$	$3.00 \pm 0.74_a$	$1.94 \pm 0.05_{ab}$
	NFSH	$10.61 \pm 0.09_b$	$5.90 \pm 0.29_{bc}$	$5.30 \pm 0.23_{bc}$	$8.97 \pm 0.08_c$	$4.43 \pm 1.00_b$	$7.36 \pm 0.07_{bc}$
	NFSH 2	$11.08 \pm 0.11_b$	$6.96 \pm 0.27_c$	$6.22 \pm 0.20_c$	$8.94 \pm 0.12_c$	$5.54 \pm 1.4_c$	$0.00 \pm 0.03_c$
September	FSH 1	$11.23 \pm 0.31_a$	$8.12 \pm 0.32_a$	$7.83 \pm 0.32_a$	$8.91 \pm 0.27_a$	$10.56 \pm 1.11_a$	$3.30 \pm 1.4_a$
	FSH 2	$8.95 \pm 0.33_b$	$8.18 \pm 0.31_b$	$6.86 \pm 0.28_b$	$9.28 \pm 0.30_{bc}$	$4.95 \pm 0.85_a$	$0.00 \pm 0.00_{ab}$
	NFSH 1	$10.97 \pm 0.27_b$	$5.94 \pm 0.28_{bc}$	$5.30 \pm 0.33_{bc}$	$10.95 \pm 0.33_c$	$4.46 \pm 0.90_b$	$8.09 \pm 2.20_{bc}$
	NFSH 2	$10.38 \pm 0.30_b$	$6.84 \pm 0.34_c$	$6.67 \pm 0.31_c$	$9.70 \pm 0.18_c$	$6.68 \pm 0.78_c$	$2.81 \pm 1.20_c$
October	FSH 1	$10.38 \pm 0.24_a$	$8.00 \pm 0.31_a$	$7.71 \pm 0.27_a$	$7.04 \pm 0.29_a$	$10.43 \pm 0.99_a$	$3.30 \pm 1.00_a$
	FSH 2	$9.00 \pm 0.20_b$	$8.25 \pm 0.33_b$	$6.86 \pm 0.32_b$	$9.28 \pm 0.40_{bc}$	$5.02 \pm 0.90_a$	$0.00 \pm 0.00_{ab}$
	NFSH 1	$10.89 \pm 0.22_b$	$6.00 \pm 0.27_c$	$5.30 \pm 0.31_{bc}$	$8.80 \pm 0.27_c$	$4.52 \pm 0.81_b$	$7.45 \pm 1.9_{bc}$
	NFSH 2	$10.10 \pm 0.30_b$	$7.40 \pm 0.31_c$	$6.61 \pm 0.31_c$	$8.36 \pm 20_c$	$6.68 \pm 0.60_c$	$4.42 \pm 1.06_c$
November	FSH1	$10.59 \pm 0.25_a$	$9.48 \pm 0.46_a$	$7.90 \pm 0.66_a$	$10.10 \pm 0.22_a$	$8.30 \pm 0.48_a$	$3.30 \pm 0.93_a$
	FSH 2	$8.86 \pm 0.27_b$	$8.09 \pm 0.44_b$	$6.86 \pm 0.64_b$	$9.20 \pm 0.20_{bc}$	$4.86 \pm 0.54_a$	$0.00 \pm 0.00_{ab}$
	NFSH 1	$10.73 \pm 0.30_b$	$5.85 \pm 0.48_{bc}$	$3.00 \pm 0.60_{bc}$	$10.90 \pm 0.15_c$	$4.20 \pm 0.42_b$	$6.73 \pm 1.11_{bc}$
	NFSH 2	$10.06 \pm 0.22_b$	$6.27 \pm 0.42_c$	$5.92 \pm 0.62_c$	$10.06 \pm 0.27_c$	$5.76 \pm 0.32_c$	$4.29 \pm 0.72_c$
December	FSH 1	$9.88 \pm 0.16_a$	$8.86 \pm 0.51_a$	$0.00 \pm 0.00_a$	$9.30 \pm 0.24_a$	$7.70 \pm 0.50_a$	$0.00 \pm 0.00_a$
	FSH 2	$8.73 \pm 0.03_b$	$7.95 \pm 0.44_b$	$0.00 \pm 0.00_b$	$9.00 \pm 0.18_{bc}$	$4.72 \pm 0.75_a$	$0.00 \pm 0.00_{ab}$
	NFSH 1	$10.70 \pm 0.49_b$	$5.00 \pm 0.52_{bc}$	$0.00 \pm 0.00_{bc}$	$10.79 \pm 0.30_c$	$4.08 \pm 25_b$	$2.24 \pm 3.88_{bc}$
	NFSH 2	$9.77 \pm 0.29_b$	$9.39 \pm 054_c$	$0.00 \pm 0.00_c$	$9.67 \pm 0.21_c$	$5.50 \pm 52_c$	$0.00 \pm 0.00_c$

Figures with the different subscript across columns shows significant difference ($P < 0.05$) in the mean of microbial result from different farms within a month, while figures with same subscripts across columns shows no significant difference (at $P < 0.05$) from different farms within a month. FSH1, food safety hygiene compliance farm 1, FSH2- food safety hygiene compliance farm 2; NFSH1, food safety hygiene noncompliance farm 1, NFSH2- food safety hygiene noncompliance farm 2. TPC, total plate count; TCC, total coliform count.

Table 7. Correlation of Total Plate Counts *in* lettuce, manure and irrigation water over seasonal variation.

TPC	Lettuce	Rainfall	Temperature	RH	Manure	Water
Lettuce	1.000					
Rainfall (mm)	0.015	1.000				
Temperature (°C)	0.161	−0.207	1.000			
RH (%)	−0.144	0.326	−0.459[1]	1.000		
Manure	−0.119	−0.361[1]	−0.131	0.185	1.000	
Water	0.303	0.164	−0.014	0.016	−0.337	1.000

TPC, total plate count; RH, relative humidity.
[1]Correlation is significant at the 0.05 level (two-tailed).

load on lettuce and the pathogenic load on manure samples which can be attributed to disinfection of the manure with synthetic fertilizers during the application of urea and NPK fertilizers by the lettuce farmers to increase plant yield because nitrogen and phosphorus are usually the most limiting nutrients in many soils in Africa (SUGE et al. 2011). Organic inputs alone may not meet the nutritional needs of crops because they contain a comparatively less quantity of nutrients compared to inorganic fertilizers, therefore, there is no need to integrate the two forms in order to achieve better crop yields (Frankenberger and Abdelmagid 1985). As a small, uncharged molecule, ammonia can cross the bacterial membrane and cause damage to the cell either by causing rapid alkalization of the cytoplasm or through a decrease in intracellular K^+ concentration (Kadam and Boone 1996; Park and Diez-Gonzalez 2003). Furthermore, the insignificant correlation can be associated with other sources of contamination as highlighted by Quadrous Rodrigues et al. (2014) that seedlings also may be contaminated, especially when they are not treated with chemicals or have not undergone heat treatments before use, as in the case of some investigated organic farms that was studied. It can be said that this observation is a result of FSH compliance that was identified in the course of this research. FDA 2008 highlighted growing conditions and agricultural practices used by specific grower are risk factors that contribute to microbial contamination of vegetables.

Conclusion

Except for TPC and TCC, other microbial loads assessed were not significantly different at ($P < 0.05$) from one another across the farms (FSH compliance and NFSH compliance farm). It is also imperative that farmers and handlers of vegetables from irrigated fields should be educated on the measures aimed at minimizing or eliminating microbial hazards. Farmer and retailer education programs that lead to increased awareness and a change in food safety practices by lettuce value chain players in Nigeria may be an effective way of reducing the magnitude and frequency of lettuce contamination. The need for consumer awareness must be emphasized because vegetables may be affected by both microbiological and chemical contamination, and for that reason, sanitization procedures should be used to avoid food-borne illnesses.

Conflict of Interest

None declared.

References

Abreu, I. M., A. M. R. Junqueira, J. R. Peixoto, and S. A. Oliveira. 2010. Qualidademicrobiológica e produtividade de alface sob adubaçãoquímica e orgânicaCiência e Tecnologia de Alimentos. Ciência e Tecnologia de Alimentos 30:108–118.

Albrecht, J. A., F. L. Hamouz, S.S. Sumner, and V. Melch. 1995. Microbial evaluation of vegetable ingredients in salad bars. J. Food Prot. 58:683–685.

Brocklehurst, T. F., C. M. Zaman-Wong, and B. M. Lund. 1987. A note on the microbiology of retail packs of prepared salad vegetables. J. Appl. Bacteriol. 63:409–415.

Chigor, V. N., V. J. Umoh, and S. I. Smith. 2010. Occurrence of *Escherichia coli* O157 in a river used for fresh produce irrigation in Nigeria. Afr. J. Biotechnol. 2:178–182.

Chukwu, O. O. C., D. Olabode, and C. Nwosuh. 2006. *Listeria monocytogenes*: The nature, public heath aspects, and retrospective situations of anemerging infectious pathogen. Anim. Prod Res. Advan. 2:86–93.

Coelho, A. F., E. P. Gomes, A. P. Sousa, and M. B. A Gloria. 2005. Effect of irrigation level on yield and bioactive amine content of American lettuce. J. Sci. Food Agric. 85:1026–1032.

Duncan, O. D., B. Duncan. 1955. A methodological analysis of segregation indexes. American Sociological Review. 20:210–217.

Eni, A. O., A. Oibukunoluwa, and U.S. Oranusi. (2010) Microbial quality of fruits and vegetable sold in Sango Ota, Nigeria. African J. Food Science 4:291–296.

Ercolani, G. L. 1976. Bacteriological quality assessment of fresh marketed lettuce and fennel. Appl. Environ. Microbiol. 31:847–852.

FAOSTAT. 2010. Export value for vegetables 2010. Available at www.faostat3.fao.org/home/index.html> (accessed online 25.09.12).

FDA. 2008. Food and Drug Administration, Center for Food Safety and Applied Nutrition, 2008. Guidance for Industry: guide to minimize food safety hazards for fresh-cut fruits and vegetables. Fed. Reg. 72:11364–11368.

Fischer-Arndt, M., D. Neuhoff, L. Tamm, and U. Köpke. 2010. Effects of weed management practices on enteric pathogen transfer into lettuce (*Lactuca sativa* var. capitata). Food Control 21:1004–1010.

Fong, T. T., L. S. Mansfield, D. L. Wilson, D. J. Schwab, S. L. Molloy, and J. B. Rose. 2007. Massive microbiological groundwater contamination associated with a waterborne outbreak in Lake Erie, South Bass Island, Ohio.. Environ. Health Perspect. 115:856–864.

Frankenberger, W.T., and H. M. Abdelmagid. 1985. Kinetic parameters of nitrogen mineralization rates of leguminous crops incorporated into soil. Plant Soil. 87: 257–271.

Garg, N., J. J. Churey, and D.F. Splittstoesser. 1990. Effect of processing conditions on the microflora of fresh-cut vegetables. J. Food Prot. 53:701–703.

Generld, M. S., R. G. James, and E. Y. Ahmed. 2006. Microbiology of fruits and vegetables. Taylor and Francis group, Boca Raton, London, New York.

Gueye, M., and M. Diouf. 2007. Traditional leafy vegetables in Senegal: diversity and medicinal Uses. Afr. J. Tradit. Complement. Altern. Med. 4:469–475.

Health Protection Agency. 2007. Annual Report and Account.

Health Protection Agency. 2009. Guidelines for Assessing the Microbiological Safety of Ready-to-Eat Foods Placed on the Market.

Heaton, J. C., and K. Jones. 2008. Microbial contamination of fruit and vegetables and the behaviour of enteropathogens in the phyllosphere: a review. J. Appl. Microbiol. 104:613–626.

Ilic, S., A. Rajic, C. Britton, E. Grasso, W. Wilkens, and S. Totton. 2012. A scoping study characterizing prevalence, risk factor and intervention research, published between 1990 and 2010, for microbial hazards in leafy green vegetables. Food Control 23:7–19.

Ingham, S. C., J. A. Losinski, M. P. Andrews, J. E. Breuer, J. R. Breuer, J. E. Breuer, et al. 2004. *Escherichia coli* contamination of vegetables grown in soils fertilized with noncomposted bovine manure: Garden-Scale Studies. Appl. Environ. Microbiol. 11:6420–6427.

ITIS, 2010 "*Lactuca sativa* L". Integrated Taxonomic Information System. Retrieved 27 March 2010

James, J.. 2006. Microbial hazard identification in fresh fruits and vegetables. Wiley-Interscience, Dublin, Ireland.

Kadam, P. C., and D. R. Boone. 1996. Influence of pH on ammonia accumulation and toxicity in halophilic, methylotrophic methanogens. Appl. Environ. Microbiol. 62:4486–4492.

Katz, S. H., and W. W. Weaver. 2003. Encyclopedia of Food and Culture. Chicago: University of Chicago Press.

King, A. D., J. A. Magnuson, T. Torok, and N. Goodman. 1991. Microbial flora and storage quality of partially processed lettuce. J. Food Sci. 56:459–461.

Kudva, I. T., K. Blanch, and C. J. Hovde. 1998. Analysis of *Escherichia coli* O157: H7 survival in ovine or bovine manure andmanure slurry. Appl. Environ. Microbiol. 9:3166–3174.

Lejeune, J. T., and N. P. Christie. 2004. Microbiological quality of ground beef from conventionally-reared cattle and "raised withoutantibiotics" label claims. J. Food Prot. 7:1433–1437.

Levantesi, C., L. Boinadonna, R. Briancesco, E. Grohmann, S. Toze, and V. Tandoi. 2012. *Salmonella* in surface and drinking water: occurrence and water-mediated transmission. Food Res. Int. 45:587–602.

Microbiological Guidelines For Ready-to-eat Food. 2007. Center for Food Safety. Risk Assessment Section. Food and Environmental Hygiene Department. Queensway, Hong Kong.

Millner, P. 2003. Composting: improving on a time-tested technique. Agric. Res. 51: 20–21.

Mossel, D. A. A. 1982. Microbiology of Foods, 3rd ed.. Pp.96. The University of Utrecht, Faculty of Veterinary Medicine, Utrecht , The Netherlands.

Moyne, A. L., M. R. Sudarshana, T. Blessington, S. T. Koike, M. D. Cahn, and L. J. Harris. 2011. Fate of *Escherichia coli* O157:H7 in field-inoculated lettuce. Food Microbiol. 28:1417–1425.

Munuera, I., D. Garc′ia, and J. J. Iba′n˜ez. 1994. Vegetales de consumeencrudo: bu′squeda de criterios y valoresmicrobiolo′gicos de referencia que aseguren la calidad e inocuidad. Alimentaria 251:63–67.

Neto, N. J. G., R. M. L. Pessoa, M. Queiroga, I. M. B. Magnani, F. I. S. Freitas, and E. L. Souza. 2012. Bacterial counts and the occurrence of parasites in lettuce (*Lactuca sativa*) from different cropping systems in Brazil. Food Control 28:47–51.

Okafo, C. N., V. J. Umoh, and M. Galadima. 2003. Occurrence of pathogens on vegetables harvested from soils irrigated with contaminated streams. Sci. Total Environ. 1–3:49–56.

Olaimat, A. N, and R. A. Holley.2012. Factors influencing the microbial safety of fresh produce: a review. J. Food Prot., 32, 1–19.

Oliveira, M., I. Viñas, J. Usall, M. Anguera and., and M. Abadias. 2012b. Presence and survival of *Escherichia coli* O157:H7 on lettuce leaves and in soil treated with contaminated compost and irrigation water. Int. J. Food Microbiol. 156:133–140.

Pacheco, M. A. S. R., Y. S. K. Fonseca, H. G. G. Dias, V. L. P. Cândido, A. H. S Gomes, andI. M. Armelin. 2002. Condiçõeshigiênico-sanitárias de verduras e legumes comercializados no CEAGESP de Sorocaba – SP. Hig. Alimentar 16:50–51.

Park, G. W., and F. Diez-Gonzalez. 2003. Utilization of carbonate and ammonia-based treatments to eliminate *Escherichia coli* O157:H7 and *Salmonella typhimurium* DT104 from cattle manure. J. Appl. Microbiol. 94:675–685.

Quadrous Rodrigues, R., M. R. Loiko Cheila, M. D. de Paula, C. T. Hessel, L. L. Jacxsens, M. Uyttendaele, et al. 2014. Microbiological contamination linked to implementation of good agricultural practices in the production of organic lettuce in Southern Brazil. Food Control 42:152–164.

Richardson, H. Y., G. Nichols, C. Lane, I. R. Lake, and P. R. Hunter. 2009. Microbiological surveillance of private water supplies in England: the impact of environmental and climate factors on water quality. Water Res. 43:2159–2168.

Rodr′iguez de lecea, J., andT. Soto Esteras. 1981. Microbiolog′ıa de, las ensaladasfrescas I. Flora microbiana de lechugas (*Lactuca.sativa, L.*). Anal. Bromatol. 33:329–338.

Ruiz, B. G. V., R. Galvez Vargas, and R. Garcia-Villanova. 1987. Contamination on fresh vegetables during cultivation and marketing. Int. J. Food Microbiol. 4:285–291.

Salem, I. B., I. Ouardani, M. Hassine, and M. Aouni. 2011. Bacteriological and physico-chemical assessment of wastewater in different region of Tunisia: impact on human health. BMC Res. Notes 4:144.

Solberg, M., J. J. Buckalew, C. M. Chen, D.W. Schaffer, K. O'NEILL, J. Mcdowell, et al. 1990. Microbiological safety assurance system for foodservice facilities. Food Technol. 12:68–73.

Soriano, J. M., H. Rico, J. C. Moltó, and J. Mañes. 2000. Assessment of the microbiological quality and wash treatments of lettuce served in University restaurants. Int. J. Food Microbiol. 58:123–128.

Suge, J. K, M. E. Omunyin, and E. N. Omami. 2011. Effect of organic and inorganic sources of fertilizer on growth, yield and fruit quality of eggplant (*Solanum Melongena*L). Appl. Sci. Res. 3:470–479.

USFDA 2012. "Chapter IV. Outbreaks Associated with Fresh Vegetables, and Cancer Prevention – A Review of the Epidemiologic Evidence. US Food and Drug Administration, New York.

World Health Organization. 1989. Health guidelines for the use of wastewater in agriculture and aquaculture. World Health OrganizationTechnical Report Series 778. World Health Organization, Geneva. Available at: www. whqlibdoc.who.int/trs/WHO_TRS_778.pdf. (accessed 11 April 2009).

World Health Organization. 2006. WHO guide lines for the safe use of wastewater, excreta and greywater: wastewater use in agriculture.Volume II, World Health Organization, France. Available at www.whqlibdoc.who.int/ publications/2006/9241546832_eng.pdf. (accessed11 April 2009).

13

Stabilization of sunflower oil with pussy willow (*Salix aegyptiaca*) extract and essential oil

Zahra Sayyari[1] & Reza Farahmandfar[2]

[1]Department of Food Science and Technology, Savadkooh branch, Islamic Azad University, Savadkooh, Iran
[2]Department of Food Science and Technology, Sari Agricultural Sciences & Natural Resources University (SANRU), Sari, Iran

Keywords
antioxidant activity, oxidative stability, pussy willow, sunflower oil, total phenolic content

Correspondence
Reza Farahmandfar, Department of Food Science and Technology, Sari Agricultural Sciences & Natural Resources University (SANRU), Sari, Iran.
E-mail: re1farahmand@gmail.com

Funding Information
No funding information provided.

Abstract

The aim of present study was to evaluate antioxidant efficacy of pussy willow extract (PWE) and essential oil (PWEO) in stabilization of sunflower oil (SFO) during ambient storage (60 days at 25°C). Initially, total phenolic (TP) and total flavonoid (TF) contents were evaluated. Then, PWE, PWEO, and TBHQ were added to SFO. Peroxide value (PV), carbonyl value (CV), total polar compound (TPC), acid value (AV), and Oxidative stability index (OSI) were measured every 15 days. The results showed that PWE had higher TP and TF than PWEO (TP: 966.72 mg GAE/g and 355.8472 mg GAE/g, respectively; TF: 619.45 mg/100 g and 195.45 mg/100 g, respectively). Furthermore, according to all stabilization parameters, PWE had higher antioxidant efficacy followed by TBHQ, PWEO, and control, respectively. Therefore, PWE has antioxidant activity and it may be recommended as natural strong antioxidants to suppress lipid oxidation.

Introduction

Sunflower oil (SFO) is an edible oil has been widely used due to its nutritional and medicinal value. sunflower oil is one source of linoleic acid (9 *cis*, 12 *cis* oxtadecadienoic) which has so many health beneficial effects (Hashemi et al. 2015). Autoxidation or oxidative rancidity is the major cause of quality losses in crude as well as refined oils during storage (Asnaashari et al. 2014a,b). When the crude and refined oils are exposed to factors such as heat, high temperatures, light, trace metals, or oxygen, the problem get more exacerbated (Crapiste et al. 1999; Sikwese and Duodu 2007; Farahmandfar et al. 2015a).

The use of antioxidants is the most appropriate way of stabilizing oils, preventing the autoxidation or oxidative rancidity, and protecting oils from the damages inflicted by free radicals (Farhoosh et al. 2016). The addition of synthetic antioxidants has been one of the most effective and popular method to prevent oxidative rancidity and development of off-flavors (Eshghi et al. 2014). Investigations have demonstrated that synthetic antioxidants are toxic and carcinogenic for humans (Iqbal et al. 2008). Recently, there has been increased interest in identifying potential sources in order to obtain natural antioxidants (Poiana 2012; Farahmandfar et al. 2015b). Essential oil (EO) and extracts from spices, fruits, herbs, and hull contain effective compounds that prevent from the undesirable oxidative process in foodstuff (Asnaashari et al. 2015a).

Salix aegyptiaca L. (pussy willow) is generally cultivated in some provinces of Iran for hedge and ornamental purposes. The distillate obtained from male inflorescences of plants, with the common local name of "Araghe Bidmeshk" and English name of "Egyptian willow distillate," in most parts of Iran have long been applied in folk medicine as cardiotonic (Sonboli et al. 2010). The aqueous extract and EO of *S. aegyptiaca* L. are being used in confectionery and flavorful syrups. In Iranian traditional medicine, *S. aegyptiaca* has been employed as laxative, cardioprotective, sedative, hypnotic, somnolent, aphrodisiac, orexigenic, carminative, gastroprotectant, anthelmintic, and vermifuge (Karimi et al. 2011). A number of chemical constituents such as flavonoids and volatile substances have been isolated from different parts of the plant (Enayat and Banerjee 2009; Karimi et al. 2011). From current pharmaceutical studies, additional pharmaceutical applications of *S. aegyptiaca* have revealed antioxidant, anti-inflammatory, analgesic, anxiolytic, and antihypercholesterolemic effects among others (Hifnawy et al. 2010; Sonboli et al. 2010; Karimi et al. 2011; Rabbani et al. 2011).

Although previous studies have presented the antioxidant properties of pussy willow (PW) extract and EO, there are no reports on the antioxidant efficacy for the stabilization of SFO been shown so far. The purpose of this study was to estimate the antioxidant efficacy of PW flower extract and EO against oil oxidative rancidity and to compare their antioxidant activity with commercially available antioxidant (TBHQ).

Materials and Methods

Materials

Refined, bleached, deodorized SFO without any synthetic antioxidants was obtained from Ghoncheh Co. (Sari, Iran). The flowers of PW were purchased from the Ghamsar botanical garden at Kashan, Iran, during March 2014, and authenticated by the Medicinal Plant Incubator Center (Islamic Azad University, Ayatollah Amoli Branch, Amol, Iran). They were washed, air dried in the shade, and then powdered utilizing an electric device and stored in refrigerator (4°C) until use. TBHQ was prepared and purchased from Sigma-Aldrich (St. Louis, MO). All other chemicals were of analytical grade and purchased from Merck Co., Frankfurt, Germany.

Preparation of PWE and PWEO

The solvent (ethanol) was added to the powdered PW in the ratio of 10:1 (w:v) and the resulting mixture was shaken overnight. After 24 h, for separating the PW particles, the extract was filtered through Whatman No. 42 filter paper. The solvent was completely evaporated in an oven at 40°C. Finally, the obtained extract was stored in a dark container in refrigerator (4°C) until use (Esmaeilzadeh Kenari et al. 2014). EOs were extracted by hydrodistillation from the powdered PW by the Clevenger-type apparatus, and the obtained oil was stored in a dark container in refrigerator (4°C) until use.

Total phenolic content

The total phenolic (TP) content of PW extracts (PWE) and PWEO was determined according to the Folin–Ciocalteu reagent as described by Pourmorad et al. (2006) and the results were expressed as mg/g gallic acid equivalents (GAE). At a concentration of 1 mg/mL, PWE and PWEO were prepared in their own solvents, and 0.5 mL of each sample was mixed with 2.5 mL of a 10-fold diluted Folin–Ciocalteu reagent and 2 mL of 7.5% sodium carbonate solution. After the samples were kept for 30 min at room temperature, the absorbance was measured at 760 nm in a UV-Vis spectrophotometer (PG Instrument, T80, London, England).

Determination of total flavonoid content

The total flavonoid (TF) content of PWE and PWEO was quantified according to the method described by Dewanto et al. (2002) and the results were determined as catechin equivalents (mg/100 g of dry weight). At a concentration of 1 mg/mL, PWE and PWEO were diluted with water (4 mL) in a 10 mL volumetric flask. Initially, 5% $NaNO_2$ solution (0.3 mL) was added to each volumetric flask; at 5 min, 10% $AlCl_3$ (0.3 mL) was added; and at 6 min, 1.0 mol/L NaOH (2 mL) was added. Water (2.4 mL) was then added to the reaction flask and mixed well. Absorbance of the reaction mixture was read at 510 nm.

Preparation of SFO samples for oxidative stability determination

PWE and PWEO were added to SFO at 1200 ppm. Synthetic antioxidant (TBHQ) was employed at a limit of 100 ppm to compare the efficacy of natural antioxidants (Fki et al. 2005). All the samples (120 mL each) were placed in dark brown colored reagent bottles with narrow necks, without stoppers, and stored at ambient conditions (25°C for 60 days) (Anwar et al. 2007). Control samples were also placed under the same storage conditions. Samples (20 g) were removed periodically every 0, 15, 30, 45, and 60 days for analysis. Immediately after storage period, oil samples were withdrawn for triplicate analysis. The oils were sampled for each measurement from separate bottles.

Analytical procedures

Peroxide value (PV) was measured according to the spectrophotometric method of the International Dairy Federation as described by Shantha and Decker (1994). The carbonyl value (CV) of the oils was measured according to the method developed by Endo et al. (2001), using 2-propanol and 2,4-decadienal as solvent and standard, respectively. AOCS Official Method Cd 3d-63 (AOCS 1990) was used to determine the acid value (AV). Total polar compounds (TPC) content was determined according to the economical micromethod developed by Schulte (2004). Oxidative stability index (OSI) is a method whereupon air passes through a lipid under a specific temperature, at which point volatile acids decomposed from lipid peroxidation are driven out by the air and subsequently dissolved in water, thereby increasing its conductivity. The conductivity of the water is constantly measured, and the OSI value is defined as the hours required for the rate of conductivity to reach a predetermined level (Liu et al. 2014).

Statistical analysis

All analyses were performed in triplicate and data reported as means ± standard deviation (SD). Statistical analyses were conducted using SPSS (Statistical Program for Social Sciences, SPSS Corporation, Chicago, IL) version 18.0 for Windows. Data were subjected to analysis of variance. Significant differences ($P < 0.05$) were calculated using Duncan's multiple range tests.

Results and Discussion

TP and TF contents

Phenolic component is one of the major groups of phytochemicals ubiquitously present in the plant kingdom, and they have received much attention in the recent years due to their potential health benefits as an antioxidant and protective agents against cancer and several other diseases (Plumb et al. 1997).

Flavonoids are the most abundant polyphenols in plants, and they have been shown to have potent antioxidant and anticancer activities (Adom and Liu 2002; Dykes and Rooney 2007).

Results of the TP in PWE and PWEO are presented in Table 1. The differences between the content of TP between PWE and PWEO were statistically significant ($P < 0.05$). The PWE gives higher content of TP (966.72 ± 44.27 mg GAE/g sample) than TP of PWEO (355.84 ± 27.53 mg GAE/g sample). Similar results were also observed related to TF (Table 1). These data suggested that PWE is valuable source of phenolic and flavonoid compounds that might be extracted and used in the food and drug industries.

Table 1. Total phenolic (TP) and total flavonoid (TF) contents of pussy willow extract and PW essential oil.

Extraction	Total phenolic content (mg GAE/g samples ± SD)	Total flavonoid content (mg/100 g samples ± SD)
Pussy willow extract	966.72 ± 44.27^{a}	619.45 ± 12.2^{a}
Pussy willow essential oil	355.84 ± 27.53^{b}	195.45 ± 9.12^{b}

Means ± SD (standard deviation) within a column with the same lower-case letters are not significantly different at p<0.05.

A linear correlation between the antioxidant activity and polyphenolic contents of the plant extracts has been reported by other researchers (Luximon-Ramma et al. 2002; Karimi et al. 2014). Kamkar et al. (2010), which showed that *Mentha pulegium* extracts had more antioxidant activity than *M. pulegium* EO. They stated that the lower antioxidative activity of the *Mentha pulegium* EO can be due to the lack of some of the different antioxidants in the EO.

Stability of SFOs as affected by the addition of PWE and PWEO

Peroxide value and carbonyl value

PV was used as indicators for the primary oxidation of oil and lipids. Hydroperoxide is the primary oxidation product produced as a result of lipid oxidation (Asnaashari et al. 2015b). The quality of the oil may be decreased if it breaks down into nonvolatile and volatile secondary products (Poiana 2012; Mei et al. 2014). By increasing the storage period time, a continuous increase in PV was observed in all the samples (Fig. 1A). The rise of PV amount was very slow, at the beginning, but it started increasing by 15th day of storage and continued to increase further with the increase in storage period, reaching a maximum value after 60 days storage. A significant difference ($P < 0.05$) in PV was observed between the control and SFO samples containing PWE and PWEO, which slowed the rate of peroxide formation revealing good antioxidant efficacy in stabilizing oil (Ben-Ali et al. 2014). Highest PV was observed for control followed by SFO containing PWEO, TBHQ, and PWE, respectively. Such pattern was presented by Kamkar et al. (2010) on the methanol extract and EO of *Mentha pulegium* compared to the butylated hydroxytoluene (BHT) when added to SFOs.

According to Woyewoda et al. (1986), primary oxidation products (peroxides) are converted into secondary products that contain carbonyl groups. These compounds are more stable than hydroperoxides and are considered to be a good index of oxidative changes in lipids. A similar trend was also observed about CV in all treatments (Fig. 1B). Thus, the lowest PV and CV were observed in SFO containing PWE. It may be attributed as a higher antioxidant ability of PWE which is related to its polyphenol component. The formation of fatty acid free radicals, which react with or absorb oxygen in the autoxidation process, was prevented by them. This delays

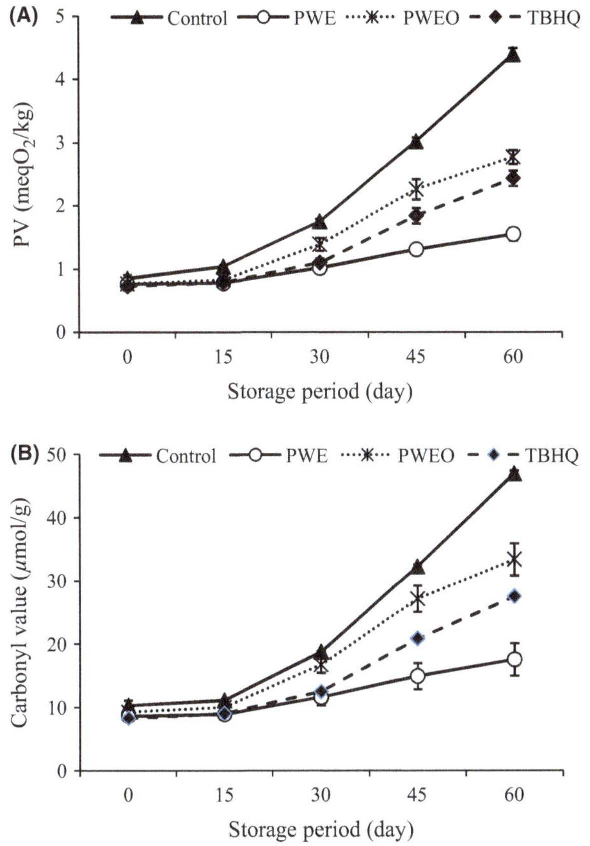

Figure 1. Effect of pussy willow extract (PWE) and PW essential oil (PWEO) on peroxide value (A) and carbonyl value (B) of sunflower oil during ambient storage. Error bars show the variations of three determinations in terms of standard deviation.

the onset of the autoxidative process in oil (Turhan et al. 2009). These results are in agreement with that described previously (Iqbal et al. 2008; Ben-Ali et al. 2014; Mei et al. 2014).

Acid value

Acid value has become a good indicator of the quality. AV is the *number* that expresses, in *milligrams*, the quantity of KOH (in mg) necessary to neutralize free fatty acids in 1 g of oil (Ban and Kang 2014). AV contents of the SFO as affected by the TBHQ, PWE, and PWEO during ambient condition are given in Figure 2. By increasing the storage period, a continuous increase in AV was observed in all the samples. The steady increase in the AV can be attributed partly to hydrolysis of triacylglycerols and partly to the component carboxyl groups present in autoxidative process (Petukhov et al. 1999; Nasirullah 2001). Control exhibited the highest AV at all the stages of analyses during storage. There was no statistically

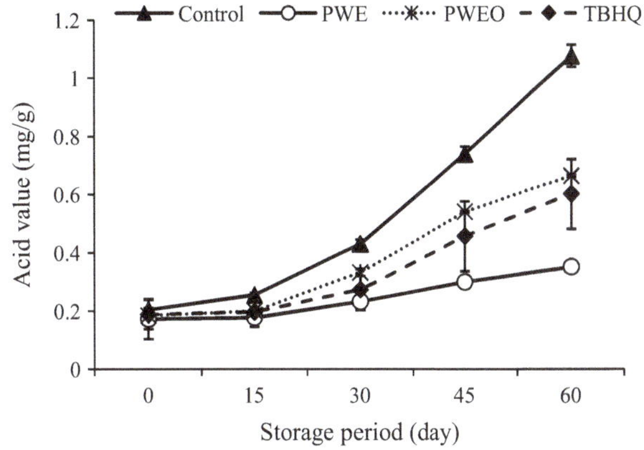

Figure 2. Effect of pussy willow extract (PWE) and PW essential oil (PWEO) on acid value of sunflower oil during ambient storage.

significant difference between SFOs that contain PWEO and TBHQ ($P > 0.05$). The oil samples stabilized with PWE showed lowest levels of AV compared to the other, which suggests the superiority of the PWE over the other antioxidants, such as PWEO and TBHQ, in delaying oxidation in SFO.

Total polar compounds

Polar compounds is an important indicator of oil quality of used oils, giving information of the total amount of newly formed compounds having higher polarity than that of triacylglycerols (Li et al. 2015). The TPC of treatments during the ambient storage are presented in Figure 3. The TPC content increased until the end of the storage period (in all samples). The TPC content of SFO contain antioxidants significantly ($P < 0.05$) lower than the control

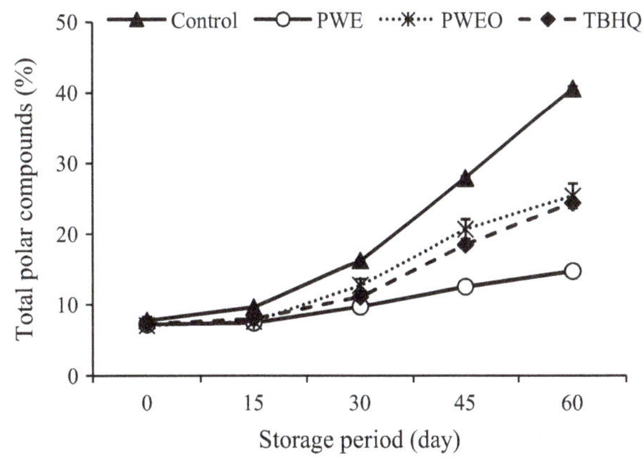

Figure 3. Effect of pussy willow extract (PWE) and PW essential oil (PWEO) on total polar compounds of sunflower oil during ambient storage.

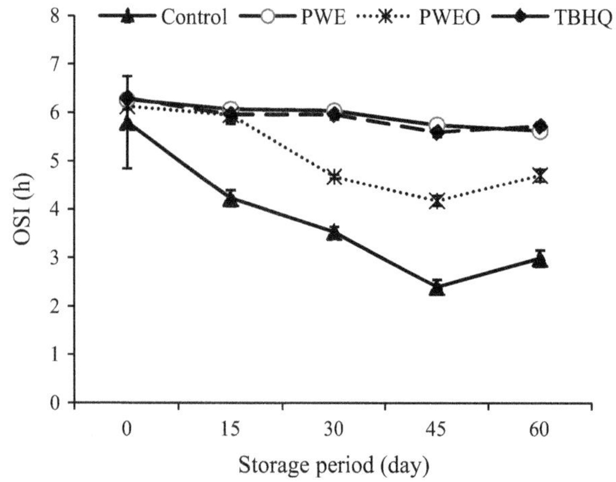

Figure 4. Effect of pussy willow extract (PWE) and PW essential oil (PWEO) on oxidative stability index of sunflower oil during ambient storage.

samples during the storage time. Literature has shown that the fractions of TPC isolated from oxidized oils are toxic to laboratory animals (Pantzaris 1998). Therefore, it has been purposed that frying oils containing more than 24–27% of TPC content should be discarded (Firestone 1993). Only the control among all the samples reached the discarding range of TPC content during storage condition.

The lowest TPC content at the end of storage period was observed in SFO containing PWE. Farhoosh and Kenari (2009) stated that canola oils containing sesame and rice bran oils were more stable than the canola oils without additives during frying, based on TPC formation.

Oxidative stability index

The OSI is an American Oil Chemists' Society approved method that determines the relative resistance of oils to oxidation. Oxidative stability instrument can be employed to determine OSI of oil samples and it is the commercial piece of equipment for the automated determination of oxidative resistance as well as it is well-known by the fats and oils industries (Shahidi and Zhong 2005; Senanayake 2013). Changes in the OSI of the SFO affected by the PWE, PWEO, and TBHQ during the ambient storage are shown in Figure 4. A continued decrease in OSI with the increase in storage period was observed in all the samples. But in control, the rate of decrease was higher than others. There was no statistically significant difference between SFOs containing PWE and TBHQ ($P > 0.05$). The rate of decrease in OSI throughout the storage period indicates higher efficiency of PWE for the stabilization of SFO than PWEO.

Conclusion

The results of the present study apparently demonstrated that the PWE had high TP and TF contents. Moreover, PWE exhibited strong antioxidant activity in stabilizing SFO during ambient storage, which was almost more effective than the antioxidant activity of synthetic antioxidants (TBHQ) as well as PWEO. Therefore, it is suggested that the PWE could be safely used for the stabilization of food systems instead of synthetic antioxidants.

Conflict of Interest

None declared.

References

Adom, K. K., and R. H. Liu. 2002. Antioxidant activity of grains. J. Agric. Food Chem. 50:6182–6187.

Anwar, F., A. Siddiq, S. Iqbal, and M. R. Asi. 2007. Stabilization of sunflower oil with *Moringa oleifera* leaves under ambient storage. J. Food Lipids 14:35–49.

Aocs, O. 1990. Tentative methods of the American Oil Chemists' Society. American Oil Chemists Society Press, Champaign.

Asnaashari, M., R. Farhoosh, and A. Sharif. 2014a. Antioxidant activity of gallic acid and methyl gallate in triacylglycerols of Kilka fish oil and its oil-in-water emulsion. Food Chem. 159:439–444.

Asnaashari, M., R. Tajik, and M. H. H. Khodaparast. 2014b. Antioxidant activity of raspberry (*Rubus fruticosus*) leaves extract and its effect on oxidative stability of sunflower oil. J. Food Sci. Technol. 52:5180–5187.

Asnaashari, E., M. Asnaashari, A. Ehtiati, and R. Farahmandfar. 2015a. Comparison of adaptive neuro-fuzzy inference system and artificial neural networks (MLP and RBF) for estimation of oxidation parameters of soybean oil added with curcumin. J. Food Meas. Charact. 9:215–224.

Asnaashari, M., B. Hashemi, S. Mohammad, H. M. Mehr, and S. H. Asadi Yousefabad. 2015b. Kolkhoung (Pistacia khinjuk) Hull oil and Kernel oil as antioxidative vegetable oils with high oxidative stability and nutritional value. Food Technol. Biotechnol. 53:81–86.

Ban, G.-H., and D.-H. Kang. 2014. Effects of gamma irradiation for inactivating Salmonella Typhimurium in peanut butter product during storage. Int. J. Food Microbiol. 171:48–53.

Ben-Ali, M., K. Dhouib, M. Damak, and N. Allouche. 2014. Stabilization of sunflower oil during accelerated storage: use of basil extract as a potential alternative to synthetic antioxidants. Int. J. Food Prop. 17:1547–1559.

Crapiste, G. H., M. I. Brevedan, and A. A. Carelli. 1999. Oxidation of sunflower oil during storage. J. Am. Oil Chem. Soc. 76:1437–1443.

Dewanto, V., X. Wu, K. K. Adom, and R. H. Liu. 2002. Thermal processing enhances the nutritional value of tomatoes by increasing total antioxidant activity. J. Agric. Food Chem. 50:3010–3014.

Dykes, L., and L. Rooney. 2007. Phenolic compounds in cereal grains and their health benefits. Cereal Foods World 52:105–111.

Enayat, S., and S. Banerjee. 2009. Comparative antioxidant activity of extracts from leaves, bark and catkins of *Salix aegyptiaca* sp. Food Chem. 116:23–28.

Endo, Y., C. M. Li, M. Tagiri-Endo, and K. Fujimoto. 2001. A modified method for the estimation of total carbonyl compounds in heated and frying oils using 2-propanol as a solvent. J. Am. Oil Chem. Soc. 78:1021–1024.

Eshghi, N., M. Asnaashari, M. H. Haddad Khodaparast, and F. Hosseini. 2014. Evaluating the potential of natural curcumin for oxidative stability of soybean oil. Nat. Prod. Res. 28:1375–1378.

Esmaeilzadeh Kenari, R., F. Mohsenzadeh, and Z. R. Amiri. 2014. Antioxidant activity and total phenolic compounds of Dezful sesame cake extracts obtained by classical and ultrasound-assisted extraction methods. Food Sci. Nutr. 2:426–435.

Farahmandfar, R., M. Asnaashari, and R. Sayyad. 2015a. Comparison antioxidant activity of Tarom Mahali rice bran extracted from different extraction methods and its effect on canola oil stabilization. J. Food Sci. Technol. 52:6385–6394.

Farahmandfar, R., R. Safari, F. Ahmadi Vavsari, and T. Bakhshandeh. 2015b. The effect of Ajwain (Trachyspermum ammi) extracted by ultrasound-assisted solvent on quality properties of silver carp (Hypophthalmichthys molitrix) surimi stored at 4C. J. Food Process. Preserv. 40:291–297.

Farhoosh, R., and R. E. Kenari. 2009. Anti-rancidity effects of sesame and rice bran oils on canola oil during deep frying. J. Am. Oil Chem. Soc. 86:539–544.

Farhoosh, R., S. Johnny, M. Asnaashari, N. Molaahmadibahraseman, and A. Sharif. 2016. Structure–antioxidant activity relationships of o-hydroxyl, o-methoxy, and alkyl ester derivatives of p-hydroxybenzoic acid. Food Chem. 194:128–134.

Firestone, D. 1993. Worldwide regulation of frying fats and oils. Inform-Int. News Fats Oils Related Mater. 4:1366–1386.

Fki, I., N. Allouche, and S. Sayadi. 2005. The use of polyphenolic extract, purified hydroxytyrosol and 3, 4-dihydroxyphenyl acetic acid from olive mill wastewater for the stabilization of refined oils: a potential alternative to synthetic antioxidants. Food Chem. 93:197–204.

Hashemi, S. M. B., A. M. Khaneghah, Y. Tavakolpour, M. Asnaashari, and H. M. Mehr. 2015. Effects of ultrasound treatment, UV irradiation and Avishan-e-Denaei essential oil on oxidative stability of sunflower oil. J. Essent. Oil Bearing Plants 18:1083–1092.

Hifnawy, M. S., N. M. Ammar, and M. S. Karawya. 2010. Phytochemical study and evaluation of the anti-inflammatory activity of some medicinal plants growing in Egypt. Med. J. Islamic World Acad. Sci. 18:139–150.

Iqbal, S., S. Haleem, M. Akhtar, M. Zia-Ul-haq, and J. Akbar. 2008. Efficiency of pomegranate peel extracts in stabilization of sunflower oil under accelerated conditions. Food Res. Int. 41:194–200.

Kamkar, A., A. J. Javan, F. Asadi, and M. Kamalinejad. 2010. The antioxidative effect of Iranian Mentha pulegium extracts and essential oil in sunflower oil. Food Chem. Toxicol. 48:1796–1800.

Karimi, I., H. Hayatgheybi, A. Kamalak, M. Pooyanmehr, and Y. Marandi. 2011. Chemical composition and effect of an essential oil of *Salix aegyptiaca* L., Salicaceae, (musk willow) in hypercholesterolemic rabbit model. Revista Brasileira de Farmacognosia 21:407–414.

Karimi, E., P. Mehrabanjoubani, M. Keshavarzian, E. Oskoueian, H. Z. Jaafar, and A. Abdolzadeh. 2014. Identification and quantification of phenolic and flavonoid components in straw and seed husk of some rice varieties (Oryza sativa L.) and their antioxidant properties. J. Sci. Food Agric. 94:2324–2330.

Li, J., W. Cai, D. Sun, and Y. Liu. 2015. A quick method for determining total polar compounds of frying oils using electric conductivity. Food Anal. Methods 9:1444–1450.

Liu, P., B. Kerr, C. Chen, T. Weber, L. Johnston, and G. Shurson. 2014. Methods to create thermally oxidized lipids and comparison of analytical procedures to characterize peroxidation. J. Anim. Sci. 92:2950–2959.

Luximon-Ramma, A., T. Bahorun, M. A. Soobrattee, and O. I. Aruoma. 2002. Antioxidant activities of phenolic, proanthocyanidin, and flavonoid components in extracts of Cassia fistula. J. Agric. Food Chem. 50:5042–5047.

Mei, W. S. C., A. Ismail, N. M. Esa, G. A. Akowuah, H. C. Wai, and Y. H. Seng. 2014. The effectiveness of rambutan (Nephelium lappaceum L.) extract in stabilization of sunflower oil under accelerated conditions. Antioxidants 3:371–386.

Nasirullah. 2001. Development of deep frying edible vegetable oils. J. Food Lipids 8:295–304.

Pantzaris, T. 1998. Comparison of monounsaturated and polyunsaturated oils in continuous frying. Grasas Aceites 49:319–325.

Petukhov, I., L. Malcolmson, R. Przybylski, and L. Armstrong. 1999. Frying performance of genetically modified canola oils. J. Am. Oil Chem. Soc. 76:627–632.

Plumb, G. W., K. R. Price, M. J. Modes, and G. Williamson. 1997. Antioxidant properties of the major polyphenolic compounds in broccoli. Free Radic. Res. 27:429–435.

Poiana, M.-A. 2012. Enhancing oxidative stability of sunflower oil during convective and microwave heating using grape seed extract. Int. J. Mol. Sci. 13:9240–9259.

Pourmorad, F., S. Hosseinimehr, and N. Shahabimajd. 2006. Antioxidant activity, phenol and flavonoid contents of some selected Iranian medicinal plants. Afr. J. Biotechnol. 5:12–15.

Rabbani, M., G. Vaseghi, S. Sajjadi, and B. Amin. 2011. Persian herbal medicines with anxiolytic properties. Journal of Medicinal Plants. 10:7–11.

Schulte, E. 2004. Economical micromethod for determination of polar components in frying fats. Eur. J. Lipid Sci. Technol. 106:772–776.

Senanayake, S. N. 2013. Green tea extract: chemistry, antioxidant properties and food applications–a review. J. Funct. Foods 5:1529–1541.

Shahidi, F., and Y. Zhong. 2005. Lipid oxidation: measurement methods. Bailey's Ind. Oil Fat Prod. John Wiley & Sons, Inc. 357–385.

Shantha, N. C., and E. A. Decker. 1994. Rapid, sensitive, iron-based spectrophotometric methods for determination of peroxide values of food lipids. J. AOAC Int. 77:421–424.

Sikwese, F., and K. G. Duodu. 2007. Antioxidant effect of a crude phenolic extract from sorghum bran in sunflower oil in the presence of ferric ions. Food Chem. 104:324–331.

Sonboli, A., M. Mojarrad, S. N. Ebrahimi, and S. Enayat. 2010. Free radical scavenging activity and total phenolic content of methanolic extracts from male inflorescence of *Salix aegyptiaca* grown in Iran. Iran. J. Pharm. Res. 9:293.

Turhan, S., I. Sagir, and H. Temiz. 2009. Oxidative stability of brined anchovies (Engraulis encrasicholus) with plant extracts. Int. J. Food Sci. Technol. 44:386–393.

Woyewoda, A., S. Shaw, P. Ke, and B. Burns. 1986. 143. Recommended laboratory methods for assessment of fish quality, numeral 1448: canadian technical report of fisheries and aquatic sciences. Minister of Supply and Services Canada, Halifax, Canada.

14

Nutritional composition, quality, and shelf stability of processed *Ruspolia nitidula* (edible grasshoppers)

Geoffrey Ssepuuya, Ivan Muzira Mukisa & Dorothy Nakimbugwe

Department of Food Technology and Nutrition, School of Food Technology, Nutrition and Bio-Engineering, College of Agricultural and Environmental Sciences, Makerere University, P.O. Box, 7062 Kampala, Uganda

Keywords
Acceptability, edible insects, nutritional value, processing, *Ruspolia nitidula*, shelf stability

Correspondence
Nakimbugwe Dorothy, Department of Food Technology and Nutrition, School of Food Technology, Nutrition and Bio-Engineering, College of Agricultural and Environmental Sciences, Makerere University, P.O. Box, 7062 Kampala, Uganda.
E-mail: dnakimbugwe@gmail.com

Funding Information
No funding information provided.

Abstract

The nutritional and commercial potential of the edible grasshopper (*Ruspolia nitidula*, *nsenene* in *Luganda*), a delicacy in Uganda and many East African tribes, is limited by a short shelf life and unverified nutritional value. This research established that *R. nitidula* is nutritious with 36–40% protein, 41–43% fat, 2.5–3.2% carbohydrate, 2.6–3.9% ash, 11.0–14.5% dietary fiber, and 900–2300 μg/100 g total carotenoids on a dry matter basis. Sautéing was the most preferred processing method resulting in grasshoppers with a notably better aroma and flavor. After 12 weeks of storage at room temperature, processed and vacuum packed, ready-to-eat grasshoppers maintained their edible quality with an acid value of 3.2 mg KOH/g, a total plate count of log 1.8 cfu/g, and an overall acceptability of 6.7–7.2 on a 9-point hedonic scale. Further research is required for extending the shelf stability beyond 12 weeks and characterizing the profile of major nutrients.

Introduction

Entomophagy (the practice of eating insects) as well as their use in livestock and pet feeds are increasing worldwide (Durst et al. 2010; Van Huis et al. 2013; Bosch et al. 2014; Kenis et al. 2014; Kelemu et al. 2015). While edible insects were formerly consumed as a cultural delicacy mostly in developing countries, they are gaining recognition as important sources of nutrients (Belluco et al. 2013; Mlcek et al. 2014; Shockley and Dossey 2014).

Edible insects are highly nutritious. According to Capinera (2008) and a review of the nutritional composition of 236 edible insects (Rumpold and Schluter 2013), insects are high in energy, with 2–60% fat on a dry matter basis, which has a high proportion of mono- and polyunsaturated fatty acids, provide satisfactory protein (20–80%) which meets the human amino acid requirements, are high in minerals such as calcium, copper, iron, phosphorus, magnesium, manganese, and potassium, have an abundance of vitamin A and carotenoids, and though in low amounts, they can contain B vitamins such as riboflavin, pantothenic acid, and some times, folic acid. Using two nutrient profiling models developed to combat over- and undernutrition, Payne et al. (2015) concluded that insects' contribution to health is not significantly lower than that of meat products, and can actually be significantly higher. Besides their potential contribution to dietary nutrient intakes, thus improving health, insects are also important for improving and conserving the environment as well as contributing to incomes and livelihoods (Morales and Wolff 2010; Ferraro and Andreatta 2014; Halloran and Vantomme 2014). However, more research and documentation are needed on their nutritional values in order to more efficiently promote insects as healthy food (Van Huis et al. 2013).

Research on edible insects in the United States and Western Europe is only starting to advance (Morales-Ramos et al. 2013) with Europe focusing more on the use of insects as feed and less as food (Van Huis et al. 2013). In all regions of the world, long-term preservation of edible insects has not been given much attention by both researchers and the food industry (Chidumayo and Gumbo 2010; Ferraro and Andreatta 2014) possibly because of their seasonal availability, and the small quantities harvested are consumed fresh. In sub-Saharan Africa, many types of edible insects continue to be processed on a small scale by women and children for home consumption normally just before eating or sale in markets (Chidumayo and Gumbo 2010). However, there is growing interest in domesticating and making insects for food and feed readily available throughout the year.

Ruspolia nitidula, the edible grasshopper native to Uganda, has a nutritional and cherished cultural and economic importance (Van Huis et al. 2013; Martin 2014) to people of diverse cultures. In Uganda, *R. nitidula* is processed by either sautéing, deep frying, or boiling followed by drying. Processed *R. nitidula* are either consumed at home or commercially traded on a small scale mainly in the streets of Kampala city and other towns such as Masaka (Ageya et al. 2008). While small-scale processing of grasshoppers in Uganda increases dietary diversity and nutrient intake and also contributes to incomes (Capinera 2008; Fellows 2009), it preserves the *R. nitidula* for only about 24 h.

This research, therefore, aimed at establishing the nutritional value of *R. nitidula* and developing preservation methods that extend its shelf life. The study specifically assessed the effect of harvesting season, geographical source area, and subtype on the nutritional composition of *R. nitidula*, and compared the effectiveness of two methods for preserving the sensory, microbiological, and chemical shelf stability of *R. nitidula*.

Materials and Methods

Sample preparation

Fresh *R. nitidula* was collected from Masaka and Kampala districts of Uganda in two subsequent swarming seasons of November–December and March–May. For each season, a 500-g sample was washed using running portable tap water, thoroughly drained using a plastic colander, sorted based on subtype (color), and stored in clean and dry plastic containers at −18°C until further analyses.

Nutritional composition analyses

Moisture content was determined by the draft oven method (Nielsen 2010), crude protein by the Kjeldahl (Horwitz 2001) method, fat content by the Soxhlet method (Nielsen 2010), total mineral content by ashing the *R. nitidula* in a carbolite furnace at 500 °C (Nielsen 2010), dietary fiber content by the acid detergent fiber assay, carbohydrate content by difference in nitrogen-free extract (NFE) (Nielsen 2010), carotenoid content by the spectrophotometric method described in the HarvestPlus handbook of carotenoid analysis (Rodriguez-Amaya and Kimura 2004), and potassium and phosphorus contents by wet digestion followed by spectrophotometry.

Choice of the preferred cooking method

Ruspolia nitidula was prepared by sautéing, boiling, and deep frying. For each method, a different set of ingredients were added resulting in nine samples (Table 1), which were screened for sensory acceptability on a 9 point hedonic scale.

Preparation of boiled and sautéed *R. nitidula* for shelf-stability studies

To 500 g of raw *R. nitidula*, 10 g salt and 40 g onion were added followed by boiling at 100°C for 30 min to a golden yellow color. A half of the boiled *R. nitidula* was sautéed without adding oil in a stainless steel pan over gentle heat for 30 min. The boiled and sautéed samples were separately dried at 80°C for 10 h in an air convection dryer (Innotech, D-7115 Altdorf, Germany) to a moisture content of about 5%, allowed to cool to room temperature, and vacuum sealed. The vacuum packs for both types of samples were stored at room temperature in opaque paper bags to eliminate light. At 2-week intervals, samples were monitored for stability over 12 weeks.

Stability monitoring

Sensory stability of boiled and sautéed *R. nitidula*

Sensory acceptability of the sautéed and dried *R. nitidula* (A) and the boiled and dried *R. nitidula* (B) were evaluated by a panel of 30 regular consumers of *R. nitidula*. Each panelist was provided with five pieces of *R. nitidula* (A and B) to rate their acceptability of each attribute (aroma, color, taste, flavor, texture, appearance, and overall acceptability) on a 9-point hedonic scale. This was done on a biweekly basis for 12 weeks.

Microbiological stability of boiled and sautéed *R. nitidula*

Total plate count (TPC) of boiled and sautéed *R. nitidula* samples was determined. A 30-g sample was weighed aseptically, mixed with 90 mL of peptone water, and homogenized in a stomacher (Seward Stomacher, 400 circulator, England) to make a 10^{-1} dilution which was used to make subsequent dilutions. Each dilution was

Table 1. Effect of preparation methods on the consumer acceptability of *Ruspolia nitidula*.

Sample	Ingredients	Mean overall acceptability	Most frequent comments
Sautéed and dried			
A	Salt	5.667	Was dry
B	Salt, onion	**6.848**	The best, well spiced
C	Salt, onion, curry powder	6.121	Tastes good, dry, fatty
D	Salt, onion, curry powder, tomatoes	6.272	Well flavored
E	Salt, onion, curry powder, tomatoes, garlic	**6.576**	Sweet/good smell Bad garlic smell
Deep fried			
F	Salt, onion	5.272	Too oily
G	Salt	**5.515**	Very dry and no flavor
Boiled and dried			
H	Salt	6.709	So dry, but tasty
I	Salt, onion	7.000	Soft, tasty
J	Salt, onion, tomato	**7.226**	Best of all, well prepared

NB: 30-panellist members were used.

plated on sterile plate count agar (PCA) media in duplicate and incubated at 37 °C for 48 h.

Fat rancidity monitoring based on acid value

Free fatty acids accumulation was determined (Nielsen 2010). A 5-g sample was weighed into a clean conical flask and 50 mL 1:1 neutral mixture of ethanol–petroleum ether was added to dissolve the fat. The mixture was titrated with 0.07 mol/L ethanolic sodium hydroxide until the colorless phenolphthalein indicator turned pink. The titer value obtained was used to calculate the acid value expressed in mg KOH/g of the *R. nitidula* fat.

Statistical analyses

IBM SPSS statistics for windows (Version 16, IBM Corporation, Armonk, NY) statistical software was used to compute the mean scores of the sensory quality and nutritional attributes. The 9-point hedonic scale was used in the interpretation of the computed mean scores. ANOVA was used to determine the effect of season, sourcing geographical location, and subtype of nutritional composition at an alpha level of 0.05. Turkey's test was used for comparisons of the levels of the different factors where ANOVA indicated a significant difference. Excel (2007) was used to generate the graphs from results of microbial and chemical analyses.

Results

Effect of season on nutritional composition of *R. nitidula*

The nutritional composition of green and brown *R. nitidula* for the two harvesting seasons is presented in Table 2. Season had an effect ($P < 0.001$) on moisture, dry matter, ash, fiber, and total carotenoids' content of *R. nitidula*. Green and brown *R. nitidula* from the March–May season had a significantly lower moisture content (47–52%) and significantly higher dry matter content (48–52%) than brown and green *R. nitidula* from the November–December season, that is, 52–55% for moisture and 45–47% for dry matter. Green *R. nitidula* in the March–May season had the lowest moisture content and highest dry matter content, both of which were significantly different from the rest. *Ruspolia nitidula* from the March–May season had a significantly lower dietary fiber (11–12.2%) and significantly higher total carotenoids content (2084.8–2273.1 μg/100 g) than *R. nitidula* from November to December season (13–14.5% for dietary fiber and 913.7–1389.4 μg/100 g for total carotenoids). The ash content of green *R. nitidula* in the November–December season was the highest (3.97%) and significantly different from brown *R. nitidula* from the Kampala and green *R. nitidula* from the two geographical sourcing regions in the March–May season. Generally, protein (39–40.4%) content in the March–May season was slightly higher than that of the November–December season, 37.0–39.2%.

Effect of subtype on nutritional composition of *R. nitidula*

Ruspolia nitidula subtype did not have an effect on macro- and micronutrient compositions except moisture and dry matter. Brown *R. nitidula* had a significantly lower dry matter (48–49%, $P = 0.018$) and higher moisture (51–52%, $P = 0.021$) content compared to green *R. nitidula* (~48% for moisture and ~52% for dry matter).

Table 2. Proximate, mineral, and total carotenoid contents of the green and brown *Ruspolia nitidula* subtypes for two swarming seasons.

Subtype and Origin	Moisture	Nutritional components (% dry matter)							
		Crude protein	Crude fat	Carobhydrate	Dietary fiber	Ash	Phosphorus (mg/kg)	Potassium (mg/kg)	Carotenoids (μg/100 g)
KGN	53.41 ± 0.9^{b}	39.12 ± 1.5^{a}	41.17 ± 0.7^{a}	2.64 ± 0.8^{a}	13.06 ± 0.8^{a}	3.96 ± 0.4^{b}	4.96 ± 0.3^{a}	4.94 ± 0.4^{a}	1267.1 ± 0.6^{a}
KGA	47.63 ± 0.3^{a}	40.08 ± 0.5^{a}	42.37 ± 1.6^{a}	3.02 ± 0.5^{a}	11.89 ± 0.8^{b}	2.67 ± 0.4^{a}	4.96 ± 0.3^{a}	5.08 ± 0.3^{a}	2164.9 ± 3.1^{b}
MGN	52.97 ± 1.0^{b}	37.92 ± 1.4^{a}	41.81 ± 2.2^{a}	2.50 ± 0.4^{a}	14.34 ± 0.5^{a}	3.41 ± 0.7^{a}	4.75 ± 0.2^{a}	5.25 ± 0.1^{a}	1389.4 ± 2.2^{a}
MGA	47.56 ± 0.7^{a}	40.30 ± 1.2^{a}	42.23 ± 0.7^{a}	3.21 ± 1.0^{a}	11.32 ± 0.8^{b}	2.60 ± 0.1^{a}	4.75 ± 0.2^{a}	4.80 ± 0.2^{a}	2156.8 ± 2.5^{b}
KBN	55.39 ± 2.4^{b}	38.49 ± 0.7^{a}	41.41 ± 1.0^{a}	2.96 ± 1.6^{a}	13.85 ± 1.3^{a}	3.27 ± 0.5^{a}	4.66 ± 0.4^{a}	5.04 ± 0.3^{a}	1224.5 ± 0.8^{a}
KBA	51.60 ± 0.7^{c}	39.73 ± 0.8^{a}	42.38 ± 1.7^{a}	2.96 ± 0.8^{a}	12.19 ± 0.5^{b}	2.74 ± 0.1^{a}	4.85 ± 0.5^{a}	5.55 ± 0.6^{a}	2084.8 ± 2.8^{b}
MBN	54.55 ± 2.7^{b}	36.99 ± 0.9^{a}	43.04 ± 1.5^{a}	2.92 ± 1.6^{a}	13.14 ± 0.9^{a}	3.75 ± 0.1^{a}	4.22 ± 0.4^{a}	4.57 ± 0.5^{a}	913.7 ± 0.1^{c}
MBA	50.93 ± 0.9^{c}	40.38 ± 2.6^{a}	41.94 ± 2.0^{a}	3.06 ± 0.4^{a}	11.34 ± 0.7^{b}	3.05 ± 0.5^{a}	4.37 ± 0.3^{a}	4.88 ± 0.6^{a}	2273.1 ± 1.4^{b}

Figures having the same superscripts in a column are not significantly different ($P \geq 0.05$, three replicates).
M, Masaka; K, Kampala; G, green; B, brown; A, March–May season; N, November–December season.

Effect of sourcing geographical location on nutritional composition of *R. nitidula*

Ruspolia nitidula sourcing geographical location did not have any effect on nutrient composition except for phosphorus content ($P = 0.001$). Brown *R. nitidula* from the Kampala harvested in the November season had a significantly higher phosphorus content (5.55 mg/kg) than brown *R. nitidula* from the Masaka in the April season (4.56 mg/kg). However, phosphorus content of the above was not different from that of other brown and green subtypes in the two seasons.

Sensory preference of *R. nitidula* processed by three methods

Acceptability can be an indirect measure of preference, implying that the sample with a higher acceptability is preferred. Generally, for both sautéed and boiled samples, the mean overall acceptability increased as the number of spices added increased (Table 1). In general, boiled and dried samples were most preferred and had the highest mean overall acceptability scores (6.7–7.2), followed by sautéed and dried samples (6.1–6.85), and finally deep fried samples (5.2–5.5). The boiled and dried samples with salt, onions, and tomatoes had the highest mean overall acceptability score of 7.2, followed by another boiled and dried sample with salt and onions only, with a similar overall acceptability score of 7. The two were followed by the sautéed and dried subsample with salt and onions only, with an overall acceptability score of 6.85. On the 9-point hedonic scale, these three samples with the highest mean overall acceptability were liked moderately.

Shelf life of processed *R. nitidula*

Sensory stability

Sensory acceptability scores of sautéed and boiled dried samples during the 12 weeks are presented in Tables 3 and 4. Sensory acceptability of sautéed and dried *R. nitidula* did not change significantly over the 12 weeks (Table 3). On the other hand, sensory acceptability of the boiled and dried *R. nitidula* dramatically and significantly decreased by the second week (Table 4) to about 5 (indifferent) which was maintained until week 12.

Microbiological stability

The microbiological quality of *R. nitidula* with time was monitored by the TPC (Fig. 1). From week 4 onward, boiled and dried samples had a slightly higher total plate

Table 3. Changes in mean attribute scores of sautéed and dried *Ruspolia nitidula* flavored with salt and onions over 12 weeks of storage.

Attribute	Biweekly mean attribute score						
	0	2	4	6	8	10	12
Aroma	6.9 ± 2.34[a]	6.8 ± 1.21[a]	6.9 ± 1.25[a]	7.3 ± 1.17[a]	6.6 ± 1.52[a]	7.3 ± 0.99[a]	6.6 ± 1.52[a]
Taste	7.6 ± 1.4[a]	7.1 ± 1.36[a]	7.2 ± 1.37[a]	7.6 ± 1.13[a]	7.3 ± 1.02[a]	7.9 ± 0.86[a]	7.3 ± 1.02[a]
Flavor	7.7 ± 1.92[a]	7.0 ± 1.18[a]	7.0 ± 1.18[a]	7.4 ± 1.28[a]	6.9 ± 1.14[a]	7.0 ± 1.44[a]	6.9 ± 1.14[a]
Texture	7.0 ± 2.13[a]	6.5 ± 1.72[a]	6.5 ± 1.50[a]	6.7 ± 1.81[a]	6.6 ± 1.61[a]	7.0 ± 1.21[a]	6.6 ± 1.61[a]
Appearance	6.8 ± 2.41[a]	6.2 ± 1.89[a]	6.6 ± 1.74[a]	6.8 ± 1.72[a]	6.9 ± 1.35[a]	7.3 ± 1.84[a]	6.9 ± 1.34[a]
Color	7.1 ± 1.16[a]	7.4 ± 1.22[a]	7.0 ± 1.07[a]	7.1 ± 0.77[a]	6.9 ± 1.31[a]	7.7 ± 1.23[a]	6.9 ± 1.30[a]
Overall acceptability	7.2 ± 1.18[a]	6.8 ± 1.33[a]	6.9 ± 1.46[a]	7.2 ± 1.39[a]	6.9 ± 1.28[a]	7.3 ± 1.18[a]	6.9 ± 1.40[a]

Results are mean ± standard deviations of 30 panelists per sitting for a period of 12 weeks.
Figures having the same superscripts are not significantly different ($P \geq 0.05$, three replicates).

Table 4. Changes in mean attribute scores of boiled and dried *Ruspolia nitidula* flavored with salt and onions over 12 weeks of storage.

Attribute	Biweekly mean attribute score						
	0	2	4	6	8	10	12
Aroma	5.8 ± 1.32[a]	5.0 ± 2.52[b]	5.1 ± 1.98[b]	5.0 ± 1.47[b]	5.3 ± 1.56[b]	5.7 ± 1.44[a]	5.3 ± 1.78[b]
Taste	6.6 ± 1.68[a]	5.2 ± 1.92[b]	6.0 ± 1.82[b]	5.2 ± 1.61[b]	5.0 ± 2.12[b]	5.7 ± 1.55[b]	5.5 ± 1.81[b]
Flavor	6.5 ± 1.51[a]	5.4 ± 1.69[b]	5.1 ± 1.79[b]	5.0 ± 1.83[b]	5.7 ± 1.69[b]	5.6 ± 1.30[b]	5.0 ± 2.22[b]
Texture	6.2 ± 1.43[a]	5.5 ± 2.33[b]	5.9 ± 2.04[b]	5.7 ± 1.58[b]	5.7 ± 1.78[b]	5.9 ± 2.08[a]	5.2 ± 1.95[b]
Appearance	6.8 ± 1.52[a]	4.7 ± 1.95[b]	6.0 ± 1.85[b]	5.2 ± 1.79[b]	5.1 ± 1.99[b]	5.5 ± 1.87[b]	5.1 ± 2.10[b]
Color	6.4 ± 1.99[a]	5.4 ± 1.96[b]	5.4 ± 1.92[b]	5.7 ± 1.76[b]	5.3 ± 1.89[b]	5.8 ± 1.69[b]	5.2 ± 1.93[b]
Overall acceptability	6.4 ± 1.59[a]	5.2 ± 1.71[b]	5.6 ± 1.62[b]	5.3 ± 1.58[b]	5.4 ± 1.86[b]	5.7 ± 1.43[b]	5.1 ± 1.91[b]

Results are mean ± standard deviations of 30 panelists per sitting for a period of 12 weeks.
Figures having the same superscripts are not significantly different ($P \geq 0.05$, three replicates).

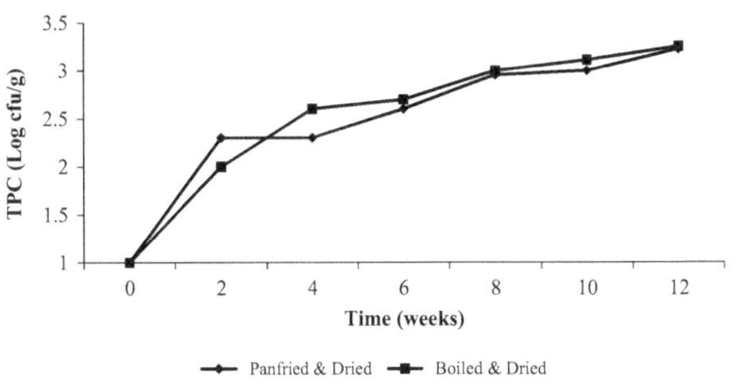

Figure 1. Changes in the total plate count of *Ruspolia nitidula* during 12 weeks of storage at ambient temperature.

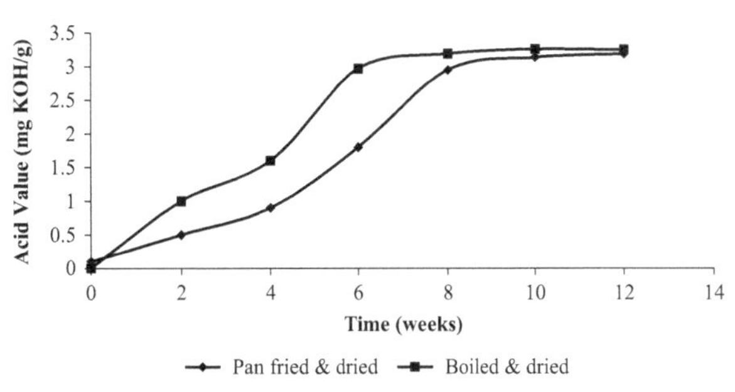

Figure 2. Changes in the acid value of *Ruspolia nitidula* during 12 weeks of storage at ambient temperature.

count than sautéed and dried *R. nitidula*. The highest count observed was 3.2 log cfu/g.

Chemical stability (acid value)

The acid values of both boiled and dried and sautéed and dried *R. nitidula* increased with time and stabilized at about 3.3 mg KOH/kg (Fig. 2). For boiled and dried *R. nitidula*, the acid value stabilized by 6th week, while for sautéed and dried *R. nitidula* it stabilized by the 8th week.

Discussion

Effect of harvesting season on the nutritional composition of *R. nitidula*

Season had an effect on moisture, dry matter, dietary fiber, and total carotenoid content of *R. nitidula*. Being herbivores (Hahn and Orrock 2015; Lenhart et al. 2015), *R. nitidula* feed on crops and grass, implying that their nutritional composition is affected by their feed among other factors. *Ruspolia nitidula* normally swarms in the rainy seasons of March–May and November–December. It is therefore possible that the effect of season on moisture, dry matter, dietary fiber, and total carotenoid was due to differences in the type of feed sources available and fed on by the *R. nitidula* in these seasons. Due to the absence of conclusive research on factors affecting feed intake and nutritional composition of *R. nitidula*, the effect of feed and other factors affecting nutritional composition are not clearly known.

Effect of sourcing geographical location and subtype on the nutritional composition of *R. nitidula*

Subtype had a significant effect on moisture and dry matter content, while sourcing geographical location had a significant effect on mineral content, particularly phosphorus. The observed differences were inconsistent with regard to the macronutrients and minerals. It is therefore possible that these differences in phosphorus, moisture, and dry matter content are purely due to individual differences and not necessarily the influence of the subtype or sourcing geographical location. The fact that the differences in the moisture and dry matter content did not induce a change in the macronutrient composition (protein, fat, carbohydrate, and dietary fiber) substantiates the possibility that the observed differences are random and individual. There is therefore no conclusive evidence that subtype and sourcing geographical location have an influence on the nutritional composition of *R. nitidula*.

Nutrient composition of *R. nitidula*

Ruspolia nitidula are very nutritious with 36–40% protein, 41–43% fat, 10–13% dietary fiber, 900–2300 μg/100 g carotenoids, 3–4% ash, and 4–6 mg/kg potassium and phosphorus (Table 2). The moisture content (47–55%) is less than other major protein sources such as fish with 80% and meat muscle with 62–70%. Thus, *R. nitidula* has a much higher dry matter content (45–53). This implies that on a dry matter basis, *R. nitidula* does not only contain more edible nutrient percent, it is also a more concentrated source of nutrient than meat and fish.

The protein content (36–40.4%) recorded for *R. nitidula* is higher than that of the small grasshopper (14.6%) and the large grasshopper (20.6%) species; quite close to *Ruspolia differens* (43–44%) in Kenya; comparable to winged termites (33.51–39.74%) in western Kenya and other edible insects. Notably, the protein content of *R. nitidula* is higher than that of commonly consumed animal and plant protein sources such as veal, lamb, chicken, and herring fish (7.5–23%); milk and milk products (3–26%); whole eggs (13%); common beans (~24%); peas (~23%); and comparable to that of soy beans ~38%. Insects are therefore high-potential sources of protein to the population. While meat, milk, and egg protein are of higher biological value and digestibility compared to plant protein, the biological value and digestibility of *R. nitidula* have not been determined and therefore, need to be established for an informed comparison.

The fat content (41–43%) is also higher than that of other grasshopper species such as small (6.1%) and large grasshoppers (3.3%), as well as the 14 edible insects in western Nigeria including a grasshopper species, *Zonocerus variegatus* (3.8%), but comparable to the winged termites (44–47%) in Kenya. *Ruspolia nitidula* also has a markedly higher fat content than that of meat, pork, and fish, all of which average less than 22% fat. Mbabazi et al. (2009) reported that the lipid/fat from *R. nitidula* consist of over 58% unsaturated fatty acids with oleic acid (41%) and linolenic acid being the predominant mono- and polyunsaturated fatty acids, respectively. Although no further studies have confirmed these findings, the high content of unsaturated fatty acids indicates that *R. nitidula* not only contains predominantly healthy fat, but it is also highly likely to suffer spoilage from oxidative rancidity.

The carbohydrate content (2.5–3.06%) is comparable to the small grasshoppers (3.9%), the large grasshopper (2.2%), and the winged termites (0.72–8.73%) in Kenya, but lower than that of *Z. variegatus* (63.2%), a grasshopper species in south-western Nigeria. Like animals and fish, *R. nitidula*'s carbohydrate content is much lower than that of plant food sources such as pulses and legumes that average between 24–68% and 68–80% for cereals.

Ruspolia nitidula contains 11–13% dietary fiber, higher than the 14 edible insects (1.68–3.40%) in south-western Nigeria and 4 winged termites (6.37–7.21%) in Kenya. Dietary fiber is normally found in only plant foods such as fruits, vegetables, nuts, and grains and not in meat, milk, or eggs. The dietary fiber of *R. nitidula* is higher than that of common plant sources such as peas (4.7%), sesame seeds (7.9%), and fruits such as mango (2.4%), guava (3.7%), and avocado (3.4%). Dietary fiber is important for normal bowel function and may play a role in the prevention of chronic diseases such as cancer, coronary artery disease, and diabetes mellitus. Being both a good source of dietary fiber and protein is a unique and excellent nutritional property compared to plant and animal nutrient sources.

Two minerals were analyzed, potassium and phosphorus with amounts ranging from 4 to 6 mg/kg. These values are much less than those of major plant and animal sources. The total carotenoid content ranged from 900 to 2300 μg/100 g or 75 to 192 RE/100 g based on retinol equivalents (RE) of 12 μg for α-carotene, β-cryptoxanthin, and other provitamin A carotenoids. This is generally much higher than that of other edible grasshopper species such as *Z. variagatus* (6.8 μg/100 g). Compared to other animal sources, muscle meats hardly contain any vitamin A except in the liver (~13,877 μg/100 g) to which *R. nitidula* can only be compared. This implies that *R. nitidula* is a potential source of carotenoids and thus vitamin A.

Screening for the best preparation method of *R. nitidula*

The hedonic scale is normally used for expression of opinion/preference through acceptance testing. From Table 1, the mean overall acceptability on a 9-point hedonic scale generally increased on addition of spices from only salt to onions, tomatoes, curry powder, and garlic. However, there was a notable exception in the sautéed samples, where addition of onions to *R. nitidula* already containing salt increased the acceptability from 5.7 to 6.8. Further addition of curry powder and tomatoes did not lead to any further increment in the mean overall acceptability, but rather a decrease from 6.8 to 6.1 and 6.3. Addition of garlic seemed to reverse the trend (6.6), but could not elicit the same effect as salt and onion alone. This suggests that adding curry powder and tomatoes probably did not suit the expected sensory characteristics and therefore scored less than the samples to which they were not added. For both boiled and sautéed samples, subsamples with salt and onions had almost the same score (I = 7 and B = 6.8), and close to the highest score. Unlike samples with salt and onions only, further addition of spices elicited mixed responses that could possibly be due to a mere expression of liking or disliking of the spices rather than the products. Therefore, sample B (sautéed and dried) and I (boiled and oven dried) were chosen for shelf-life testing. This is because they were liked by both consumers who enjoy spices and those who do not. According to comments from panelists (Fig. 3), being moderately dry, quite soft, and not oily were some of the characteristics associated with the products' preference.

Shelf life of processed *R. nitidula* products

Sensory acceptability and shelf stability of *R. nitidula*

Loss of consumer acceptance is a common criteria used to monitor shelf life of foods. Often, the shelf life of products stored at ambient temperature is based on sensory quality (Kilcast 2010). During the 3 months of evaluation, both sautéed (A) and boiled (B) *R. nitidula* with salt and onion were all liked moderately, and none was disliked on average. None of the sensory attributes was on average liked extremely for both preservation methods.

Generally, the sautéed and dried *R. nitidula* scored higher (6.5–7.6) for each attribute on average and had the highest mean overall acceptability score (6.9–7.2) compared to boiled and dried *R. nitidula* (5.1–6.4). The sautéed and dried *R. nitidula* (A) remained acceptable throughout the testing period with a mean overall acceptability score ranging between 6.8 and 7.2, that is, generally liked moderately. Texture was the least liked attribute scoring averagely, 6–7. Majority of the sensory panelists commented that sautéed and dried *R. nitidula* had a golden

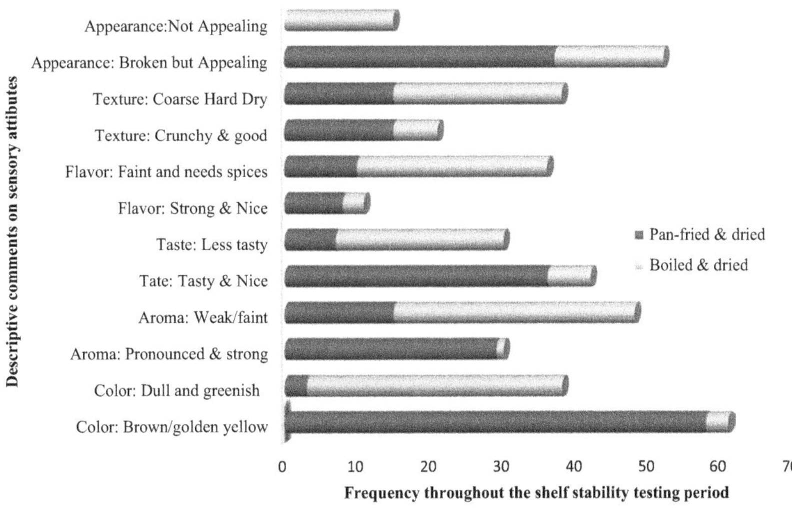

Figure 3. Frequency of descriptive comments given by panelists on each attribute during shelf-life testing of *Ruspolia nitidula*.

yellow appearance, marked/strong flavor, was tasty, coarse and crunchy, and dry/not oily (Fig. 3). Although some liked the crunchiness, they did not like the other texture attributes such as being coarse and dry. These could be the reasons as to why sautéed and dried *R. nitidula* never attained a score of 8 (like very much) or 9 (like extremely). Appearance could have scored less because the sautéed and dried *R. nitidula* were broken. This was due to pressure applied during vacuum packaging of the dried samples. The breakage was worsened by double packing, that is, use of double polyethylene packs, one inserted into another. The double packing was necessary because a single pack was often pierced by the *R. nitidula* mandibles leading to loss of vacuum.

Boiled and dried *R. nitidula* had the least mean overall acceptability scores ranging between the "indifferent" (5.0) to "almost like moderately" (6.6). Notably, all the attributes were initially scored about 7 (like moderately), quite close to the sautéed and dried scores, but by the second week, the scores declined and stabilized at about 5. This trend can be partly explained by panelists' comments about the different sensory attributes. The color of the boiled and dried *R. nitidula* remained greenish and dull. This was disliked by many panelists compared to the brown (golden yellow) color of sautéed and dried *R. nitidula*. This could have influenced the scoring of other attributes as well, because color is known to affect the consumers' perception of all the other sensory attributes (Lawless and Heymann 2010). Color is a key factor in consumers' perception, choice, and preference for food as it predetermines the expected perception of flavor and taste (Socaciu 2007; Lamb et al. 2008). This is probably contributed to the majority of the panelists commenting that boiled and dried R. *nitidula* had a faint aroma and flavor, was less tasty, and not appealing.

In general, the sautéed and dried *R. nitidula* was preferred to the boiled and dried *R. nitidula* because of the differences in color, aroma, taste, and appearance. The difference in preference of the sautéed and dried *R. nitidula* compared to boiled and dried *R. nitidula* can be attributed to the method of preparation and its effect on final product sensory quality. Frying operations normally produce food with an attractive color, well-developed flavor, and good aroma (Keeling and Ridout 2002; Du Toit and Botha 2007), consistent with panelists' comments in Figure 3. Sautéing is most likely to have led to the more pronounced/strong good flavor and aroma, the golden brown color, and good taste.

None of the samples had attribute scores below 5, however, sautéed and dried *R. nitidula* was preferred to boiled and dried *R. nitidula*. Sautéed and dried *R. nitidula* can therefore be improved to eliminate the undesirable coarseness, hardness, and dryness (Fig. 3), possibly by optimizing the drying temperature–time combination. In light of this, there is need to establish a sensory quality specification such as a cut-off point or a defined point on a hedonic scale to cater for product quality and the effects of processing changes on shelf life (Hough 2010).

Microbial stability of *R. nitidula*

Ready-to-eat dried *R. nitidula* remained microbiologically stable during the 12 weeks. The Canadian guidelines for microbiological quality of ready-to-eat foods that need no further preparation prior to consumption recommends a TPC of less than 10^5 log cfu/g for a food to remain acceptable. A similar guideline by the New South Wales state's (2009) permits the same value but for fully cooked foods for immediate sale or consumption. In view of the above criteria, the highest count observed was 3.2 log cfu/g (Fig. 1), a value less than 5 log cfu/g, and hence regarded safe for human consumption. Although the United Kingdom and Hong Kong microbiological criteria recommend the same threshold value (5 log cfu/g), but disregard TPC as an applicable criteria for judging the quality of dried foods (HPA 2009, Centre for Food Safety, Food and Environmental Hygiene Department 2014). The available guidelines are based on meat and fish products, whose nutritional composition (intrinsic environment) differs from that of *R. nitidula* (exemplified by the high protein [36–40%], fat [41–43%], and low carbohydrate [2–3%] contents) implying that also the microbial ecology is different (Ray and Bhunia 2013). There is need therefore to study *R. nitidula*'s microbial ecology and set microbiological limits regarding the different types of microorganisms in ready-to-eat *R. nitidula* that are of concern in guaranteeing its quality and safety as food (King 2013).

Chemical stability of *R. nitidula*

Hydrolytic rancidity results into formation of free fatty acids which can contribute to objectionable doors and flavors (O'Brien 2008). The acid value increased for the first 3 weeks, stabilizing by the 6th week at about 3.2 mg KOH/g of sample. Generally, high acid values above 2 mg KOH/g are correlated with rancidity, since the free fatty acids may have off odors or may undergo auto oxidation to produce off flavors and odors (Fennema 1996; Nielsen 2010).

However, though the amount of free fatty acids was high, rancid flavors or aromas were not detected or reported by the sensory panelists. *Ruspolia nitidula* fat has 41% linolenic acid, 31% palmitic acid, and 13% linolenic acid all of which have carbon atom number greater than 12–14 carbon atoms known to contribute to off flavors upon hydrolysis. Even though the contribution of free fatty acids to autoxidation is insufficient and contradictory, inability of panelists to detect rancid flavors and aromas may not necessarily imply its absence. This is because there was no direct measurement of primary and secondary auto-oxidative products responsible for off flavors and aromas. It is possible that by this time, they existed in lower concentrations than the sensory thresholds detectable by panelists. This possibly explains why FFA is only used to accompany other auto-oxidative and stability measurements. Therefore, in any further attempts to determine shelf life of the highly fatty *R. nitidula*, measurements of primary and secondary oxidation products should be considered.

Conclusion

Ruspolia nitidula is highly nutritious compared to conventional foods and has potential to significantly contribute to food and nutrition security. Proper processing methods can guarantee *R. nitidula* consumers a safe and a tasty product beyond the harvesting season.

Recommendation

There is need to fully profile and characterize the nutrients in *R. nitidula* so as to understand their functionality and bioactivity, as well as characterize its microbial ecology. Alternatives to vacuum packaging should be investigated to better preserve the structure of processed *R. nitidula* products and extend the shelf life beyond the 3 months attained in this work. Primary and secondary oxidation products measurements should be done to directly account for oxidative rancidity and its contribution to sensory quality and stability.

Conflict of Interest

None declared.

References

Ageya, G. J., D. Biryomumaisho, M. Buyinza, and N. G. Nabanoga. 2008. Commercialization of *R. nitidula* (Nsenene Grasshoppers) in central Uganda. Afr. J. Food Agric. Nutr. Dev. 3:319–332.

Alters, S., and W. Schiff. 2011. Pp 600 Essential concepts for healthy living update. Jones & Bartlett Publishers, MA.

Belluco, S., C. Losasso, M. Maggioletti, C. C. Alonzi, M. G. Paoletti, and A. Ricci. 2013. Edible insects in a food safety and nutritional perspective: a critical review. Compr. Rev. Food Sci. Food Saf. 12:296–313.

Bosch, G., S. Zhang, D. G. A. B. Oonincx, and W. H. Hendriks. 2014. Protein quality of insects as potential ingredients for dog and cat foods. J. Nutr. Sci. 29:1–4.

Capinera, J. L. 2008. Pp. 4346 Encyclopedia of entomology. Springer Science+Business Media LLC, Heidelberg, Germany.

Centre for Food Safety Food and Environmental Hygiene Department. 2014. Microbiological guidelines for food; for ready-to-eat foods in general and specific food items. Centre for Food Safety, Food and Environmental Hygiene Department, Queensway, Hong Kong.

Chidumayo, E. N., and D. J. Gumbo. 2010. Pp 304. The dry forests and woodlands of Africa: managing for products and services. Earthscan Publishers, New York, NY.

Du Toit, T., and L.Botha. 2007. Pp. 252 FCS food preparation L2. South African Pearson Press, Cape Town, South Africa.

Durst, B. P., V. D. Johnson, N. R. Leslie, and K. Shono. 2010. Forest insects as food: humans bite back. Pp. 241 Asia-Pacific resources and their potential for development. Food and Agricultural Organization of the United Nations, Chiang Mai, Thailand.

Fellows, P. J. 2009. Food processing technology: principles and practice. Woodhead Publishing, FL

Fennema, O. 1996. Pp. 1067 Food chemistry, 3rd ed. Marcel Dekker Inc. Publishers, New York, NY.

Ferraro, G., and S. Andreatta. 2014. Pp 30 Cultural anthropology: an applied perspective.Cengage Learning, Stamford, CT

Hahn, P. G., and J. L. Orrock. 2015. Land-use history alters contemporary insect herbivore community composition and decouples plant–herbivore relationships. J. Anim. Ecol. 3:745–754

Halloran, A., and P. Vantomme. 2014. Pp. 4 The contribution of insects to food security, livelihoods and the environment. FAO Report. Food and Agriculture Organization, Rome.

Horwitz, W. 2001. AOAC official method 2001.11 protein (crude) in animal feed, forage (plant tissue), grain, and oilseeds. (2000):29–30C.

Hough, G. 2010. Pp. 264 Sensory shelf life estimation of food products. CRC Press, Taylor and Francis Group, FL

HPA, Health Protection Agency. 2009. Guidelines for assessing the microbiological safety of ready-to-eat foods placed on the market. Health Protection Agency, London, U.K.

Keeling, W., and M. Ridout. 2002. Pp. 223 People, places and themes. Heinemann Educational Publishers, Oxford, UK.

Kelemu, S., S. Niassy, B. Torto, K. Fiaboe, H. Affognon, H. Tonnang, et al. 2015. African edible insects for food and feed: inventory, diversity, commonalities and contribution to food security. J. Insects Food Feed 2:103–119.

Kenis, M., N. Kone, C. A. A. M. Chrysostome, E. Devic, G. K. D. Koko, V. A. Clottey, et al. 2014. Insects used for animal feed in West Africa. Entomologia 2:104–114.

Kilcast, David. 2010. Sensory analysis for food and beverage quality control: a practical guide. Woodhead Publishing Limited, Cambridge.

King, H. 2013. Pp 130 Food safety management: implementing a food safety program in a food retail business. Springer Science and Business Media Publishers, NY

Kumar, M. D. 2011. Pp. 567 Pulse crop production: principles and technologies. PHI Learning Pvt. Ltd, New Delhi, India.

Lamb, C., J. Hair, and C. McDaniel. 2008. Pp 672 Essentials of marketing.Cengage Learning Press, OH.

Lawless, H. T., and H. Heymann. 2010. Pp 827 Sensory evaluation of food: principles and practices. Springer Science+Business Media, LLC, New York, NY.

Lenhart, P. A., M. D. Eubanks, and S. T. Behmer. 2015. Water stress in grasslands: dynamic responses of plants and insect herbivores. Oikos 124:381–390.

Martin, D.. 2014. Pp 250. Edible: an adventure into the world of eating insects and the last great hope to save the planet. Houghton Mifflin Harcourt Publishers, New York, NY

Mbabazi, M., Y. B. Byaruhanga, and T. Omara-Alwala. 2009. Proximate composition and effect of processing on fatty acid profiles in edible grasshoppers (*Ruspolia Nitidula*) and white ants (*Macrotermes bellicosus*) in Uganda. Masters' Thesis Report, Kampala: Makerere University.

Mlcek, J., O. Rop, M. Borkovcova, and M. Bednarova. 2014. A comprehensive look at the possibilities of edible insects as food in Europe – a review. Pol. J. Food Nutr. Sci. 3:147–157.

Morales, G. E., and M. Wolff. 2010. Insects associated with the composting process of solid urban waste separated at the source. Revista Brasileira de Entomologia 4:645–653.

Morales-Ramos, J. A., M. Guadalupe Rojas, and D. I. Shapiro-Ilan. 2013. Pp. 711 Mass production of beneficial organisms: invertebrates and entomopathogens. Academic Press, London.

Nielsen, S.. 2010. Pp 620 Food analysis manual. Springer Science+Business Media, LLC Publishers, New York, NY.

O'Brien, R. D.. 2008. Pp 680 Fats and oils: formulating and processing for applications. 3rd ed. CRC Press, Taylor & Francis Group, FL.

Payne, C. L. R., P. Scarborough, M. Rayner, and K. Nonaka. 2015. Are edible insects more or less 'healthy' than commonly consumed meats? A comparison using two nutrient profiling models developed to combat over-and undernutrition. Eur. J. Clin. Nutr.. doi:10.1038/ejcn.2015.149.

Ray, B., and A. Bhunia. 2013. Fundamental food microbiology, 5thed. CRC Press, Taylor and Francis Group, FL.

Rodriguez-Amaya, B. D., and M. Kimura. 2004. Pp. 59 HarvestPlus handbook for carotenoid analysis. International Food Policy Research Institute (IFPRI), Washington DC.

Rumpold, B. A., and K. O. Schluter. 2013. Nutritional composition and safety aspects of edible insects. Mol. Nutr. Food Res. 57:802–823.

Shockley, M., and A. T. Dossey. 2014. Insects for Human Consumption. Pp 617–651 *in* J. A. Morales-Ramos, M. Guadalupe Rojas, D. I. Shapiro-llaneds. Mass production of beneficial organisms: invertebrates and entomopathogens. Academic Press, San Diego

Socaciu, C.. 2007. Pp. 648. Food colorants: chemical and functional properties. CRC Press, Taylor and Francis Group, FL

Van Huis, A., J. Van Itterbeeck, H. Klunder, E. Mertens, A. Halloran, G. Muir, et al. 2013. Pp. 201 Edible insects: future prospects for food and feed security. FAO Publication, Rome, Italy.

15

Removal of cadmium from contaminated *Lentinula edodes* by optimized complexation and coagulation

Yi Wang[1], Chen Wang[1], Wei Cheng[1], Yinbing Bian[2] & Peng Guo[1]

[1]Hubei Academy of Agricultural Sciences, Institute of Agricultural Products Processing and Nuclear Agriculture Technology Research, Wuhan 430064, China
[2]Institute of Applied Mycology, Huazhong Agricultural University, Wuhan 430070, China

Keywords
Cadmium, heavy metal pollution, lentinan, *Lentinula edodes*

Correspondence
Peng Guo, Institute of Agricultural Products Processing and Nuclear Agriculture Technology Research, Hubei Academy of Agricultural Sciences, Wuhan 430064, China.
E-mail: gpeng_2008@cau.edu.cn

Funding Information
This work was supported by the Special Fund for Agro-scientific Research in the Public Interest of China (No. 201303080), the National Key Technology Research and Development Program of China during the 12th Five-Year Plan Period (2012BAD36B05), and Science-Technology Support Plan Projects of Hubei Province (No. 2013BBB06).

Abstract

Heavy metal pollution is a serious problem for *Lentinula edodes*; however, the treatment of contaminated *L. edodes* has seldom been studied. This study investigated the removal of cadmium (Cd) from contaminated *L. edodes* and its lentinan by complexation and coagulation. Some influencing factors, such as pH, medical dosage, and preoxidation were examined. Cd complexation from contaminated *L. edodes* was shown to be more efficient under acidic conditions (pH 5.0), with a clearance rate of 80.47% in 25 mmol/L EDTA and 78.45% in 25 mmol/L sodium citrate. The Cd content in the lentinan of the contaminated *L. edodes* was markedly lower than that in the powdered mushroom (2.77 mg/kg vs. 19.49 mg/kg) and was easier to remove. The maximum Cd clearance rate (96.3%) for lentinan was obtained using an optimized process that involved preoxidation with 0.5 mg/L $KMnO_4$, complexing with 25 mmol/L EDTA and 25 mmol/L sodium citrate, and coagulation with 50 mg/L activated carbon (AC) at pH 10.0.

Introduction

Recently, with rapid industrial development, heavy metal pollution has become an increasing problem, leading to serious food security risks (Campanella et al. 1994). *Lentinula edodes*, commonly known as the shiitake mushroom, is one of the most popular edible mushrooms and the second most cultivated mushroom in the world (Breene 1990). It is highly nutritious with a characteristic fragrance and important medical value (Bisen et al. 2010). Heavy metal pollution is an even more serious problem in *L. edodes* because the mushroom tends to accumulate heavy metals (Melgar et al. 1998; Thomet et al. 1999; Demirbas 2001). It has been documented that *L. edodes* and other saprophytic mushrooms can be used to remove heavy metals efficiently (Gabriel et al. 1996; Melgar et al. 2007; Chen et al. 2008), which reflects the strong heavy metal sorption capability of *L. edodes*. Thus, purifying heavy metal–contaminated *L. edodes* would be a challenging endeavor.

Cadmium (Cd) is one of most notoriously toxic heavy metals and is included in the Environmental Protection Agency's list of priority pollutants (Cameron 1992). It combines with sulfhydryl groups in proteins and inhibits enzyme activity, which is detrimental to humans (Thomet et al. 1999). The famous itai-itai disease in Toyama Prefecture was caused by Cd poisoning (Murata et al. 1971). One recent investigation indicated that over 50%

of the Cd content of the *L. edodes* cultivated in Hubei province of China exceeded the limit (Yang et al. 2014).

Fungal interactions with toxic heavy metals have been investigated previously. It was speculated that accumulation of heavy metals by mushrooms involves two processes. One possible mechanism is the bioaccumulation process in which essential metal ions are substituted by heavy metals (Brunnert and Zadrazil 1985). The other mechanism is biosorption, such as adsorption, ion exchange processes, and complexation with functional groups (Płaza et al. 1996; Mar'in et al. 1997). It has been proposed that one possible way of removing the heavy metals may be to release them through competitive binding by other strong metal-binding agents.

Various methods, such as chemical precipitation (Ku and Jung 2001), ion exchange (Alyüz and Veli 2009), membrane filtration (Landaburu-Aguirre et al. 2009), and adsorption and coagulation using polymer materials (Dias et al. 2007) have been employed for the removal of heavy metal contamination. Complexing agents, such as EDTA (Peters 1999; Zou et al. 2009) and sodium citrate (Gao et al. 2003; Yuan et al. 2007), have been used to leach heavy metals from contaminated soil, and have also been used as food additives. However, many methods are not suitable for purifying contaminated *L. edodes*, for food safety reasons.

Another restriction is the insolubility of the mushroom, which limits the use of an identical insolubility adsorbing material and coagulating agents. Moreover, the complex composition of *L. edodes* makes heavy metal removal challenging. Lentinan is one of the most important active constituent of *L. edodes*, which has many biological effects, such as antiviral, immune regulatory, and antitumor effects, etc. (Sasaki and Takasuka 1976; Zhang et al. 2011).

The aim of this study was to explore processes for removing toxic heavy metal (Cd) from polluted *L. edodes*. Complexing agents (EDTA and sodium citrate) were used to leach heavy metal from contaminated *L. edodes*. Lentinan was then extracted, and complexing and coagulating agents (active carbon, polyaluminium chloride, and chitosan) were applied to remove the heavy metal. Some factors that can affect the binding capacity, such as pH, the dosage of agents used, and the initial valence state of Cd (by addition of oxidant), were investigated in the course of optimizing this process. This work filled the gaps in the study of dealing with heavy metal–polluted mushroom, with regard to potential use in treating of heavy metal–polluted food or medicinal sources.

Materials and Methods

Assays of Cd accumulation by L. edodes

L. edodes (L26) was obtained from the Institute of Applied Mycology, Huazhong Agricultural University, Wuhan, China. It was maintained on a medium containing malt extract (20 g/L), yeast extract (1 g/L), peptone (1 g/L), and glucose (20 g/L). The cultivation substrate contained 80% sawdust, 19% wheat bran, 1% gypsum ($CaSO4{\cdot}2H_2O$), and had a water content of about 60%. $Cd(NO_3)_2$ was added to the cultivation substrate to a final Cd concentration of 0, 0.5, 1, 2, 2.5, 5, 7.5, or 10 (mg/kg dry weight). Twelve replicates were performed for each concentration. Once grown, the mushroom cap was collected for further investigations. Cd contents in the compost and the cap were examined to calculate the Cd enrichment factor, as described in "Determination of Cd concentration".

Determination of Cd concentration

Cd concentrations were determined by atomic absorption spectrometry (AAS) after dry-ashing pretreatment, using a carbon rod atomizer (Gast et al. 1988). Duplicates of *L. edodes* samples were prepared independently.

Treatment of polluted L. edodes to remove Cd

Cd-polluted *L. edodes* was ground in a high-speed disintegrator to a particle size of 800 μm and dried to a constant weight at 55°C. Two grams of *L. edodes* powder was leached using 50 mL deionized water containing disodium-EDTA or sodium citrate at various concentrations, as indicated. After 1 h incubation at 25°C on a rotary shaker at 100 rpm, the mixtures were centrifuged at 12000 g for 10 min. The precipitates were collected, and the Cd concentration was determined after drying to a constant weight. Each sample was prepared in triplicate. The effect of pH was investigated by using different volumes of acid (1 mol/L HCl) or alkali (1 mol/L NaOH) to adjust the pH of the mixture.

Extraction of lentinan

Dried *L. edodes* powder was extracted with deionized hot water (powder:water ratio of 1:25 [v/v]) at 120°C and 0.1 Mpa for 1 h. After centrifuging at 12000 g for 10 min, the aqueous phase was collected and concentrated to about half the initial volume under reduced pressure. Four volumes of precooled 95% ethanol were added to the solution and the mixture was stored overnight at 4°C. The precipitates were collected by centrifugation at 12000 g for 10 min, and then washed with 75% ethanol. The crude lentinan obtained in this way was dried to a constant weight at 55°C (Ye and Jiang 2011).

Treatment of the lentinan to remove Cd

Complexation and coagulation were carried out to remove Cd in the lentinan prior to ethanol precipitation. For complexation, various concentrations of disodium EDTA or sodium citrate were added to the aqueous phase containing the lentinan described in "Extraction of lentinan". After a 1-h incubation at 25°C while shaking at 100 rpm, followed by 20 min centrifugation at 12000 g, the supernatant was collected, ethanol precipitated, and later process was performed as described in "*Extraction of lentinan*". For coagulation, various amounts of activated carbon (AC), polyaluminium chloride (PAC), or chitosan was added to the aqueous phase containing lentinan. After incubation for 1-h incubation at 25°C while shaking at 100 rpm, the coagulation precipitate was removed by 20 min centrifugation at 12000 g, and ethanol precipitation was performed subsequently as described in "*Extraction of lentinan*". The effect of pH, by using 1 mol/L HCl or 1 mol/L NaOH, and the concentrations of the complexation or coagulation agents were investigated.

Preoxidation by $KMnO_4$

The effect of preoxidation was investigated by adding 0.5 mg/L $KMnO_4$ to the aqueous phase described in "Extraction of lentinan", prior to the complexation and coagulation process. Preoxidation was performed at 25°C, for 30 min while shaking at 100 rpm.

Results and Discussion

Cd accumulation by L. edodes

L. edodes has been reported to accumulate heavy metals from the environment (Holan and Volesky 1995; Demirbas 2001). Here, we deliberately contaminated *L. edodes* with Cd by adding Cd to the compost, and investigated the enrichment factor. Figure 1 shows that the Cd content in the *L. edodes* cap and in the compost was significantly positively correlated, corresponding to the formula $y = 3.655x - 0.678$ ($R^2 = 0.997$), in which x was the practical Cd content in the compost and y was the Cd content in the *L. edodes* cap (Fig. 1). This indicated that *L. edodes* had a strong capacity for Cd accumulation. A sample containing 19.49 mg/kg Cd was used in the later Cd removal experiment.

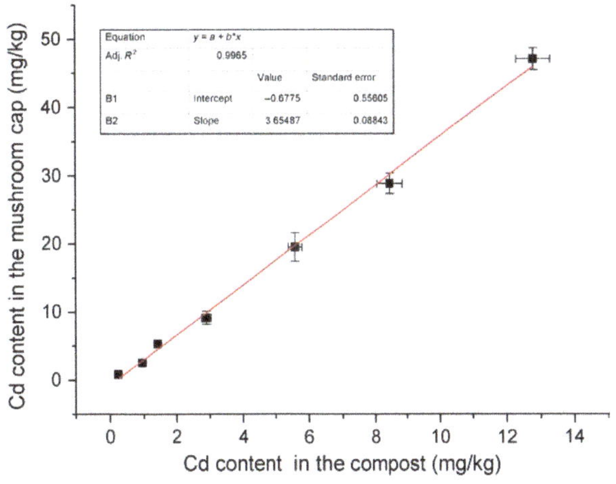

Figure 1. Cadmium (Cd) accumulation by *Lentinula edodes*. Cd was added to the mushroom cultivation substrate to a theoretical value of 0, 0.5, 1, 2, 2.5, 5, 7.5, or 10 mg/kg dry weight. The correlation between the actual Cd content in the compost and the mushroom cap was determined, and it corresponded to the formula $y = 3.655x - 0.678$ ($R^2 = 0.997$). Bars represent the standard deviation of 12 replicates.

Removal of Cd from polluted L. edodes by complexation

EDTA and sodium citrate are known to be efficient chelating agents that can form strong metal-ligand complexes, and they are widely used in restoring heavy metal–contaminated soil (Peters 1999; Gao et al. 2003). In this study, 10 mmol/L EDTA or sodium citrate was used to complex Cd from contaminated mushrooms. As shown in Figure 2, the Cd clearance rate (denoted as the ratio of Cd content of the treated sample to the initial Cd content in the contaminated mushrooms) at pH 7.0 was 72.65% and 68.41% for EDTA and sodium citrate, respectively (Fig. 2).

As it is known that pH is a very important factor affected complexing (EDTA, e.g., $EDTA^{4-} + nH^{+} \leftrightarrow H_nEDTA^{(n-4)+}$ [n = 1, 2, 3, 4]; $EDTA^{4-} + nH^{+} + Cd^{2+} \leftrightarrow CdH_nEDTA^{(n-2)+}$ [n = 0,1]). Moreover, $Cd(OH)_2$ precipitation occurred in an alkaline solution ($Cd^{2+} + 2OH^{-} \leftrightarrow Cd(OH)_2$), which might be adsorbed by the mushroom biomass and may obstruct Cd removal (Basta and Tabatabai 1992; Nastaran et al. 2011). When the effect of pH was examined, including an acidic condition at pH 5.0, a neutral condition at pH 7.0, and an alkaline condition at pH 9.0, respectively, Cd was found to be more easily removed under acidic conditions. At pH 5.0, the Cd clearance rate was the highest; that is, 80.47% in EDTA and 78.45% in sodium citrate. This complemented the report of Melgar and others who found that mushroom biomass could absorb most heavy metal from a solution at an alkaline pH (Melgar et al. 2007).

Extraction of lentinan

So far, we had shown that EDTA and sodium citrate could remove a fair amount of Cd from contaminated mushrooms; however, approximately 20% of the Cd remained, which might exceed the safety limit under heavily polluted conditions. Thus, a more efficient process was needed. Nevertheless, the insolubility of the mushroom

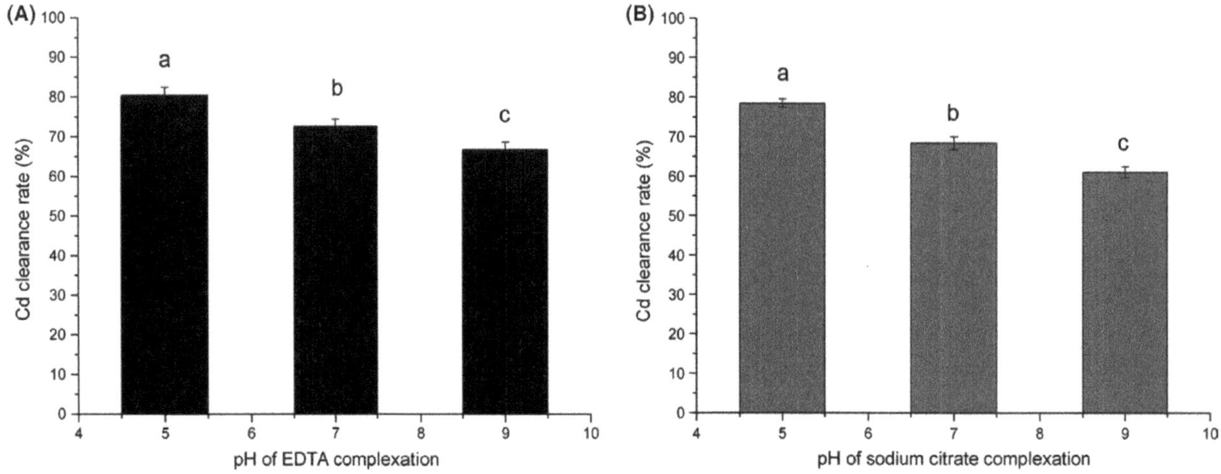

Figure 2. Effect of pH on cadmium (Cd) removal from polluted *Lentinula edodes* by complexation. A solution of 10 mmol/L EDTA (A) or 10 mmol/L sodium citrate (B) was used, and the effect of pH effect on them was detected independently. Bars represent the standard deviation of the set of values. Values (means of three replicates) not sharing common letters are significantly different (one-way ANOVA with the Student-Newman-Keuls method, $P < 0.05$).

powder excluded the use of many insolubility additives that are typically used to remove heavy metals. Moreover, the complex physical structure and multiplicity of functional groups in the mushroom components are the main reason for its heavy metal accumulation (Volesky 2007). Therefore, we speculated that preparing simple soluble components might allow us to address this issue. As lentinan is the most important active constituent of this mushroom, we chose it as a candidate component.

Crude lentinan was extracted as described in "Extraction of lentinan". The Cd content in the lentinan extract was markedly less than that in the mushroom per se (19.49 mg/kg vs. 2.77 mg/kg; data not shown). This indicated that Cd adsorption capacity of the lentinan was lower than that of the mushroom, which might be due to its simple physical structure and low number of functional groups. We then attempted to remove Cd from the lentinan in subsequent experiments.

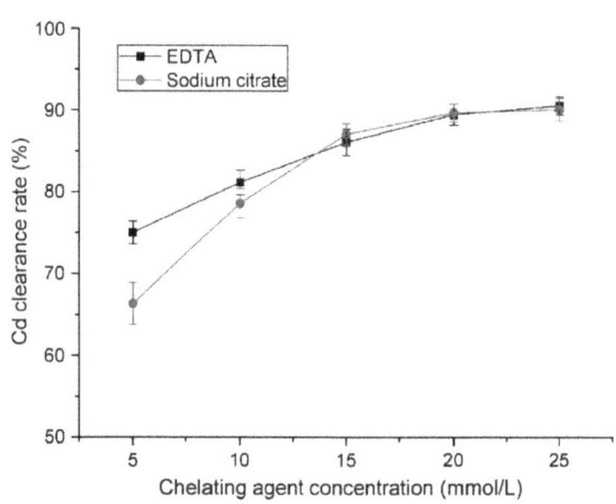

Figure 3. Effect of dosage on cadmium (Cd) removal from lentinan by complexation. The effect of the concentration of EDTA or sodium citrate was examined independently using a concentration series (5, 10, 15, 20, and 25 mmol/L). Means of three replicates are presented, and bars represent the standard deviation of the set of values.

Cd removal of lentinan by complexation

The chelating agents, 10 mmol/L EDTA or 10 mmol/L sodium citrate, were applied individually during lentinan extraction at pH 7.0, and the Cd-chelate complex would remain in the aqueous phase and could be removed from the lentinan after ethanol precipitation. The Cd clearance rate was denoted as the ratio of the Cd content of the treated lentinan to the Cd content of untreated lentinan. We showed that the Cd clearance with 10 mmol/L EDTA and 10 mmol/L sodium citrate in lentinan was 81.10% and 78.58%, respectively (Fig. 3), which was even higher than that in the mushroom powder. This was probably due to the weaker Cd adsorption capacity of lentinan. The mechanism of heavy metal removal was mainly via competitive binding; therefore, it was easier for the chelating agents to compete with lentinan than with the mushroom powder.

Effect of dosage

The effect of the concentration of EDTA and sodium citrate (5, 10, 15, 20, and 25 mmol/L) was examined at pH 7.0. For EDTA, the Cd clearance rate was 74.96% at

5 mmol/L, and clearance was positively correlated with the EDTA concentration. The maximum clearance rate of 90.49% was obtained at an EDTA concentration of 25 mmol/L (Fig. 3). Similar findings were achieved for sodium citrate. At 5 mmol/L sodium citrate, the Cd clearance rate was 66.31%, and this increased as the sodium citrate concentration increased. The maximum clearance rate of 90.01% was obtained at 20 mmol/L sodium citrate (Fig. 3).

Effect of pH

As previously described, pH is a crucial factor that affects the complexing between Cd and chelating agents (Nastaran et al. 2011). The effect of pH was examined individually when various additives were used. As shown in Figure 4, the Cd clearance rate slightly decreased as pH increased from 5 to 7. Zou et al. had studied the pH effect when using EDTA to leach heavy metal from polluted soil, and found that the efficiency of heavy metal removal decreased as pH increased (Zou et al. 2009). Moreover, it has been reported that the heavy metal removal efficiency follows the order of H_4-EDTA > Na_2EDTA > Na_4EDTA (Papassiopi et al. 1999). Thus, it was reasonable that the Cd clearance would decrease from pH 5 to pH 7. However, when the pH was higher than 7, the removal of Cd showed a marked increment. It is known that Cd tends to form a hydroxide, $Cd(OH)_2$, at pH >7 (Basta and Tabatabai 1992). During soil washing, $Cd(OH)_2$ precipitates would be absorbed and will not be removed; however, in our study, lentinan was present in the aqueous phase. Thus, $Cd(OH)_2$ precipitation actually facilitated Cd removal, so that Cd clearance would increase when pH >7. Moreover, the polysaccharide structure is unstable under alkaline conditions (Cintra and Takagi 2015), which may destabilize its binding to Cd. Additionally, it was noted that excessively high alkaline pH should be avoided so as not to damage the lentinan.

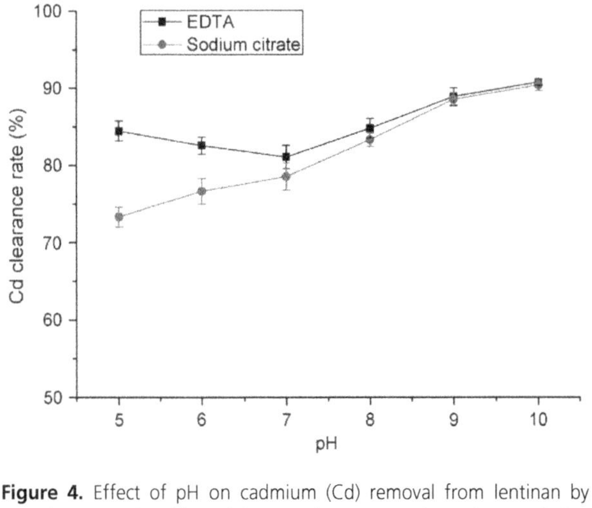

Figure 4. Effect of pH on cadmium (Cd) removal from lentinan by complexation. The effect of the pH of EDTA or sodium citrate solution was examined independently using a pH series (pH 5, 6, 7, 8, 9, and 10). Means of three replicates are presented, and bars represent the standard deviation of the set of values.

The Cd clearance rate of sodium citrate increased with increasing pH in the pH 5–pH 10 range. Other than the effects of $Cd(OH)_2$ precipitation and lentinan stability, these results also corresponded to previous studies on heavy metal chelation by citrate. Citrate (denoted as H_3L) changes from H_3L, H_2L^-, and HL^{2-}, to L^{3-} as the pH increases. HL^{2-} and L^{3-} show greater chelating ability for heavy metals than do H_3L and H_2L^- (Martell and Smith 1977). Thus, the Cd clearance under alkaline conditions in the presence of HL^{2-} and L^{3-} was greater than that under acid conditions in the presence of H_3L and H_2L^-.

Cd removal from lentinan by coagulation

Activated carbon was used as adsorbent because of its large surface area (Jusoh et al. 2007). PAC is a commercial coagulant widely used in wastewater treatment (El-Sikaily et al. 2007). Chitosan is a natural polymer used as a new type of heavy metal flocculant (Bratskaya et al. 2009). These agents were added individually to the lentinan aqueous phase before ethanol precipitation, at pH 7.0. In the process, Cd would be absorbed and coagulated, and then removed by centrifugation. The Cd clearance rates with 90 mg/L activated carbon, 90 mg/L PAC, and 90 mg/L chitosan were 59.21%, 51.87%, and 48.13%, respectively (Fig. 5A). Coagulation agents could thus remove Cd from lentinan. No significant difference was detected between PAC and chitosan (P = 0.142), whereas AC showed the strongest competitive force among these agents. A mixture of AC, PAC, and chitosan showed a Cd clearance rate of 59.3%, which was not significantly different from that achieved by AC alone (P = 1.000). This implied that the mechanisms of action of these agents are likely to be similar and not cumulative. Thus, AC was used as the only coagulating agent in later experiments.

The effect of the concentration of AC was investigated using a concentration series (50, 70, 90, 110, and 130 mg/L); however, the Cd clearance rate was not significantly different (data not shown), which suggested that 50 mg/L was already a saturated concentration of AC for Cd coagulation. We did not investigate concentrations of less than 50 mg/L. The influence of pH on the Cd removing efficiency of AC was also examined. The Cd clearance rate of AC was positively correlated with the pH value (Fig. 5B). Under alkaline conditions, $Cd(OH)_2$ precipitates were absorbed by the AC and facilitated the coagulation process.

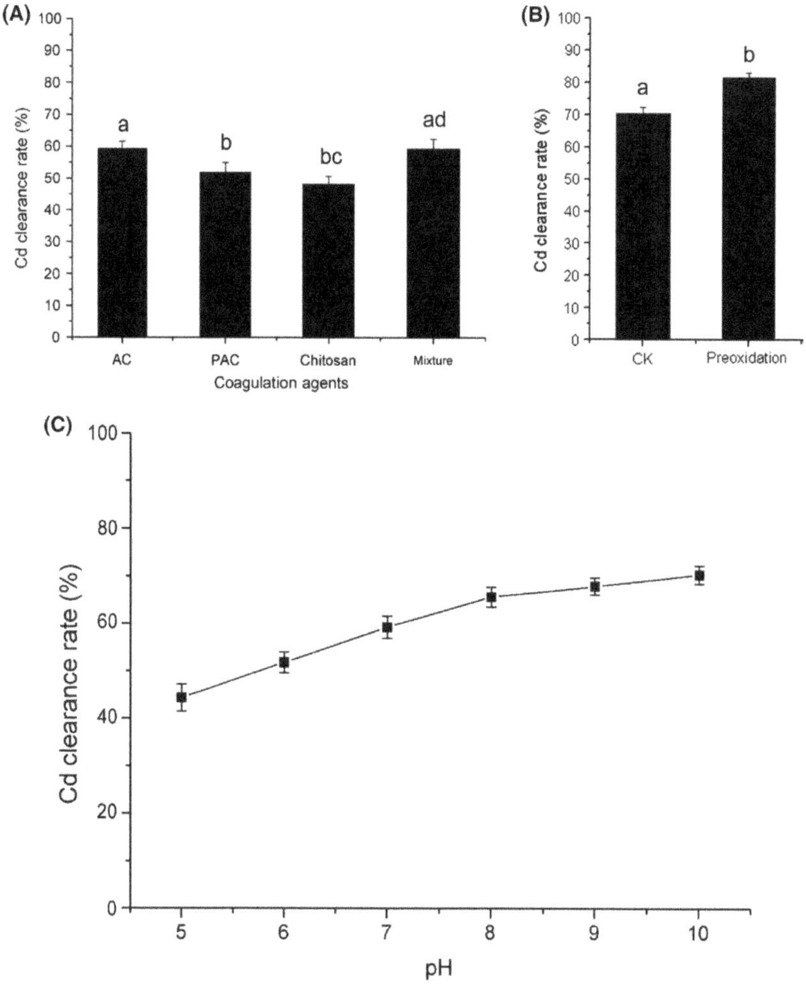

Figure 5. Cadmium (Cd) removal from lentinan by coagulation. (A) Use of different coagulation agents; (B) Effect of different pH (pH 5, 6, 7, 8, 9, and 10); (C) Effect of preoxidizing with 5 mg/L $KMnO_4$. Means of three replicates are presented. Bars represent the standard deviation of the set of values. Values (means of three replicates) not sharing common letters are significantly different (one-way ANOVA with Student-Newman-Keuls method, $P < 0.05$).

Preoxidation is one of the principal methods for improving the coagulation process by destroying the organic coating on the surface of particles. $KMnO_4$ preoxidation was performed prior to coagulation. Figure 5C shows that preoxidation with $KMnO_4$ greatly improved Cd removal by coagulation (from 71.40% to 81.59%). Ma and Li reported that preoxidation is particularly effective for enhancing the coagulation of waste waters with a relatively high organic content (Ma and Li 1993), such as the lentinan solution used here.

However, it was noted that the Cd clearance with AC reached only 81.59% under these optimal conditions. Chang and Gang 2007 also considered that coagulation cannot treat the heavy metal wastewater completely. Therefore, a combination of coagulation and complexation would be a possible way around this problem.

Optimization of lentinan Cd removal

After $KMnO_4$ preoxidation, a combination of chelating agents (25 mmol/L EDTA and 25 mmol/L sodium citrate) and coagulation agents (50 mg/L AC) were used at pH 10.0. The final Cd content in the treated lentinan was 0.10 mg/kg, which was 3.7% of that in the untreated lentinan (2.77 mg/kg) and only 0.5% of that in the initial contaminated mushroom powder (19.49 mg/kg; Fig. 6). The optimized Cd removal process was thus proven to be very efficient.

Conclusions

Here, we implemented new strategies to treat Cd-contaminated *L. edodes*. Complexing agents (EDTA and

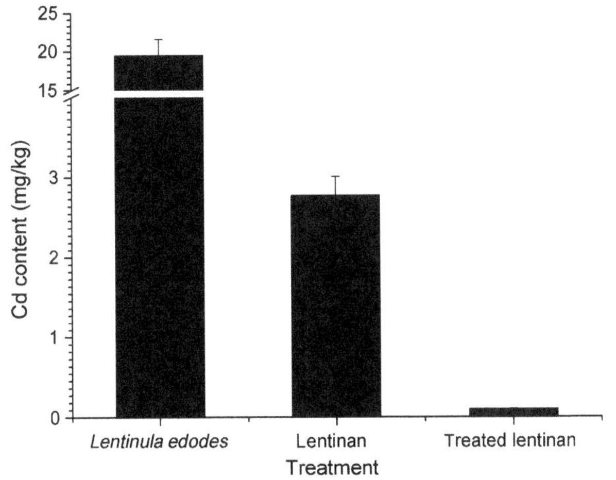

Figure 6. Optimization of lentinan Cd removal means of three replicates are presented. Bars represent the standard deviation of the set of values. Values (means of three replicates) not sharing common letters are significantly different (one-way ANOVA with Student-Newman-Keuls method, $P < 0.05$).

sodium citrate) were used to leach the metal from the contaminated *L. edodes*. The Cd clearance rate was higher under alkaline conditions, and EDTA and sodium citrate were considered competent for general removal of Cd from contaminated *L. edodes* when the Cd concentration was not excessive. For heavily polluted *L. edodes*, extraction of purified lentinan would be a superior approach. Complexing agents (EDTA and sodium citrate) and coagulating agents (AC, PAC, and chitosan) were applied to remove the residual Cd from the lentinan. The Cd extraction efficiency increased with increasing pH in the pH 5–pH 10 range for sodium citrate and all three coagulating agents, whereas it decreased slightly over the range of pH 5–pH 7 and then increased from pH 7–pH 10. In general, an alkaline condition (pH 10) was optimal for Cd removal. Preoxidation with $KMnO_4$ could enhance Cd removal by coagulation. Taking all these findings into consideration, an optimized process was developed for removal of Cd from lentinan, which involved preoxidizing with 0.5 mg/L $KMnO_4$, complexing with 25 mmol/L EDTA and 25 mmol/L sodium citrate, and coagulating with 50 mg/L AC at pH 10.0. The optimized process obtained a Cd clearance rate of 96.3% for the lentinan, and the final Cd content of the treated lentinan was only 0.5% of that in the initial contaminated mushroom (0.10 vs. 19.49 mg/kg). This new strategy for obtaining purified lentinan from contaminated *L. edodes* was demonstrated to be effective, and also indicated that it is advisable to extract purified active ingredients from polluted materials. This study provides a new approach for the treatment of heavy metal–polluted food or medicinal sources.

Acknowledgments

This work was supported by Science-Technology Support Plan Projects of Hubei Province (No. 2013BBB06), the National Key Technology Research and Development Program of China during the 12th Five-Year Plan Period (2012BAD36B05), and the Special Fund for Agro-scientific Research in the Public Interest of China (No. 201303080).

Conflict of Interest

None declared.

References

Alyüz, B., and S. Veli. 2009. Kinetics and equilibrium studies for the removal of nickel and zinc from aqueous solutions by ion exchange resins. Hazard. Mater 167:482–488.

Basta, N. T., and M. A. Tabatabai. 1992. Effect of cropping systems on adsorption of metals by soils: II. Effect of pH. Soil Sci. 153:3.

Bisen, P. S., R. K. Baghel, B. S. Sanodiya, G. S. Thakur, and G. B. Prasad. 2010. *Lentinus edodes*: a macrofungus with pharmacological activities. Curr. Med. Chem. 17:2419–2430.

Bratskaya, S. Y., A. V. Pestov, Y. G. Yatluk, and V. A. Avramenko. 2009. Heavy metals removal by flocculation/precipitation using N-(2-carboxyethyl)chitosans. Colloids & Surfaces A Physicochemical & Engineering Aspects 339:140–144.

Breene, W. M. 1990. Nutritional and medicinal value of specialty mushrooms. J. Food Prot. 53:883–899.

Brunnert, H., and F. Zadrazil. 1985. The influence of zinc on the translocation of cadmium and mercury in the fungus *Agrocybe aegerita* (a model system). Angew Bot 59:469–477.

Cameron, R. E. 1992. Guide to site and soil description for hazardous waste site characterization: Vol. 1. Metals US Environmental Protection Agency (EPA) report 600/4–91/029.

Campanella, L., E. Cardarelli, M. Cordatore, and L. Patrolecco. 1994. Mushrooms as bioaccumulators of pollutants. Med. Fac. Landbouww. Univ. Gent. 59:1883–1886.

Chang, Q., and W. Gang. 2007. Study on the macromolecular coagulant PEX which traps heavy metals. Chem. Eng. Sci. 62:4636–4643.

Chen, G., G. Zeng, L. Tang, C. Du, X. Jiang, and G. Huang. 2008. Cadmium removal from simulated wastewater to biomass byproduct of *Lentinus edodes*. Bioresour. Technol. 99:7034–7040.

Cintra, F. D. O., and M. Takagi. 2015. Study of the chemical stability of the capsular polysaccharide produced

by *Haemophilus influenzae* type b. Carbohydr. Polym. 116:167–172.
Demirbas, A. 2001. Heavy metal bioaccumulation by mushrooms from artificially fortified soils. Food Chem. 74:293–301.
Dias, J. M., M. C. M. Alvim-Ferraz, M. F. Almeida, J. Rivera-Utrilla, and M. Sánchez-Polo. 2007. Waste materials for activated carbon preparation and its use in aqueousphase treatment: a review. Environ. Manage. 85:833–846.
El-Sikaily, A., A. E. Nemr, A. Khaled, and O. Abdelwehab. 2007. Removal of toxic chromium from wastewater using green alga Ulva lactuca and its activated carbon. Hazard Mater 148:216–228.
Gabriel, J., J. Vosáhlo, and P. Baldrian. 1996. Biosorption of cadmium to mycelial pellets of wood-rotting fungi. Biotechnol. Tech. 10:345–348.
Gao, Y., J. He, W. Ling, H. Hu, and F. Liu. 2003. Effects of organic acids on copper and cadmium desorption from contaminated soils. Environ. Int. 29:613–618.
Gast, C. H., E. Jansen, J. Bierling, and L. Haanstra. 1988. Heavy metals in mushrooms and their relationship with soil characteristics. Chemosphere 17:789–799.
Holan, Z. R., and B. Volesky. 1995. Accumulation of cadmium, lead, and nickel by fungal and wood biosorbents. Appl. Biochem. Biotechnol. 53:133–146.
Jusoh, A., L. S. Shiung, and Noor M. J. M. M. AliN. 2007. A simulation study of the removal efficiency of granular activated carbon on cadmium and lead. Desalination 206:9–16.
Ku, Y., and I. L. Jung. 2001. Photocatalytic reduction of Cr (VI) in aqueous solutions by UV irradiation with the presence of titanium dioxide. Water Res. 35:135–142.
Landaburu-Aguirre, J., V. García, E. Pongrácz, and R. L. Keiski. 2009. The removal of zinc from synthetic wastewaters by micellar-enhanced ultrafiltration: statistical design of experiments. Desalination 240:262–269.
Ma, J., and G. Li. 1993. Laboratory and full-scale plant studies of permanganate oxidation as an aid in coagulation. Waterence & Technol. 27:47–54.
Mar'in, A., C. Conti, G. Gobbi. 1997. Sorption of lead and caesium by mushrooms grown in natural conditions. Resour. Environ. Biotechnol. 2:35–49.
Martell, A. E., and R. M. Smith. 1977. Other Organic Ligands. Critical Stability Constants. 3:158–167.
Melgar, M. J., J. Alonso, M. Pérez-López, and M. A. García. 1998. Influence of some factors in toxicity and accumulation of cadmium from edible wild macrofungi in nw spain. J. Environ. Sci. Health B. 33:439–455.
Melgar, M. J., J. Alonso, and M. A. García. 2007. Removal of toxic metals from aqueous solutions by fungal biomass of *Agaricus macrosporus*. Sci. Total Environ. 385:12–19.
Murata, I., S. Nakagawa, T. Hirono, and Itai itai disease. 1971. Saishin igaku. Modern Med. 26:1–2.
Nastaran, M., B. Stéphane, and B. Alain. 2011. Kinetic characterizing of soil trace metal availability using Soil/EDTA/Chelex mixture. Chemosphere 83:997–1004.
Papassiopi, N., S. Tambouris, and A. Kontopoulos. 1999. Removal of Heavy Metals from Calcareous Contaminated Soils by EDTA Leaching. Water Air Soil Pollut. 109:1–15.
Peters, R. W. 1999. Chelant extraction of heavy metals from contaminated soils. J. Hazard. Mater. 66:151–210.
Płaza, G., W. Łukasik, and K. Ulfig. 1996. Sorption of cadmium by filamentous soil fungi. Acta Microbiol. Pol. 45:193–201.
Sasaki, T., and N. Takasuka. 1976. Further study of the structure of lentinan, an anti-tumor polysaccharide from *Lentinus edodes*. Carbohydr. Res. 47:99–104.
Thomet, U., E. Vogel, and U. Krähenbühl. 1999. The uptake of cadmium and zinc by mycelia and their accumulation in mycelia and fruiting bodies of edible mushrooms. Eur. Food Res. Technol. 209:317–324.
Volesky, B. 2007. Biosorption and me. Water Res. 41:4017–4029.
Yang, D. G., Y. Wu, and G. Q. Qiu. 2014. Investigation of the cadmium content in the fruit body of the *Lentinula Edodes* grown in HuBei province. Edible and Med. Mushrooms 22:45–47. Article in China.
Ye, C. L., and C. J. Jiang. 2011. Optimization of extraction process of crude polysaccharides from *Plantago Asiatica* L by response surface methodology. Carbohydr. Polym. 84:495–502.
Yuan, S., Z. Xi, Y. Jiang, J. Wan, C. Wu, and Z. Zheng. 2007. Desorption of copper and cadmium from soils enhanced by organic acids. Chemosphere 68:1289–1297.
Zhang, Y., S. Li, X. Wang, L. Zhang, and P. C. K. Cheung. 2011. Advances in lentinan: isolation, structure, chain conformation and bioactivities. Food Hydrocolloids 25:196–206.
Zou, Z., R. Qiu, W. Zhang, H. Dong, Z. Zhao, and Z. Tao. 2009. The study of operating variables in soil washing with EDTA. Environ. Pollut. 157:229–236.

16

Nutritional quality and sensory acceptability of complementary food blended from maize (*Zea mays*), roasted pea (*Pisum sativum*), and malted barley (*Hordium vulgare*)

Obse Fikiru[1], Geremew Bultosa[2], Sirawdink Fikreyesus Forsido[3] & Mathewos Temesgen[4]

[1]Department of Food Science and Postharvest Technology, Ambo University, Ambo, Ethiopia
[2]Department of Food Science and Technology, Botswana College of Agriculture, Private Bag 0027, Gaborone, Botswana
[3]Department of Postharvest Management, Jimma University, Jimma, Ethiopia
[4]Department of Biology, Ambo University, Ambo, Ethiopia

Keywords
Complementary food, maize, malted barley, proximate composition, roasted Pea, sensory quality

Correspondence
Obse Fikiru, Department of Food Science and Postharvest Technology, Ambo University, Ambo, Ethiopia.
E-mail: obsemaatii@yahoo.com

Funding Information
We would thank CIDA and Jimma University for financial, laboratory, and material support.

Abstract

The aim of this study was to evaluate the effect of blending ratio of malted barley, maize, and roasted pea flour on complementary food quality and sensory acceptability. D- Optimal mixture design was used to generate 14 formulations. Each ingredient had 55–90% maize, 20–35% pea and 4–12% malted barley. Pretreatments like debranning of maize, roasting of pea and dehusking of malted barley were done. The three component-constrained mixture design was conducted using Design-Expert® 6 (Stat-Ease). Ash, protein, fat, fiber, moisture, and carbohydrate contents were found in between range of 1.5–2.5%, 13.0–18.5%, 1.8–2.5%, 3.06–4.45%, 5.0–6.5%, and 68.9–74.1%, respectively. Significant difference ($P < 0.05$) among the treatments was observed for protein, moisture, odor, flavor and sensory overall acceptability. Lack-of-fit was significantly different only for fat ($R^2 = 0.90$). Thus, the model generated can predict all attributes except for fat. The optimum values of high nutrient content and sensory acceptability were observed in the range of 55.0–68.5%, 27.5–35.0%, and 4.0–10.0% for maize, pea, and malted barley respectively.

Introduction

Complementary foods are any nutrient-containing foods or liquids other than breast milk given to young children during the period of complementary feeding (6–24 months) (WHO 2001). The growth of an infant in the first 2 years is very rapid and breast feeding alone will not meet the child nutritional requirements. The ability of breast milk to meet the requirements for macronutrients and micronutrients becomes limited with the increasing age of infants (Agostoni et al. 2008). Thus, timely introduction of complementary foods during infancy is necessary for both nutritional and developmental reasons (Agostoni et al. 2008; Kamchan et al. 2004). However, the capacity of a complementary diet to meet the protein-energy requirements of infants depends on its nutritional quality (Kamchan et al. 2004).

It is well known that high cost of fortified complementary foods in many parts of developing countries is beyond the reach of most families (Amankwah et al. 2009; Muhimbula et al. 2011). Hence, many families depend on inadequately processed and low-quality traditional complementary foods for their children. That is why protein-energy malnutrition is a major infant problem in the developing countries (WHO 2001). Therefore, inadequate complementary food is a major cause for the high incidence of child malnutrition, morbidity, and mortality in many developing countries (Krebs and Westcott 2002). To reduce these problems, low-cost indigenous and unexploited legumes which can be processed and when properly complemented with commonly available carbohydrate sources will provide relatively affordable complementary foods that will help to alleviate protein-energy malnutrition and improve infants' nutrition (Amankwah et al.

2009; Mbata et al. 2009; Muhimbula et al. 2011). Legumes are known to contain lysine in a quantity that exceeds the requirements for human nutrition, but are with the low content of sulfur-containing amino acids (Davidson et al. 1980). According to Davidson et al. (1980), cereals also have sulfur amino acids but, deficient in lysine. A mutual complementation of amino acids and consequent improvement in protein quality is therefore achieved when legumes are blended with cereals in the right proportions (Gibson and Hotz 2001).

In Ethiopian, complementary foods given to infants by mothers or caretakers are deficient both in macronutrients (protein, carbohydrates, and fat) and micronutrients (minerals and vitamins) (Zewditu et al. 2001). Therefore, adequate nutrition and health care during the first 2 years of infant life is very essential to prevent this malnutrition (Temesgen 2013). Some researchers tried to improve these problems, but still the protein-energy-malnutrition remains a serious problem (Zewditu et al. 2001). Generally, the use of low price and locally available foods formulated in the home has high potential to supplement breast feeding. These are also very important to address the limitation of complementary foods in developing countries (Dewey and Brown 2003; Muhimbula et al. 2011). Therefore, here we aim to evaluate the effect of blending a ratio of maize as a source of starch, roasted pea as a source of protein and malted barley as a source of enzymes and carbohydrates on nutritional and sensory quality of complementary foods was evaluated.

Materials and Methods

The experiment was conducted at Jimma University, College of Agriculture and Veterinary Medicine (JUCAVM), Postharvest laboratory in 2012 which is located at the south western part of Ethiopia 345 km from Addis Ababa. Samples were collected from three different organizations. Maize (*Zeamays* var., BH660) (50 kg) was taken from Ethiopian seed enterprise Nekemte Branch, Barley (*Hordium vulgare* var., Miscal 21) (20 kg) and peas (*Pisum Sativum* var.,adi) (30 kg) were from Holota Agricultural research center, Ethiopia.

Sample preparation

Maize, pea and malt barley were processed into their respective flour prior to conducting the experiments as follows.

Maize grain flour production

The maize grain was hand sorted and cleaned. The grains were washed with tap water and rinsed in deionized water and finally soaked for 10 min (Mehra and Eckhoff 1996) and debranned using a traditional Ethiopian wooden pestle and mortar. Thereafter, the bran and grits were dried under the sun for easy separation and to reduce the moisture in the grits. Finally, the grits were grain milled (KARLKOLB D-6072, Dreich, West Germany) and passed through the 0.5 mm sieve. The milled samples were packed in airtight sealed polythene bags and stored in a refrigerator for later use (about 5°C).

Barley grain malt flour production

The barley grains were cleaned manually and sieved to remove impurities and dockages. Malt was prepared under controlled steeping, germination, and kilning conditions as described in Galano et al. (2011). The cured sample was polished to remove the dried rootlets and acrospires and milled (KARLKOLB D-6072, Dreich, West Germany) to pass through the 0.5 mm sieve. The flour was packed in airtight polythene bags and stored in a cool place (about 5°C) until used.

Pea grain flour production

Pea grain was cleaned, sorted, washed in tap water and rinsed with deionized water and soaked in water for two hours (Gibson and Hotz 2001). The soaking water was removed and rinsed with fresh water again and then sun dried. Finally, 100 g of the dried samples was roasted (350°C) on stainless steel iron pan, using an electric heating appliance according to the Ethiopian shiro processing method with some modification, that is, by reducing the roasting time to only 5 min. Then the roasted pea was milled (KARLKOLB D-6072, Dreich, West Germany) to pass through the 0.5 mm sieve, packed in an airtight polythene bags and stored in a cool place (about 5°C) until used.

Experimental design and treatment combinations

The experimental design was generated using D-Optimal mixture design (Table 1) and the constrained region was indicated on Table 2. A mixture design is appropriate when the response depends on the component proportions of the mixture and not on the component quantities. The treatment consists of three mixtures: 55 < maize <90, 20 < pea <35, and 4 < malted barley <12 (maize + pea + malted barley = 100%). Accordingly, 14 samples as treatment combinations were generated.

Proximate composition analysis

Nutritional composition of the experimental flour: moisture, crude fat, crude protein, crude fiber, and total ash

Table 1. Ratios obtained by mixture design for the fourteen formulations of flour.

Run	Maize (%)	Pea (%)	Barley (%)
1	67.5	24.3	8.2
2	55.0	35.0	10.0
3	61.0	35.0	4.0
4	61.0	35.0	4.0
5	76.0	20.0	4.0
6	68.0	20.0	12.0
7	68.5	27.5	4.0
8	59.0	31.3	9.0
9	63.0	28.6	8.4
10	76.0	20.0	4.0
11	72.0	20.0	8.0
12	61.0	26.5	12.0
13	55.0	35.0	10.0
14	68.0	20.0	12.0

Table 2. Constraint region of maize, pea, and barley taken by mixture design.

Low	≤Constraint	≤High
0.55	≤A: Maize	≤0.95
0.20	≤B: Pea	≤0.35
0.04	≤C: Barley	≤0.12

A + B + C = 1.

were determined, using the AOAC Official Method Nos: 925.09, 4.5.01, 979.09, 962.09, and 923.03, respectively (AOAC 2000). The total carbohydrate was determined by FAO, 1998 was included in the reference list difference (FAO, 1998) based on the following formula. Results were expressed per 100 g of the flour.

Carbohydrate (%) = 100 − (% Protein + % Moisture + % Crude fat + % Crude fiber + % Ash).

Sensory analysis

Porridge was prepared from flour to water ratio (1:3), 10 g sugar was also added to all samples (Owino et al. 2007) and worked to uniform consistency for about five 5 min. The product was assessed for their color, texture, flavor, odor, and overall acceptability on 5- point hedonic scales.

Statistical analysis

The three component constrained mixture design was conducted using Design-Expert® 6 (Stat-Ease) Minneapolis MN, USA. Regression models, contour plot, and response surface were obtained using Minitab 16 statistical package. The significance test was set at $P < 0.05$. The fitted models for all parameters were generated in three-dimensional contour plots. Graphical optimization was done to determine the optimum formulation point of maize, pea, barley, and carrot flour.

Results and Discussion

Proximate composition of the complementary foods

The moisture content, crude protein, crude fiber, crude fat, ash, and carbohydrate content of the complementary food flour formulations ranged between 5.0–6.6%, 13.0–18.5%, 3.06–4.45%, 1.8–2.5%, 1.5–2.5%, and 68.9–74.1% respectively (Table 3). Except for fat, the lack-of-fit was not significantly different ($P < 0.05$) (Table 4).

Moisture content

The moisture content for the 14 treatments of complementary food samples was ranged between 5.0 and 6.6%. The highest moisture content was recorded in blend of 76% maize, 20% pea and 4% malted barley while the least moisture content was observed in blend of 55% maize, 35% pea and 10% malted barley (Table 3). Moisture content was increased when the proportion of maize increased and roasted pea decreased in the blend. Our finding is in the range of Nelson (1992) who reported 3–8% of moisture content as a quality factor for the food prepared from cereals. It is also very close to that of Amankwah et al. (2009) report (5.0–6.0%) who formulated complementary foods from fermented maize, rice, soybean and fishmeal. However, the result is below the Ahmad et al. (2008) report (7.2–8.7%) who formulated complementary food from wheat and soybean flour. However, our result is slightly greater than the recommended moisture content (<5%) by CODEX CAC/GL 08. 1991) except in the blend of 55% maize, 35% pea and 10% malted barley flour. This may be because of steeping and drying methods employed during the preparation of flour (Gausman et al. 1951).

Crude protein content

The protein content for the 14 treatments of complementary food samples had ranged from 13.0–18.5%. The highest protein content was recorded in blend of 55% maize, 35% pea, and 10% malted barley and the least was found in 76% maize, 24% pea, and 4% malted barley blend. Protein content was increased with increasing of pea and decreased with increasing of maize proportion in the blend (Table 3). The result is similar with Saeeda et al. (2009) who reported 14.4% of crude protein from rice, mong, potato and poppy seeds blend; 17.5% crude protein from wheat, pea, cabbage and groundnut blends, and 14.5% of crude protein from maize, lentil, carrot, and sesame blend. But, the result is less than that of Ijarotimi and Keshinro (2012) report (23.85–28.84%) who

Table 3. Proximate composition and energy contents of the 14 different complementary food flour formulations.

Ingredients in a mixture (%)				Proximate composition						
Run	M	P	B	MO %	CP%	CF%	Fat%	Ash%	CHO%	Energy (kcal/100 g)
1	67.5	24.3	8.2	5.8	14.0	4.1	2.4	1.9	72.2	366.4
2	55.0	35.0	10.0	5.0	18.0	3.5	1.8	2.3	69.5	366.2
3	61.0	35.0	4.0	5.4	17.00	3.26	2.1	2.5	69.16	365.15
4	61.0	35.0	4.0	5.4	17.05	3.21	2.1	2.5	69.10	365.11
5	76.0	20.0	4.0	6.4	13.0	3.4	2.5	1.6	73.2	367.3
6	68.0	20.0	12.0	5.6	13.8	4.0	2.2	1.5	74.1	371.0
7	68.5	27.5	4.0	5.9	15.0	3.8	2.2	2.5	71.2	364.4
8	59.0	31.3	9.7	5.2	16.0	3.4	2.0	2.4	71.1	366.4
9	63.0	28.6	8.4	5.5	15.5	3.1	2.1	2.0	72.4	370.5
10	76.0	20.0	4.0	6.5	13.0	3.3	2.5	1.6	73.4	368.2
11	72.0	20.0	8.0	6.0	13.5	3.7	2.5	1.5	73.1	368.4
12	61.5	26.5	12.0	5.5	14.5	3.8	2.1	1.5	72.6	367.5
13	55.0	35.0	10.0	5.0	18.5	3.3	1.9	2.4	68.9	366.7
14	68.0	20.0	12.0	5.6	13.8	4.0	2.2	2	72.7	365.6

M, maize; P, pea, B, barley; MO, moisture; CP, crude protein; CF, Crude fat; CHO, total carbohydrate.

Table 4. Predicted model for the proximate content analysis.

Approximates	Model	R^2 value
Moisture	$Y = 7.9X_1 - 5.79X_2 + 26.58 X_3 + 11.76X_1X_2 - 41.88 X_1 X_3 + 1.95X_2 X_3$	0.987
Crude protein	$Y = 16.4 X_1 + 106.9 X_2 - 60.5 X_3 - 138.5 X_1X_2 + 96.1 X_1 X_3 - 27.9X_2 X_3$	0.988
Flavor	$Y = 4.06X_1 + 10.29X_2 - 39.3X_3 - 12.24X_1X_2 + 46.34 X_1 X_3 + 59.55X_2 X_3$	0.997
Overall acceptability	$Y = 4.12X_1 + 8.11X_2 - 12.39X_3 - 8.27X_1X_2 + 12.23 X_1 X_3 + 40.01X_2 X_3$	0.958

X_1 = maize, X_2 = Pea and X_3 = Barley.

formulated from germinated and fermented popcorn but, higher than that of Bojňanská et al. (2012) report (12.57–16.28%) who formulated from wheat, lentil and chickpea flour (10–50%). The difference could be due to the difference in blending ratio and crop types used during the formulation. According to Gibson and Hotz (2001), blending of cereal-based foods and their processing methods can improve the protein content of the flour. The required daily allowance for protein contents in the complementary foods is ≥15% (WHO/ FAO 2004). However, in our finding, this result can be satisfied when the proportion of pea in the blend is greater than 27%. This suggests that increasing of the pea can improve the protein content of complementary processed foods (Barac et al. 2010).

Crude fat

The fat content for the 14 treatments of complementary food samples had ranged from 1.8 to 2.51%. The highest fat content was recorded in the blend of 76% maize, 20% pea and 4% malted barley and the least was found in 55% maize, 35% pea and 10% malted barley blend ratios. The crude fat content was increased with the increasing of maize and decreased with the increasing of malted barley proportion in the blend (Table 3). The result is similar with that of Ghavidel and Davoodi (2011) who reported 1.36% crude fat in complementary food processed from Wheat and Green gram, and 1.27% crude fat from Wheat and Lentil seed flour composites. However, the result is lower than that of Solomon (2005) report (11.5–24.8%) who processed complementary food from rice, maize, acha grains, soya beans, bambara nut, benniseed, carrot, garden egg, and crayfish. In addition, our result is less than the daily recommended fat content in complementary foods range from 10 to 25% (WHO/ FAO 2004). This is may be due to the differences in crop types used and the processing methods employed during the formulation of the flour. For instance, the processing methods (removal of outer part of maize and germ) have significant effect on reduction in fat content (Arif et al. 2011). In case of our finding, increasing the maize content can improve the fat content of complementary processed food.

Crude fiber

The crude fiber content in the complementary food processed was ranged from 3.1–4.1%. The high crude fiber content was recorded in the blended ratio of 67.5% maize, 34.3% pea and 8.2% malted barley while the least fiber content was recorded in 63% maize, 28% pea and 8.4% malted barley blended ratio (Table 3). This is similar with the investigations of Hussain et al. (2012) who reported fiber content from 1.36–1.81% in a formulation of wheat and lentil-based complementary food flour. The daily recommended allowance of crude fiber in the complementary food is <5%. Thus, all the complementary foods processed in this study meet this requirement.

Total ash

The total ash content in the complementary foods processed was ranged in between 1.5% and 2.5%. The highest ash content was recorded in the blended ratio of 61% maize, 35% pea and 4% malted barley and least ash content was observed in 72% maize, 20% pea and 8% malted barley blends respectively (Table 3). The ash content has increased with increasing the proportion of pea in the blend. Similar results were reported by Bojňanská et al. (2012) and Gibson and Hotz (2001) when legumes (lentil and chick pea) are included into cereal-based complementary foods. All the complementary foods processed in this study meets the recommended ash content by WHO/FAO (2004) in the complementary food (<5 g/100 g).

Carbohydrates

The carbohydrate contents in the complementary food processed had ranged from 68.9–74.1%. The highest carbohydrate content was observed in the blended ratio of 68% maize, 20% pea and 12% malted barley. The least carbohydrate content was seen in the blended ratio of 55% maize, 35% pea and 10% malted barley (Table 3). With the increasing of maize content in the blend, the carbohydrate content was found to be increased. Processing method like dehusking may increases carbohydrates content in the diet (Abiodun and Adepeju 2011). Similar results were reported by Elemo et al. (2011) and Hussain et al. (2012) who reported 63.7%–77.4% of carbohydrate content in complementary food processed from sorghum and cowpea, and 61.24–70.73% from wheat and lentil composite flour, respectively. All the complementary foods processed in this work meet the carbohydrate content recommended by WHO/ FAO (2004) in the complementary food (≥65 g/100 g).

Energy

The energy (caloric) content of the 14 complementary foods processed was ranged between 364.4–371.0 kcal/100 g. The highest energy content was observed in 68.5% maize, 27.5% roasted pea and 4% malted barley blended ratio and the least energy content was observed in the blend of 68% maize, 20% roasted pea and 12% malted barley (Table 3). Energy content increased with the increasing of malted barley in the complementary processed food. Similar result (376.23–376.27 kcal/100 g) was reported by Hussain et al. (2012) who formulated complementary food from wheat and lentil composite flour. However, the result is less than the recommended energy content by WHO/ FAO (2004) in the complementary foods (400–425 kcal/100 g). This may be due to the less fat content of the raw materials used in the formulation of the food.

Sensory evaluations

Sensory attributes of the blended flour products were assessed by 50 untrained panelists. Of these, 18 were mothers and females of reproductive age of Jimma University. The score values were found in between range of 3.51–4.10, 3.59–4.20, 3.69–4.30, 3.00–4.20 and 3.68–4.25 for odor, flavor, texture, color, and overall acceptance of the porridge, respectively (Table 5). Lack-of-fit for all sensory attributes were not significant ($P \geq 0.05$) and the model is predictable.

Odor

The sensory score of odor for the 14 treatments of complementary food samples had ranged from 3.51 to 4.10. The highest score was recorded in the blending ration of 55% maize, 35% roasted pea and 10% malted barley, and the least score was found in 76% maize, 20% roasted pea, and 4% malted barley (Table 5).

Flavor

The flavor acceptance of complementary processed food was found in between 3.58 and 4.20%. The highest flavor acceptance was scored in 55% maize, 35% roasted pea, and 10% malted barley composite and the least was scored in 76% maize, 20% roasted pea, and 4% malted barley blended ratio (Table 5). The flavor acceptance was increased when the proportion of pea was increased and maize was decreased. These could be because of release of flavor compounds by nonenzymatic (Maillard and caramelization) reactions during roasting of pea (Muhimbula et al. 2011). The process enhances the acceptability of porridge made from roasted flour, because of dextrinization, and starch breakdown (Mensah and Tomkins 2003). Germination is also known to enhance flavor acceptability of food products (Inyang and Zakari 2008).

Color

The color acceptance of complementary processed food in this study was found in range of 3.65–4.30%. The

Table 5. Sensory analysis of the 14 different complementary food flour porridges.

	Ingredients in a mixture (%)			Sensory evaluation result on 5-point hedonic scale				
Run	M	P	B	Texture	Odor	Color	Flavor	Overall acceptability
1	67.50	24.30	8.20	3.80	3.80	3.76	3.77	3.83
2	55.00	35.00	10.00	4.20	4.00	4.20	4.20	4.45
3	61.00	35.00	4.00	3.60	3.80	4.05	3.86	3.94
4	61.00	35.00	4.00	3.59	3.80	4.00	3.85	3.93
5	76.00	20.00	4.00	3.00	3.51	3.69	3.59	3.68
6	68.00	20.00	12.00	3.70	3.86	3.75	3.65	3.80
7	68.50	27.50	4.00	3.50	3.66	3.92	3.68	3.82
8	59.00	31.30	9.70	4.00	3.89	4.02	4.00	4.19
9	63.00	28.60	8.40	3.58	3.85	3.94	3.87	3.98
10	76.00	20.00	4.00	3.00	3.51	3.70	3.60	3.69
11	72.00	20.00	8.00	3.50	3.76	3.65	3.70	3.75
12	61.50	26.50	12.00	3.75	3.82	3.9	3.82	3.98
13	55.00	35.00	10.00	4.00	4.10	4.30	4.18	4.25
14	68.00	20.00	12.00	3.72	3.87	3.67	3.66	3.77

M, maize; P, pea, B, barley.

highest color acceptance was recorded in 55% maize, 35% roasted pea, and 10% malted while the least color acceptance was recorded in 70% maize, 20% roasted pea, and 8% malted barley blended ratio (Table 5). Color acceptance of the porridge was increased with the increasing of proportion of roasted pea in the composite flour. Similar results were reported by Pelembe et al. (2002) who studied sorghum– cowpea instant porridge by extrusion cooking.

Texture

The texture acceptance of the porridge of complementary processed food was found in the range of 3.00–4.20%. The highest texture acceptance was recorded in the composite flour of 55% maize, 35% roasted pea and 10% malted barley blended ratio and the least was recorded in 76% maize, 20% roasted pea, and 4% malted barley blended ratio (Table 5). The highest texture acceptance was recorded when the proportion of malted barley and roasted pea increased. This may be because of roasting and malting effects in the processing of pea and barley. According to Shim and Lim (2013), cooking and mixing cereals with legumes increases the porridge texture.

Overall acceptability

The overall acceptability of the 14 treatments of complementary food samples had ranged from 3.68 to 4.45. The highest score had recorded in the proportion of 55% maize, 35% roasted pea, and 10% malted barley blended ratio and the least score was observed in 76% maize,

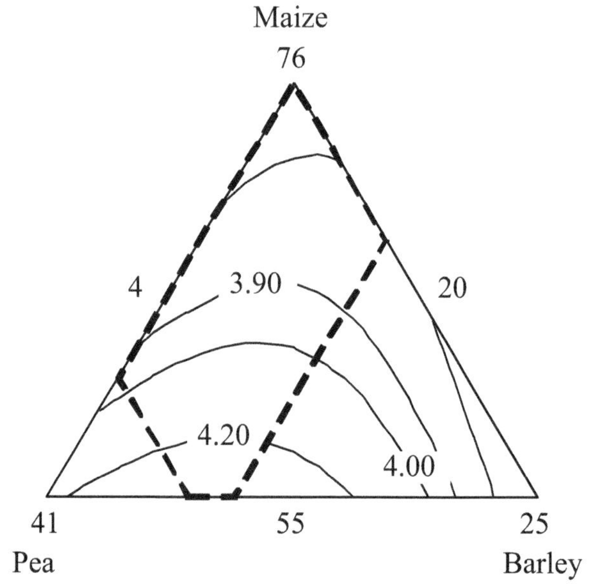

Figure 1. Mixture contour plot of overall acceptance.

20% roasted pea, and 4% malted barley blended ratio (Table 5). The overall sensory acceptability of the porridge increased with the increasing of roasted pea (Fig.1). This result was in agreement with the investigations of Mbata et al. (2009) who reported high overall acceptability of complementary processed food formulated from maize–bambara ground nut. Compaore et al. (2011) also stated that the porridge from composite flour is organoleptically acceptable by the panelists in addition to its nutrient improvement.

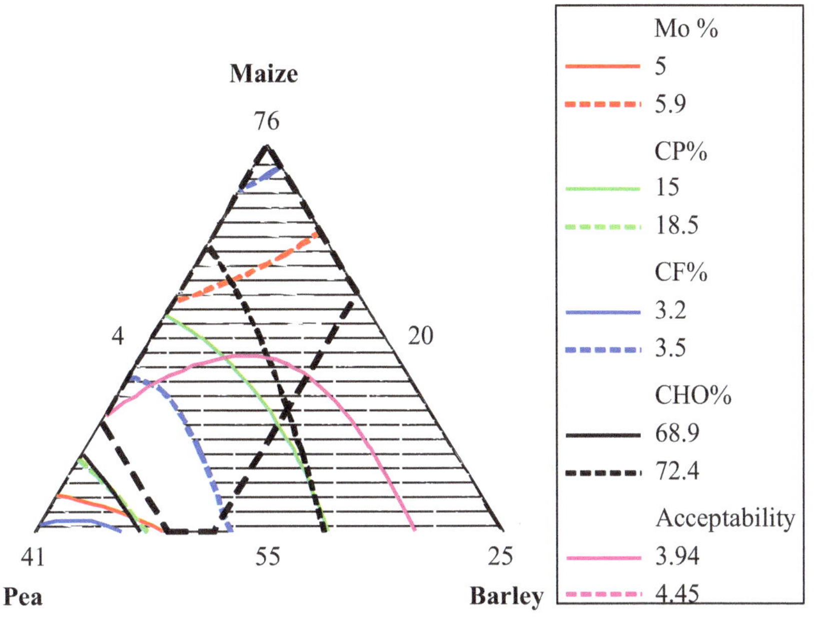

Figure 2. Overlaid contour plot of moisture content, protein, crude fiber, carbohydrate, and overall acceptability.

Superimposition of proximate composition and overall acceptability

This study focused on determining the optimal formulation ratio of individual food source that can be suited to produce flour with desirable nutrient compositions. In order to determine the optimum formulation, the regions of acceptability in the contour plot for moisture content, protein, crude fiber, carbohydrate, and overall acceptability sensory attribute were superimposed looking at the daily recommendation of WHO/FAO (2004) for complementary foods. The sweet point of complementary food blended in this study (5.0–5.9% for moisture content, 15.0–17.5% for protein, 3.2–4.1% for fiber, 68.9–72.4% for Carbohydrate, and 3.94–4.45 for overall acceptability) was found in the flour samples prepared within the range of 55.0–68.5% for maize, 27.5–35.0% for roasted pea, and 4–10% for malted barley, respectively (Fig. 2).

Conclusions

Based on our finding, the total moisture content, crude protein, crude fiber, crude fat, ash and carbohydrate of the complementary food flour had ranged between 5.3–5.7%, 13–18.5%, 3.06–4.45%, 1.8–2.5%, 1.5–2.5% and 68.9–74.1%, respectively. The sensory acceptability was found in between 3.51–4.10, 3.59–4.20, 3.69–4.30, 3.00–4.20, and 3.68–4.25 for odor, flavor, texture, color and overall acceptance of the porridge. In general, the optimum nutrient quality of the complementary food prepared from the flour of maize, pea, and malted barley was found to be in the range of 55.0–68.5% maize, 27.5–35.0% pea, and 4–10% malt barley. Such blending would lead to the complementary food contents to have 5.0–5.9% moisture content, 15.0–17.5% crude protein, 3.2–4.1% fiber, 68.9–72.4% carbohydrate content, and 3.94–4.45 of the overall acceptability.

Acknowledgments

The authors acknowledge the Ethiopian seed enterprise Nekemte Branch, Ambo University, and the Holota Agricultural Research Center for their assistance by granting seeds used for the study. We also thank CIDA and Jimma University for financial, laboratory, and material support. Finally, all authors in this study are duly acknowledged.

Conflict of Interest

None declared.

References

Abiodun, A. O., and A. B. Adepeju. 2011. Effect of processing on the chemical, pasting and anti-nutritional composition of Bambara Nut (*Vigna subterranea* L. Verdc) Flour. Adv. J. Food Sci. Technol. 3:224–227.

Agostoni, C., F. Marangoni, G. Stival, I. Gatelli, F. Pinto, P. Rise, et al. 2008. Whole blood fatty acid composition differs in term vs. mildly preterm infants: small versus matched appropriate for gestational age. Pediatr.Res. 64:298–302.

Amankwah, E. A., J. Barimah, R. Acheampong, L. O. Addai, and C. O. Nnaji. 2009. Effect of fermentation and malting on the viscosity of maize-soyabean weaning blends. Pak. J. Nutri. 8:1671–1675.

AOAC. 2000. Official methods of analysis. Vol. 2, 17th edn., Official Methods 923.03, 923.05, 4.5.01, 925.09, 962.09 and 979.09, Gaithersburg, Md. publisher, Washington, DC.

Arif, M., J. A. Bangash, F. Khan, and H. Abid. 2011. Effect of soaking and malting on the selected nutrient profile of barley. Pak. J. Biochem. Mol. Biol. 44:18–21.

Barac, M., S. Cabrilo, M. Pesic, S. Stanojevic, and O. Macej. 2010. Profile and functional properties of seed proteins from six pea(*Pisum sativum*) genotypes. Int. J. Mol. Sci. 11:4973–4990.

Bojňanská, T., H. Frančáková, M. Líšková, and M. Tokár. 2012. Legumes – the alternative raw materials for bread production. J. Microbiol. Biotechnol Food Sci. 1:876–886.

Compaore, W. R., P. A. Nikiema, H. I. N. Bassole, A. Savadogo, D. J. Hounhouigan, J. Mouecoucou, et al. 2011. Nutritional properties of enriched local complementary flours. Adv. J. Food Sci. Technol. 3:31–39.

Davidson, S., S. Passmore, J. F. Brock, and A. S. Truswell. 1980. Human nutrition and dietetics. Churchill Livingstone, New York. Pp. 213–215.

Dewey, K. G., and K. H. Brown. 2003. Update on technical issues concerning complementary feeding of young children in developing countries and implications for intervention programs. Food Nutr. Bull. 24:5–28.

Elemo, G. N., B. O. Elemo, and J. N. C. Okafor. 2011. Preparation and nutritional composite of a complimentary food formulated from germinated sorghum (*Sorghum bicolor*) and steamed cooked cowpea (*Vigna unguiculata Walp*). Am. J. Food Technol. 6:413–421.

FAO. 1998. Carbohydrates in human nutrition. Report of a Joint FAO/WHO Expert Consultation. FAO Food and Nutrition Paper No.66. Rome, Italy.

Galano, T., G. Bultosa, and C. Fininsa. 2011. Malt quality of 4 barley (*Hordeum vulgare* L.) grain varieties grown under low severity of net blotch at Holetta, West Shewa, Ethiopia. Afri. J. Biotechnol. 10:797–806.

Gausman, H. W., J. H. Ramser, G. H. Diungan, F. R. Earle, M. M. Macmasters, H. H. Hall, et al. 1951. Some effects of artificial drying of corn grain. American society of plant biologists, 27(4):794–802.

Ghavidel, R. A., and M. G. Davoodi. 2011. Processing and assessment of quality characteristics of composite baby foods. World Acad. Sci. Eng. Technol. 59:2041–2043.

Gibson, R. S., and C. Hotz. 2001. Dietary diversification/ modification strategies to enhance micronutrient content and bioavailability of diets in developing countries. Br. J. Nutr. 85:S159–S166.

Hussain, M. S., M. Anjam, B. Uddin, and M. Hanif. 2012. Preparation and evaluation of complementary diets from germinated wheat and lentil for Bangladeshi children. Pak. J. Sci. 64:304–308.

Ijarotimi, O. S., and O. O. Keshinro. 2012. Formulation and nutritional quality of infant formula produced from germinated popcorn, Bambara groundnut and African locust bean flour. J. Microbiol. Biotechnol. Food Sci. 1:1358–1388.

Inyang, C. U., and U. M. Zakari. 2008. Effect of germination and fermentation of pearl millet on proximate, chemical and sensory properties of instant fura- A Nigerian cereal food. Pak. J. Nutr. 7:9–12.

Kamchan, A., P. Puwastien, P. P. Sirichakwal, and R. Kongkachuichai. 2004. In vitro calcium bioavailability of vegetables, legumes and seeds. J. Food Comp. Anal. 17:311–320.

Krebs, N. F., and J. Westcott. 2002. Zinc and breastfed infants: if and when is there a risk of deficiency? Adv. Exp. Med. Biol. 503:69–75.

Mbata, T. I., M. J. Ikenebomeh, and S. Ezeibe. 2009. Evaluation of mineral content and functional properties of fermented maize (Generic and specific) flour blended with Bambara groundnut (*Vigna subterranean* L). Afri. J. Food Sci. 3:107–112.

Mehra, S. K., and S. R. Eckhoff. 1996. Single stage short-duration tempering of corn for dry-milling. Cereal Chem. 74:484–488.

Mensah, P., and A. Tomkins. 2003. Household-level technologies to improve the availability and preparation of adequate and safe complementary foods. Food Nutr Bulle. 24:104–125.

Muhimbula, H. S., A. Issa-Zacharia, and J. Kinabo. 2011. Formulation and sensory evaluation of complementary foods from local, cheap and readily available cereals and legumes in Iringa, Tanzania. Afri. J. Food Sci. 51:26–31.

Nelson, S. S. 1992. P93—96, 137–148, 113–115.Introduction to the chemical analysis of foods. International Thomson Publishing, New York.

Owino, V. O., M. Sinkala, B. Amadi, A. Tomkins, and S. M. Filteau. 2007. Acceptability, storage stability and costing of α-amylase-treated maize-beans-groundnuts-bambaranuts complementary blend. J. Sci. Food Agri. 87:1021–1029.

Pelembe, L. A. M., C. Erasmusw, and J. R. N. Taylor. 2002. Development of a protein-rich composite sorghum-cowpea instant porridge by extrusion cooking process. Lebensm Wiss technol. 35:120–127.

Saeeda, R., N. S. Muhammad, M. Amer, S. Noumann, N. Khalid, and A. Muhammad. 2009. Preparation and quality evaluation of nutritious instant baby food from indigenous sources. Pak. J Agri. Res. 22:50–55.

Shim, S. M., and S. Y. Lim. 2013. Texture properties and radical scavenging ability of porridge products based on beans, grains, and nuts. J. Korean Appl. Biol. Chem. 56:77–82.

Solomon, M. 2005. Nutritive value of three potential complementary foods based on cereals and legumes. Afri. J. Food Agri. Nutri. Dev. 5:1–14.

Temesgen, M. 2013. Nutritional Status of ethiopian weaning and complementary foods: a review. Open Access Sci. Report 2:1–9.

WHO. 2001. P.34.Complementary feeding: report of the global consultation, and summary of guiding principles for complementary feeding of the breastfed child. Convened jointly by the Department of Child and Adolescent Health and Development and the Department of Nutrition for Health and Development, WHO Library Cataloguing-in-Publication Data, Geneva.

WHO/ FAO. 2004. Human vitamin and mineral requirements. Report of a joint FAO/WHO consultation, Bangkok, Thailand. Rome: Food and Agriculture Organization of the United Nations (FAO) and World Health Organization (WHO).

Zewditu, G., U. Kelbessa, G. Timotewos, and N. Ayele. 2001. Review of the status of malnutrition and trends in Ethiopia. Ethiopian J. Health Develop. 15:55–62.

17

Consumers' preferences for fresh yam: a focus group study

Carla Barlagne[1], Denis Cornet[2], Jean-Marc Blazy[1], Jean-Louis Diman[1] & Harry Ozier-Lafontaine[1]

[1]UR1321 ASTRO Agrosystèmes tropicaux, INRA, Petit-Bourg (Guadeloupe) F-97170, France
[2]UMR AGAP, CIRAD, Petit-Bourg (Guadeloupe) F-97170, France

Keywords
Consumer profile, focus groups, food quality, sectorial innovation, the Caribbean, yam *(Dioscorea sp.)*

Correspondence
Carla Barlagne, UR1321 ASTRO Agrosystèmes tropicaux, Domaine de Duclos, F-97170 Petit-Bourg (Guadeloupe), France.
E-mail: carla.barlagne@antilles.inra.fr

Funding Information
The first author benefited from a PhD Grant co-financed by the European Union (Fonds Social Européen), the Guadeloupe Regional Council and the INRA social science division.

Abstract

In West and Central Africa and in the Caribbean, yam is one of the most important sources of carbohydrates and has a great potential to improve food security. The yam production sector is, however, now challenged by the satisfaction of evolving consumers' preferences. Since little is known about consumers' preferences regarding yams' characteristics, product quality, and the drivers of yam purchase, six focus group discussions were conducted (for a total of 31 participants). Among the purchasing criteria, price was considered more important than the others. It was followed by the external damage, the origin, and the size of the tuber. The most frequently cited consumption criteria were the taste, the texture, and color of flesh after cooking. Taste was considered more important than the other criteria. Three consumers' profiles were established reflecting heterogeneity in preferences, especially as concerns the willingness to pay for yam and consumption habits. They were designated as the Hedonistic, the Thrifty and the Flexible. Our results suggest that innovations can be implemented to sustain and stimulate the development of the yam sector in Guadeloupe. Two main development paths were identified. The first path is the valorization of the great existing diversity of yam varieties and the increase in the level of information for consumers about product attributes such as the cooking mode, the origin, and the mode of production. Building a marketing strategy based on the valorization of this diversity can help maintain and preserve yam's agro-biodiversity and the satisfaction of rapidly evolving consumption habits. The second path is the definition of yam ideotypes that suit consumers' needs. We expect that tailoring the production to consumers' needs will have a positive impact on global food security in the Caribbean region.

Introduction

Yam (*Dioscorea* spp.) is a major source of food for millions of people in tropical and subtropical areas of the world and especially in West and Central Africa where it contributes to the income and food of more than 60 millions of people (Asiedu and Sartie 2010). In West and Central Africa and in the Caribbean, yam is one of the most important sources of carbohydrates to many people and is considered a food security crop. Global projections for root and tuber crops foresee an increase in its economic importance, through the increase in both the production and demand (Scott et al. 2000; Alexandratos and Bruinsma 2012).

Despite its nutritious value (Bradbury and D Holloway 1988) and its major contribution to the daily calorie intake of the population (Asiedu and Sartie 2010), little is known about consumers preferences regarding yams' characteristics and product quality. However, awareness has been raised that a greater integration of consumers preferences in the design of new crop management systems is necessary if sustainable food systems are to be built (Selfa et al. 2008; Rastoin and Ghersi 2010; Tsolakis et al. 2014). This question is all the more crucial, as rural exodus and fast growing urbanization are changing peoples' way of life and consumption habits. Since rural food production may strongly depends on consumers and end markets in urban areas (Campbell et al. 2009), the yam production sector is therefore challenged by the satisfaction of these evolving consumers' preferences (Hounhouigan et al. 2003; Amegbeto et al. 2008). Taking into account consumers' preferences for fresh yam can have two important implications for building sustainable food sectors. First, at the production level, it may help designing new crop varieties and crop management systems that simultaneously satisfy the needs of the farmers and the consumers' preferences (Hounhouigan et al. 2003; Amegbeto et al. 2008). Second, it may also have implications at the market level for identifying the relevant information about the product and the quality attributes that have to be given to consumers.

The aim of the study presented in this paper is to identify consumer preferences for fresh yam through focus groups. The study is conducted in Guadeloupe, a tropical island in the Caribbean where yam has a strong cultural value (Dulcire 2005) and represents the first food crop (Agreste 2009a; Agreste 2009b). Yam production is however declining, since it was 26,700 tons in 1970 and is now about 7 000 tons. The yam sector in the French West Indies has faced many hurdles that hindered its development: 1) high sensitivity to pests and diseases at the field scale (Ano et al. 2005; Arnolin and Lombion 2005); 2) long-lasting soil pollution by chlordecone, a persistent pesticide, making root and tuber production conditional to strict controls on the final level of contamination of the harvested organs (Cabidoche and Lesueur-Jannoyer 2012), and 3) poor organization of the actors within the sector. Guadeloupe relies heavily on imports for 80% of its food supply (Chambre d'Agriculture de la Guadeloupe 2014) and in order to enhance food security, research is conducted to increase the sustainability of the yam sector. Research aimed to target the biotic constraints by selecting varieties resistant to the major diseases (Onyeka et al. 2006). Although resistant and high-yield varieties have been developed, they have not been appreciated by consumers (AGRESTE 2009a,b). As a consequence, farmers have not adopted them. Therefore, a sound assessment of consumer expectations regarding yam characteristics needed to be performed.

Material and Methods

Pilot study

In a pilot study, five local experts were asked to describe the main yam varieties that can be found in Guadeloupe as well as to enumerate purchasing and consumption criteria. Among those five experts were: a cook used to experimenting new yam-based meals; two geneticists and a technician involved in yam breeding programs; and one agricultural advisor involved in participatory selection of yam testing varieties with farmers. All of them had a deep knowledge and experience of yam and were all yam consumers and purchasers. In total, those experts listed 10 purchasing and four consumption criteria. Purchasing criteria included: cooking time, cooking mode, maturity, shape, variety, freshness, origin, size, price, and external damage. Consumption criteria included: color of flesh after cooking, fibrousness, texture of flesh after cooking, and taste.

Focus group discussions

We used focus group discussions because they were identified as an efficient method to elicit the drivers of consumer choices and explore new product concepts (van Kleef et al. 2005). Focus group discussions allow access to a wealth of information and insights regarding an issue, providing a platform for interaction between the participants within a limited period of time (Morgan 1997; Kitzinger et al. 2004). They are used in market research and sensory analysis to assess consumers behaviors and perceptions (Lee and Lee 2007; Boquin et al. 2014), their attitudes toward new type of food (Wan et al. 2007; Barrios et al. 2008; Chung et al. 2011) or to define consumers' preferences regarding product quality (Cardinal et al. 2003). They provide qualitative information at the early stages of product development and are often used prior to laboratory and quantitative consumer tests, like sensory assessment and conjoint analysis (Chung et al. 2011; Boquin et al. 2014). At those early stages, they give access to participants' perceptions of new products that they describe in their own words and meanings. To this end, they provide useful information for the design of appropriate questionnaire and protocol in this field of research.

Subjects

Six focus group discussions were conducted that accounted for a total of 31 participants. The discussions lasted one hour, and each group consisted of a maximum of six participants to give people sufficient time to express themselves. The conditions for taking part in the focus groups were to be a yam consumer and purchaser. Participants were recruited at the National Institute for Agronomic Research following an email that was sent to all the employees. Participation to the focus group discussion was volunteer and not paid for. Participants were informed about the conditions for participating in the email. Participants were selected irrespective of socio-economic profiles. There were 15 women and 16 men; ages ranged between 24 and 58; and household size varied from one to six persons. We ensured participants that the results of the study would remain anonymous and would be used for the sole purpose of this study. Additionally, results of the study were fed back to the participants on two occasions.

The number of focus group discussions to be conducted was determined by the principle of data saturation: we stopped doing focus groups when we could obtain no further insight into the different themes from an additional focus group (Krueger and Casey 2009).

Procedure

One moderator led the focus group discussions, and one observer kept record of the interactions between participants and of the eventual leadership phenomenon during the discussions. The moderator was trained to do focus group discussions as part of her academic curriculum and had already conducted focus group discussions in previous studies (Barlagne 2006, 2007; unpublished). Additionally, before undertaking the study reported here, she validated the methodology and guide of interview with a consultant in polls and opinions surveys, and attended a focus group discussion led by the consultant. The observer also helped in the logistics generated by the discussions by handling the recording device and the material used as support during the discussions. The moderator used a semistructured interview guide to conduct the discussions and maintained a consistent flow of discussion while allowing the flexibility to discuss the themes raised by participants (Krueger and Casey 2009). The themes addressed in the interview guide were related to consumer behavior, purchasing and consumption criteria, the warranty regarding the origin and the mode of production of yams, and the quality of yams. The moderator followed the usual guidelines and animation techniques (Morgan 1997; Kitzinger et al. 2004; Krueger and Casey 2009)to ensure equal participation of the informants in the discussions and to avoid censoring. In particular, in an introductory phase, participants were informed about the objectives of the focus group discussions, and the moderator insisted on the fact that there were no right or wrong answers. The layout of the interview guide is presented in Table 1.

Yam tubers were used as supporting examples for the discussions after the results of the pilot study. The tubers were purposely chosen for their contrasting characteristics (variety, size, shape, weight, origin, and mode of production) to provoke participant reactions and stimulate the discussion. Participants could examine and handle the tubers. A description of the different varieties used as supporting examples for the focus group discussions or mentioned by the participants during the discussions is provided in Table 2.

The list of 10 purchasing and four consumption criteria that had previously been elicited in the pilot study was presented into a questionnaire to the participants at the end of the focus group discussions. They were first asked to select the criteria they considered important at the purchasing and consumption stages. Each participant was asked to fill out the questionnaire individually. The resulting frequencies of selection gave an understanding of the criteria that count in absolute terms for the participants. Thereafter, they were asked to rank purchasing and consumption criteria from the most important to the least important. This allowed an understanding of the relative importance of the criteria for the participants. The relative importance of the criteria was normalized as expressed in the Data Analysis section. Expressing frequencies and relative importance as percentages allowed a better comparison of the importance of the criteria in the two cases.

Table 1. Layout of the interview guide.

Introduction
1.1 Welcoming and introducing the research team
1.2 Definition of the topic of discussion
1.3 Introduction to the rules of focus groups
1.4 Taping and recording of the focus group
Warm-up and qualification of the panel of participants
2.1. State your name and describe your experience with yams
2.2. Habits regarding yam purchasing and consumption
a) How often do you eat yams?
b) Where do you buy yams?
Probing questions (yam tubers are used as supporting examples for the discussion)
3.1. Purchasing and consumption criteria
a) What do you think of these yams?
b) Would you purchase them? Why? Why not?
c) What do you think is important at the purchasing stage? Discuss each criterion.
d) What do you think is important at the consumption stage? Discuss each criterion.
3.2. Warranty on the origin and the mode of production
a) Do you care about the mode of production of yams? Why? Why not?
b) Do you care about the origin of yams? Why? Why not?
c) Would you be in favor of a warranty for the origin of yams? For the mode of production?
d) How much would you be willing to pay for it?
3.3. Definition of the quality of yams
a) What do you think is a good quality yam?
b) What do you think is a bad-quality yam?
c) Can you find good-quality yams on the market?
Conclusion
4.1. Filling out the questionnaire (individually)
a) Tick the criteria that you think are important at the purchasing and consumption stages.
b) Rank the purchasing and consumption criteria in order of decreasing importance.
4.2. Thanking participants for their involvement and concluding the discussion

Table 2. Perception of YAM varieties by local experts.

Local name	Scientific name of the specie	Colour of the flesh after cooking	Size	Fibrosity	Texture of the flesh after cooking	Cooking time	Origin	Taste	Mode of production
Kabusah	*Dioscorea alata*	White	Medium	Not Fibrous	Tender	8 to 10 min	Local or imported	Neutral	Conventional
Anba bon	*Dioscorea alata*	White to light brown	Medium or big	Fibrous	Tender and pasty	8 to 10 min	Local	Wild	Conventional
Pas Possible	*Dioscorea esculenta*	White	Small	Not Fibrous	Tender	8 to 10 min	Local	Slightly sweet and refined	Conventional
Adon	*Dioscorea bulbifera*	Grey	Small	Not Fibrous	Firm	20 to 30 min	Local	Bitter	Conventional
Cousse Couche	*Dioscorea trifida*	White	Small	Not Fibrous	Tender	8 to 10 min	Local or imported	Slightly sweet and refined	Conventional
Igname Jaune	*Dioscorea rotundata*	Yellow	Big	Not Fibrous	Firm	20 to 30 min	Local	Bitter	Conventional
Grosse caille	*Dioscorea cayenensis*	White	Medium	Not Fibrous	Firm	20 to 30 min	Local or imported	Neutral	Conventional

Focus group discussions were recorded with a video recorder. This device was important for clarifying the moments when participants designated the yam tubers for each of the activities during the discussions. We completed the focus group discussions with a sociodemographic questionnaire to keep a record of their characteristics.

Data analysis

Analysis of the focus group transcripts

The focus group discussions were fully transcribed using video records and field notes. Coding and analysis of the transcripts was performed using the content analysis software NVivo10 (QSR International, Melbourne, Australia). The codes resulted from the original research question and hypothesis and from recurring themes that emerged during the focus group discussions. The data were coded according to 14 main themes that ranged from the appreciation of yams to questions of traceability. The themes and their definition are given in Table 3.

Content analysis was performed on all themes. The "Purchasing and Consumption Criteria" theme contained 14 categories that related to the criteria that the participants selected in the questionnaire.

Consumers' profiles were established following content analysis of the theme "Attitude toward the price of yam". Transcripts coded under this theme related to participant opinions about the price of yam, their purchasing behavior, and strategies. For each profile identified, we examined the frequencies and relative importance of the purchasing and consumption criteria. We also proceeded to the content analysis of the themes "origin," "mode of production," and "traceability" to understand the heterogeneity in perception and interest in those themes. Additionally, queries were run using the "Matrix Coding Query" tool available in the software to examine the intersection between themes or between a theme and participant profiles. This allowed understanding a theme within differentiated categories.

Analysis of the questionnaire results

The frequency and the relative importance of each criterion were calculated from the questionnaire data. The frequency of a criterion was calculated as the percentage of participants selecting the criterion. The relative importance of a criterion j was $\bar{I}_j\%$, computed as in the following: $\bar{I}_j\% = 100\frac{\sum_{i=1}^{n} r_{ij}}{\sum_{j=1}^{c}\sum_{i=1}^{n} r_{ij}}$, where n is the number of participants, c is the number of criteria, and r_{ij} is the rank attributed to the criteria by participant i, $\bar{I}_j\%$ varying between 0% (i.e., the least important criteria) and 100% (i.e., the most important criteria).

Table 3. Themes highlighted in the focus group discussions and their definition.

Themes	Definition
Appreciation of yam	Consumers opinion on yam. How much they like it and how much they buy it
Procurement	How consumers get to eat yams. Which marketing chains or gift chains they go through to get yams
Attitude toward price	What consumers think of the price of yam, how they react to it when they intend to buy yam. Type of adjustments they make towards the price
Contamination by pollutants	Whether consumers are suspicious about the contamination of yam by chlordecone or not and how they adapt to it in their purchasing behavior
Knowledge of the product	Whether consumers know different varieties of yam and how they describe them
Conservation	How consumers keep yams and how the different varieties can be kept
Purchasing and consumption criteria	Criteria consumers take into account when they purchase and/or eat yams
Easiness of peeling	Easiness of peeling of the different varieties
Time of consumption	Time of the year or time of the week when people eat yams. Type of celebration they associate yams with
Losses	Losses associated with the peeling of yam or with damages caused by bugs and how consumers related to those losses
Yam quality	Definition of the quality of yams by the participants
Yam status	Perception of yam as a dish and as a cultural food product Importance in consumption habits
Processing	Type of processing of yam by the participants and their opinion about processed yams
Traceability	What do consumers think of traceability and whether they do their purchases in relation to it

Results

Purchasing and consumption criteria

Figure 1 represents the Frequency and Relative Importance ($\bar{I}_j$%) of the purchasing (1) and consumption (2) criteria of the participants.

Ten purchasing criteria were cited by participants (Fig. 1A). The most frequent criteria were the external damage and price, both of which were selected more than 80% of the time. Four more criteria were cited more than half the time: the size, the origin, the freshness, and the variety. The last criteria considered important were the cooking mode and the cooking time. Among the purchasing criteria, price was considered more important than the others ($\bar{I}$=24%). It was followed by the external damage ($\bar{I}$=17%), the origin ($\bar{I}$=15%), and the size ($\bar{I}$=12%). Price and origin were given a higher relative importance than the external damage and the size, respectively, though they were cited fewer times than those criteria.

Four consumption criteria were cited by the participants (Fig. 1B). The most frequent criteria were the taste and the texture of flesh after cooking, both of which were cited more than 80% of the time. The other two criteria, the fibrousness and the color of flesh after cooking, were cited more than 50% of the time. Among the consumption criteria, taste was considered more important than the other criteria with a relative importance ($\bar{I}$=53%). The texture of the flesh after cooking was considered the second most important criterion ($\bar{I}$=29%). The color of the flesh after cooking was given a higher importance than the fibrousness although it has been cited less.

Definition of the quality of yams and sensory preferences

Participants defined the quality of yams with a set of eight attributes (or criteria) that referred exclusively to the visual and sensory characteristics. Table 4 presents these attributes and their definition according to the participants.

The external damage is the only frequently cited criterion that made consensus (i.e., many people viewed the external damage as important, and all agreed on the expected product). The absence of external damage was associated with a healthy product in the mind of the participants, and a broken yam tuber or one that had external signs of insect bites prompted suspicion of possible rotting inside the tuber. Participants defined the other attributes using a range of values. For example, they expressed their taste preferences using not less than five different words, some of them referring to the usual taste descriptors (sweet, bitter, neutral) and some reflecting particular individual perceptions of the taste (wild and refined). To illustrate their perceptions of the taste of yam, participants referred to specific yam varieties: "the anba bon *(D. alata)* was perceived as having a wild taste" whereas "the taste of the *pas possible (D. esculenta)* was perceived as refined". The attribute "wild" recalled a woody taste while the attribute "refined" echoed to a sensation of delicacy.

Preferences for the texture were firm or tender, the common requirement being a good density of the piece of yam. Participants disliked a piece of yam that crumbles in the pan during cooking. Two yam varieties were specifically mentioned as having a firm texture: the *igname jaune*, otherwise known as the *yellow yam (D. cayenensis)*, and the *grosse caille*, otherwise known as the *white yam*

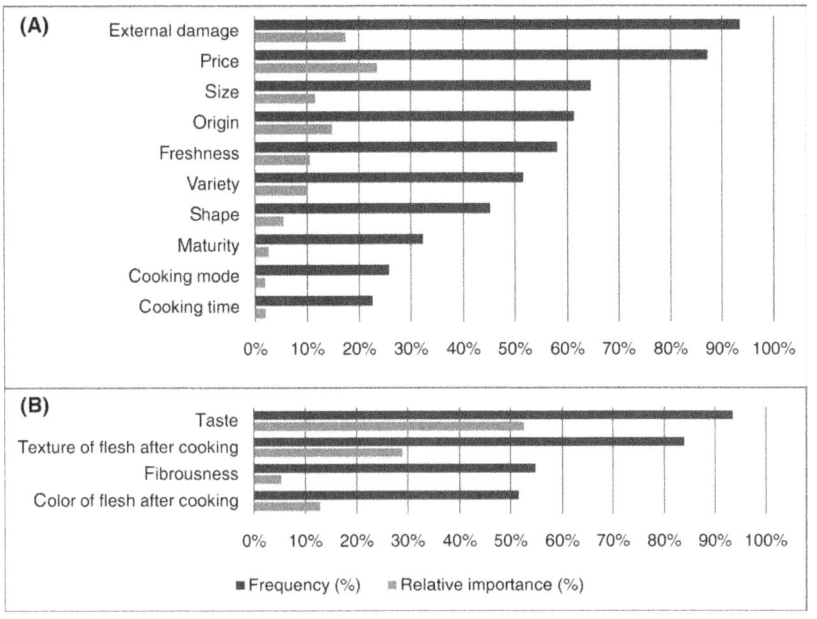

Figure 1. Frequency and relative importance ($\bar{I}$%) of the purchasing (A) and consumption (B) criteria of the participants. Frequency of the criteria represents the number of times the criteria were cited by the participants while Relative Importance represents the ranking of the criteria by the participants

Table 4. Perception of the quality of yams according to the participants (*N* = 31).

Attributes	Good-quality yam	Bad-quality yam
Sensory attributes		
Taste	Sweet, bitter, neutral, refined, wild	Undefined
Texture of flesh after cooking	Firm or tender but dense	Lack of consistency; yam that crumbles during cooking; yam that is too firm when cooled
Fibrousness	Absence of fibers	Presence of fibers
Color of flesh after cooking	Plain and clear; white or yellow	Presence of black spots or rotting; brownish; grayish
Visual attributes		
External damage	Healthy external aspect of the tuber	Presence of external damage; presence of insect bites; broken yam
Size	Small, medium, big	Undefined
Shape	Regular that facilitates the peeling	Crooked shape that entails losses when peeling
Maturity	Tuber little wrinkled, big or brown-colored; presence of buds	Tuber white-colored

(D.rotundata). Participants mentioned that these two varieties were suitable for consumption when freshly cooked but that they tended to become too hard to eat (therefore not suitable for consumption) when cooled. Additionally, the participants established the suitability of the different varieties for different modes of cooking according to texture. Thus, they stated that firm varieties were suitable for fries or gratin, while the tender varieties were more suitable for puree. They considered that both types of texture were suitable for boiling, but that the cooking time had to be adjusted to the type of texture (longer for the firm varieties). In terms of the size, the participants preferred to buy yam tubers suitable for only one meal, in general lunch. They did not eat yams for the evening meal nor on the following day because they believed that yams did not keep well.

Consumer profiles

Based on purchasing and consumption criteria, three main profiles emerged among the participants. The first two profiles were distinct: the participants were either Hedonists (23% of the participants) or Thrifty people (42% of the participants). Participants in the third profile had a mixed and changing attitude. We designated this group as Flexible (35% of the participants).We would like to draw attention to the fact that the proportions of different profiles are only indicative of the present sample and that they, by no means, intend to be representative of the global population of yam consumers. They simply reveal that different consumers' profiles do exist which are relevant in terms of market segmentation. Figure 2 represents the Frequency of the purchasing (Fig. 2A) and consumption (Fig. 2B) criteria for the different profiles of the participants, while Figure 3 represents the Relative Importance of the purchasing (Fig. 3A) and consumption (Fig. 3B) criteria according to the different profiles of the participants.

The Hedonists (23% of the participants)

Except for the first criteria (external damage) and the last three criteria (maturity, cooking mode and cooking time), the distribution of the frequencies of the purchasing criteria differed in this group from that of the whole sample. The external damage and the origin were cited more frequently than the price and the shape, respectively, but they were given a lower relative importance ($\bar{I}_J$%). As for the other criteria, the $\bar{I}_J$% they were given by the participants reflected their frequencies (i.e., the criteria were ranked in the same order after their relative importance as well as their frequencies).

Considering the $\bar{I}_J$% of the purchasing criteria, the Hedonists placed the emphasis on the price first ($\bar{I}$=23%), then on the freshness ($\bar{I}$=17%), the external damage ($\bar{I}$=14%), and the size ($\bar{I}$=12%). As for the consumption criteria, the distribution of the frequencies was similar to that of the whole sample. In spite of the fact that the relative importance of the consumption criteria reflected their frequencies, the Hedonists emphasized the taste over the other criteria ($\bar{I}$=62%).

The Hedonists found that local yams were expensive, particularly when out of the production season, but they declared that the price had no importance. "Very often, the price does not mean anything… I mean… from the moment I have decided that I want to eat yam, the price does not interest me anymore". "If I go somewhere and I buy yams and I find them good, then I'll go back to buy some more and I will not pay attention to the price". They would pay a higher price for yams in four cases: 1) the quality of the yam is perceived to be better, 2) a willingness to eat yams from organic farmers, 3) a commitment to sustaining local farmers "I buy from guadeloupean farmers and I probably pay more for it. I don't ask myself questions about it. I has never been a problem for me and I think it's good to buy from local farmers" and/or 4) greater purchasing power "Yam is not that expensive still…at 3 to 4 €/Kg, it is not a luxury product. Sometimes, you will buy tomatoes at 7€/Kg. Then it starts to be expensive but as long as it is 3 to 4 €/Kg, it does not seem expensive for me. It's what you cook yam with, that makes it expensive. It might be the fish that you cook alongside that is expensive". The participants were aware of the price hierarchy that exists between the yam species on the Guadeloupean market, and they justified this by the fact that they thought that some of them had superior sensory characteristics. "It's true that if there is some *cousse-couche (D. trifida)*, then I will buy it. It's priceless. Of course it depends on the quantity, but if it's the *cousse-couche,* I'll

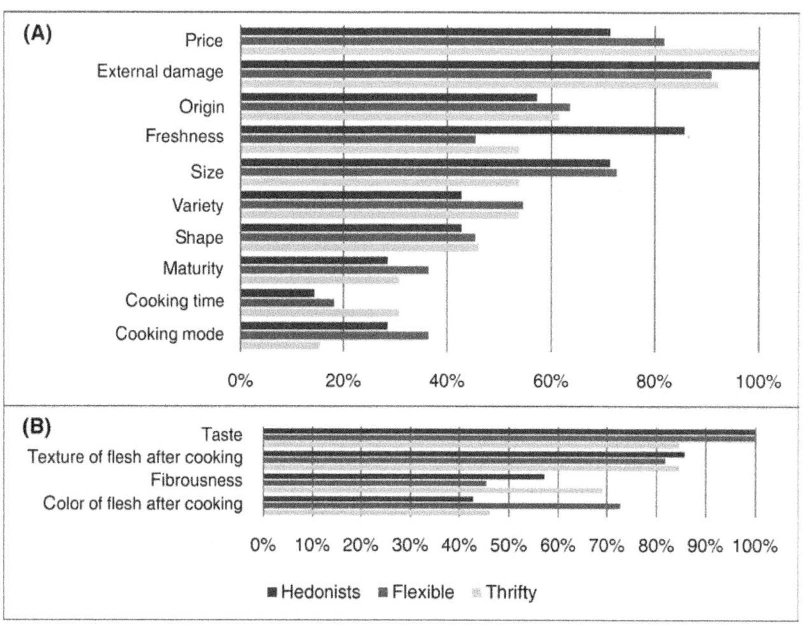

Figure 2. Frequency of the purchasing (A) and consumption (B) criteria according to the participant profiles

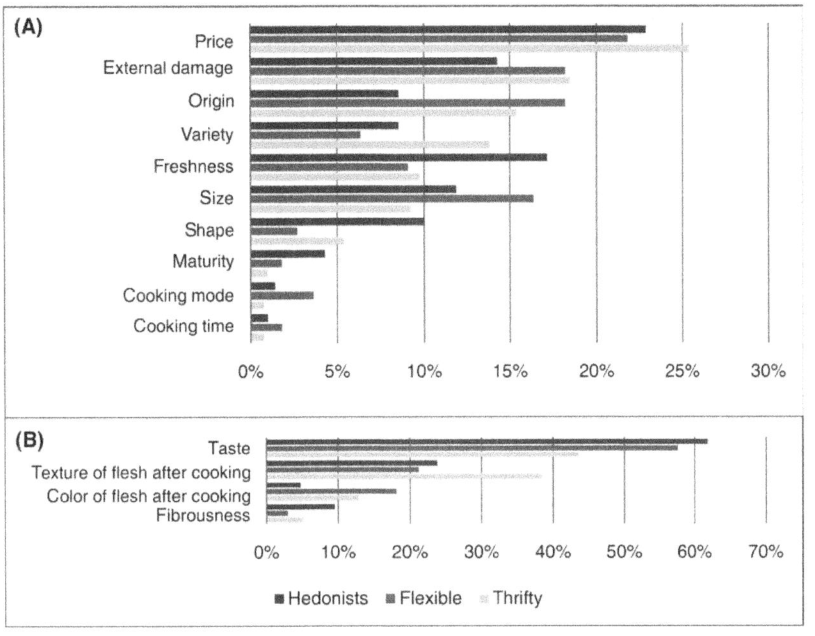

Figure 3. Relative importance of the purchasing (A) and consumption (B) criteria according to the participant profiles

do it". This highlights the importance of putting forward sensory characteristics when marketing yams.

This group expressed suspicion about yam contamination by chlordecone and would purchase yams outside the periphery of the contaminated area. They expressed the desire to eat yams produced within low-input cropping systems and were favorable toward warranties verifying the approach. In terms of the origin, this profile did not appear to be very concerned about the origin of the yams, and this criterion ranked only ninth compared to the other criteria after its relative importance. Participants of this group purchased yams in short marketing chains, that is at farms and stalls alongside the road (73% of the informants within that category), because they were viewed as strongly representative of the traditional aspects of yams.

The Flexible (35% of the participants)

In this group, the external damage was cited more frequently than the price and the origin, but it was given a lower relative importance ($\bar{I}_j$ %) than the price and an equal relative importance ($\bar{I}_j$%) to the origin. In the same way, variety and shape were cited more frequently than the freshness and cooking mode, respectively, but were given a lower ($\bar{I}_j$%). Considering the ($\bar{I}_j$%) of the purchasing criteria, the Flexible placed the emphasis on the price first ($\bar{I}=22\%$), then on the external damage and the origin ($\bar{I}=18\%$) and the size ($\bar{I}=16\%$).

As concerns the consumption criteria, the distribution of the frequencies differed from that of the whole sample for the color of the flesh after cooking and fibrousness. The relative importance of the consumption criteria reflected their frequencies, but the Flexible place more emphasis on the taste compared to the other criteria ($\bar{I}=58\%$).

This group was willing to pay between 2.50 €/Kg and 3.50 €/Kg because they thought that the sensory characteristics of the yams would be worth the price and because they believed that local farmers set fair prices. "In direct sale, I don't ask myself too many questions about the price because I trust the farmer; he knows all the production process and all he invested in the production… I trust him". Sometimes, they would even pay 4.00 €/Kg for specific varieties which are more expensive on the market. "If it's yellow yam, I know that the price is around 3.50–4.0 €/Kg. If I want to eat those yams, then, yes, I'll pay that price". They adjust the quantity of yams purchased in the cases of expensive market prices or the frequency of purchase: "If it is very expensive, then I do not buy a lot, and I will cook something else along with it". "If it is expensive, well… I will buy some now, but I won't next time". Occasionally, they would purchase imported yams as a lower priced substitute. They also purchased them when no local yams were available on the market. Nevertheless, they thought that imported yams were of a lesser sensory quality than the same local variety, and they considered the local yams purchased in short marketing chains to be to all intents and purposes organic. Participants within that group expressed a strong conviction to eat local yams and thought that three situations would justify a higher selling price of yams: 1) supporting local farmers, 2) compliance with higher quality standards through, for example, organic certification "Organic farmers (...) I prefer to pay more but to buy from them because at least, I know that there is traceability," and 3) the improved sensory characteristics of the yam varieties. They declared to be in favor of the warranty that certified the yams were produced with less inputs and were ready to pay an additional 1.00 or 2.00 €./Kg to eat organic yams, especially for their children. This group was suspicious about yam contamination by the chlordecone and would purchase yams outside the periphery of the contaminated area. They equally purchased yams in short or diversified and long marketing chains, the latter mainly for the sake of convenience.

The Thrifty (42% of the participants)

Considering the ($\bar{I}_j$%) of the purchasing criteria, the Flexible placed the emphasis on the price first ($\bar{I}$=25%), then on the external damage ($\bar{I}$=18%), the origin ($\bar{I}$=15%), and the variety ($\bar{I}$=14%).

As for the consumption criteria, the distribution of their frequencies differed from that of the whole sample aside from the texture. The relative importance ($\bar{I}$ %) of the consumption criteria show that they placed the emphasis on both the taste ($\bar{I}$=44%) and the texture of the flesh after cooking ($\bar{I}$=38%).

This profile of participants thought that a convenient price for yams was between 1.50 and 2.50 €/Kg, and they declared that they bought yams within this price range, "2.50 €/Kg is a maximum. I consider that I cannot live here and pay more than 2.50 €/Kg for yam (...) I rely all the more on this principle since I consider that I could grow some myself". Occasionally, they would concede to paying a higher price for a different variety when highly motivated by its sensory characteristics. This profile tended to consider yams a basic staple product comparable to rice or other starchy products used as substitutes when the market price of yam rises. "The price... there is a maximum when psychologically I do not purchase like 2.00 €/Kg. Above, it's excessive. I always make analogies between a yam-based and a rice-based meal, and it costs me 5 to 10 times more per kilogram for a meal when I purchase yams". They would also use imported yams as a substitute in case of expensive prices for local yams, despite imported yams being viewed as of a lesser quality. "At this time of year [when yam is expensive], people just buy yam from Costa Rica [imported yam] which is much more affordable". As a consequence, this profile would increase the consumption of yams during the production season, and some participants would even choose to store yams purchased at a good price during the season to have for future consumption. "I am not ready to pay more than 2.50–3.00 €/Kg, because I know that, at some point, in December, the price will go decrease up to 1.50 €/Kg and then I can store some since you can keep it". This group was concerned with the origin and the mode of production of local yams, but argued that they would purchase them from farmers they knew. They insisted on the importance of buying from local farmers (69% of the participants purchased yams in short marketing chains) who "would use few if any inputs". Provided with this source, participants would be sure of both the origin and the mode of production of the yams, and they did not express willingness to have an additional warranty regarding the origin and the mode of production.

Discussion

With regard to the percentage of dry matter (25–33%), a kilogram of yam is three to four times more expensive than a kilogram of rice or pasta; nevertheless, consumers sometimes prefer to keep buying yams. This indicates that there are prospects for the development of the yam sector in Guadeloupe. Market differentiation based on the sensory and cooking mode diversity of yam species and varieties, the development of new yam ideotypes, and also the provision of information about the credence attributes of yam to consumers, are promising opportunities.

Valorizing the sensory and cooking mode diversity of yams varieties

While consumers always expect quality from a product, this term was not clearly defined for yam in the literature, making it unclear as to what to focus on. In this study, we made clear what quality meant for yam consumers. Here, quality first appealed to the senses of the participants, and it referred to a wide range of attributes of yams. They also described the attributes with a range of values that reflected the heterogeneity of their preferences. Participants defined the quality of yams with several sensory and visual attributes: taste preferences (sweet, bitter, neutral), particular individual perceptions of the taste (refined, wild), an external aspect of the tuber free of damages and a small or medium size of tubers (depending on family size). Yam texture also plays an important role, for example, the firm varieties were suitable for fries or gratin, while the tender varieties were more suitable for puree. Both types of texture were suitable for boiling, but the cooking time had to be adjusted to the type of texture (longer for the firm varieties). This clearly shows the importance of the cooking mode for defining yam quality.

Because quality did not mean one standardized type of yam, it directly reflected the diversity of the yam species and varieties present in Guadeloupe, and this advocates for the valorization of that diversity on the marketing side. However, while participants mentioned the yam varieties to illustrate the specific desired traits or cooking modes, some of them were wrong in identifying the varieties used as supporting examples for the discussion. More generally, few people in Guadeloupe are aware of the diversity of yams. Therefore, improving the level of information available to the consumers might help them make choices that better suit their needs and so motivate them to purchase and eat more yams. For example, as it is made for potatoes, packaging yams and giving information regarding the suitability of the different varieties for different cooking modes (i.e., mashed, fried or boiled) would help consumers to make informed choices. As a consequence, information about the diversity of yams could also result in increased demand for yams. It appears as a promising vector of market differentiation that could help sustain and develop the sector. This can be considered an advantage because a wide range of consumer preferences offers flexibility in terms of the choice of yam varieties from the point of view of the farmer. Building a marketing strategy based on the valorization of this diversity can help maintain and preserve yam's agrobiodiversity and satisfy rapidly evolving consuming habits.

Increasing consumers' level of information about credence attributes

The different types of consumers that were highlighted in our study reflect consumer segmentation in the market and lay the foundation for addressing product differentiation in the yam sector. All the profiles considered the price as important, but they would neither be willing to pay the same price for yams given a set of attributes nor to pay the same premium to benefit from additional attributes such as warranties. Indeed, all the profiles would consider attributes such as support for local farmers, organic farming, or a lower use of inputs to produce yam to be desirable; however, only the Hedonist and the Flexible would be willing to pay for these attributes and would like to have a warranty for them. The Thrifty did not need a third party warranty because they already had an ensured intrinsic warranty as a consequence of purchasing yams from farmers they knew. Regarding the risk of pesticide contamination, it has to be noted that all the profiles had a risk avoidance strategy: they bought yams outside the contaminated area to ensure that the yams were free of contamination.

Loureiro and Hine (2002) found that sociodemographic characteristics affect consumer willingness to pay for potato attributes such as the local origin, the organic mode of production, and the absence of GMOs. The comparison of the willingness to pay for the different attributes helped them to identify the best niche market for potato growers. Similarly, the marketing of yams could also be improved by the provision of information about the credence attributes that would add value to the product and give increased guarantees for the product to consumers. In this case, we would need to assess if the added value benefits the farmers on the other side of the food supply chain. Indeed, as differentiation and labeling stand on the compliance to specifications, we have to ensure that the additional cost generated is covered by the price premium that consumers said they would be willing to pay. Laboratory experiments give a good indication for what happens in real life (Lusk and Fox 2003; Levitt and List 2007). Because the premiums in our study were declarative and might not properly reflect the real price consumers would pay for new products, this real price should be determined by the implementation of laboratory experiments.

Toward the definition of new yam ideotypes

Measuring the value of both consumption and purchasing attributes in the Guadeloupean context, as well as understanding consumer preferences using sensory data, can enable the guidance of breeding programs toward the definition of yam ideotypes, tailored to this well-defined and heterogeneous needs.

Our results indicated that all purchasing and consumption criteria were cited by the participants, but the relative importance they gave to the criteria helped to understand the one they prioritized (the four purchasing criteria: price, external damage, origin, and size; and the two consumption criteria: taste and texture). These attributes are of four different types: sensory (taste, texture), visual (external damage, size), economic (price), and credence (origin). Our results are consistent with the few reported studies, since Aidoo (2009) has shown that majority of yam consumers in Ghanaian urban communities preferred white yam to yellow and water yams, and the most important reason for their preference was taste. Amegbeto et al. (2008), by estimating market demand for fresh yam characteristics using contingent valuation in Togo, showed that producers should focus on small size, low weight, and conical-shaped tubers. Just like in Guadeloupe, cooking characteristics and esthetic qualities are preferred by urban consumers. Hounhouigan et al. (2003) have shown that culinary and organoleptic characteristics preferred by urban consumers in Benin are texture after cooking, taste, color and digestibility.

Some differences occur across the three profiles as to the composition of this minimum set of attributes. The Hedonists focused on sensory and visual attributes, while the Flexible and the Thrifty focused on the sensory and visual attributes as well as on the credence attribute (origin). The reason for which the Hedonists did not emphasize the origin to a great degree is most likely because certain varieties viewed as having a very high sensory quality can only be purchased as an imported staple today (e.g., cousse-couche). Additionally, the Thrifty emphasized two sensory attributes (i.e., taste and texture) contrary to the two other profiles.

As consumers intended to maximize their utility across a set of product attributes, they had to make trade-offs between them in relation to the price. Our results revealed the importance of the price, origin, taste, and texture as drivers of consumer choice. This is in accordance with the literature on consumer values (Lusk and Briggeman 2009) and specific to yam (Amegbeto et al. 2008). As the first step in the research process, our study revealed the trade-off that consumers made between attributes. Amegbeto et al. (2008) has measured the value of fresh yam characteristics, but he has concentrated on the attributes at the purchasing stage. Other studies have used sensory data alone or in combination with value elicitation methods to understand consumer preferences (Lee and Lee 2008; Combris et al. 2009; Chung et al. 2011).

Conclusion

Because yam research programs are generally production driven and often lack the consumer perspective, we conducted a demand-driven study to identify the levers of action for the development of the yam supply chain. We organized in Guadeloupe six focus group discussions accounting for a total of 31 participants to understand the drivers of yam purchasing and consumption. Participants considered the price, origin, taste, texture, external damage, and size as important yam attributes. They defined a good-quality yam as a regularly shaped tuber with a range of sensory attributes that revealed the diversity of their expectations and preferences. Three profiles of participants were identified, each of which were characterized by different consumer behaviors, suggesting that different yam varieties can answer different needs. Therefore, our results suggest that innovations can be implemented to sustain and stimulate the development of the yam sector in Guadeloupe. Two main development paths were identified. The first path is the valorization of the great existing diversity of yam varieties and the increase in the level of information for consumers about experience attributes such as the cooking mode and credence attributes such as the origin and the mode of production. The second path is the definition of the yam ideotypes that suit consumer needs. The next step of the research process would be to analyze deeper consumers' preferences through the implementation of sensory characterization of yam varieties and laboratory experiments. It would allow measuring quantitatively the sensory characteristics of each yam variety, the sensory and cooking preferences of consumers, and the price they would be willing to pay for the different attributes of yams. This work suggests the detailed investigation of how to best match consumer expectations with the production capacity of yam farmers.

Acknowledgments

The authors thank José Dubréas for his much appreciated comments on the interview guide and on the earlier version of this paper and Samuel Joseph for his support in the organization of the focus group discussions. They also thank the consumers who took part in this study. The first author benefited from a PhD Grant co-financed by the European Union (Fonds Social Européen), the Guadeloupe Regional Council, and the INRA social science division. Experiments and data collection were part of the AGROECOTROP project co-financed by the European Union (Fond Européen de Développement Régional) and the Guadeloupe Regional Council.

Conflict of Interest

None declared.

References

AGRESTE. 2009a. L'agriculture guadeloupéenne en 2007.Ministère de l'Agriculture de l'Agroalimentaire et de la Forêt, Basse-Terre, pp 1–28.

AGRESTE 2009b. Tubercules 1981 à 2007. Ministère de l'Agriculture de l'Agroalimentaire et de la Forêt, Basse-Terre, pp 1–2.

Aidoo, R. 2009. An analysis of yam consumption patterns in Ghanaian urban communities. PhD Thesis. In Department of Agricultural Economics, Agribusiness and Extension. pp. 180 + appendices, Kwame Nkrumah University of Science & Technology, Kumasi, Ghana.

Alexandratos, N., and J. Bruinsma. 2012. World agriculture towards 2030/2050. The 2012 Revision. ESA Working Paper No. 12-03, 1-147. Agricultural Development Economics Division, FAO United States.

Amegbeto, N. K., V. M. Manyong, O. Coulibaly, and R. Asiedu. 2008. Estimating market demand for fresh yam characteristics using contingent valuation: implications for crop breeding and production choices. Agric. Econ. 39:349–363.

Ano, G., J. Gelabale, and P. Marival. 2005. L'igname *D. alata* la génétique et l'anthracnose. Phytoma la Défense des Végétaux. 584:36–38.

Arnolin, R., and K. Lombion. 2005. L' igname cousse-couche *Dioscorea trifida* et les virus. Phytoma la Défense des Végétaux. 584:33–35.

Asiedu, R., and A. Sartie. 2010. Crops that feed the World 1 Yams. Food Sec. 2:305–315.

Barlagne, C., 2006. Impact des migrations et des transferts d'argent sur l'agriculture paysanne des communes de Telpaneca et Mozonte, Nicaragua. Ecole Nationale d'Ingénieurs des Techniques Agricoles, Clermont-Ferrand, France.

Barlagne, C. 2007. MOVE: An Evaluation of a business training program for the peri-urban poor. Thesis dissertation for the partial fulfillment for the degree of Master of Science in International Natural Resources Development, pp. 1-130, University of Wales, Bangor. Available at www.bestpracticesfoundation.org/pdf/MOVEEvaluation-Barlagne.pdf. (accessed 1 September 2015)

Barrios, E. X., S. Bayarri, I. Carbonell, L. Izquierdo, and E. Costell. 2008. Consumer attitudes and opinions toward functional foods: a focus group study. J. Sens. Stud. 23:514–525.

Boquin, M. M., H. R. Moskowitz, S. M. Donovan, and S.-Y. Lee. 2014. Defining Perceptions of Picky Eating Obtained through Focus Groups and Conjoint Analysis. J. Sens. Stud. 29:126–138.

Bradbury, J.H., and W. D Holloway. 1988. Chemistry of Tropical Root Crops: significance for nutrition and agriculture in the Pacific. ACIAR Monograph, Melbourne, pp. 1–201.

Cabidoche, Y. M., and M. Lesueur-Jannoyer. 2012. Contamination of Harvested Organs in Root Crops Grown on Chlordecone-Polluted Soils. Pedosphere 22:562–571.

Campbell, R., H. Schiff, D. Snodgrass, D. Neven, J. Downing, and D. Sturza. 2009. Global food security response: West Africa rice value chain analysis In MicroReport 161. USAID, Washington.

Cardinal, P., A. Flores, A. Contarini, and G. Hough. 2003. Focus group research on sensory language used by consumers to describe mayonnaise. J. Sens. Stud. 18:47–59.

Chambre d'Agriculture de la Guadeloupe. 2014. Les échanges agricoles contrôlés. La Note de l'Observatoire Economique et Social de la Chambre d'Agriculture. Baie-Mahault: Chambre d'Agriculture de la Guadeloupe, pp. 1–4.

Chung, H. S., H.-D. Hong, K. Kim, C.-W. Cho, H. R. Moskowitz, and S.-Y. Lee. 2011. Consumer attitudes and expectations of ginseng food products assessed by focus groups and conjoint analysis. J. Sens. Stud. 26:346–357.

Combris, P., P. Bazoche, E. Giraud-Heraud, and S. Issanchou. 2009. Food choices: what do we learn from combining sensory and economic experiments? Food Qual. Prefer. 20:550–557.

Dulcire, M. 2005. Une culture patrimoniale du mythe à la renaissance, le café "bonifieur" de Guadeloupe. In Anthropology of Food. Available at www.aof.revues.org/124. (accessed 1 September 2015)

Hounhouigan, J. D., A. P. P. Kayodé, N. Bricas, and M. C. Nago. 2003. Les caractéristiques culinaires et organoleptiques des ignames recherchées en milieu urbain au Bénin. Les Annales des Sciences Agronomiques du Bénin 4:143–160.

Kitzinger, J., I. Marková, and N. Kalampalikis. 2004. Qu'est-ce que les focus groups? Bulletin de Psychologie 57:237–243.

van Kleef, E., H. C. M. van Trijp, and P. Luning. 2005. Consumer research in the early stages of new product development: a critical review of methods and techniques. Food Qual. Prefer. 16:181–201.

Krueger, R.A., and M. A. Casey. 2009. Focus Groups: A Practical Guide for Applied Research. SAGE Publications. Thousand Oaks, London, New Delhi, pp. 1–215.

Lee, C. M., and S.-Y. Lee. 2007. Consumer insights on healthy breakfast cereal - a focus group research. J. Sens. Stud. 22:417–432.

Lee, S.-J., and K.-G. Lee. 2008. Understanding consumer preferences for rice wines using sensory data. J. Sci. Food Agric. 88:690–698.

Levitt, S. D., and J. A. List. 2007. What Do Laboratory Experiments Measuring Social Preferences Reveal About the Real World? J. Econ. Perspect. 21:153–174.

Loureiro, M. L., and S. Hine. 2002. Discovering Niche Markets: A Comparison of Consumer Willingness to Pay for Local (Colorado Grown) Organic, and GMO-Free Products. J. Agric. Appl. Econ. 34:477–487.

Lusk, J. L., and B. C. Briggeman. 2009. Food Values. Am. J. Agric. Econ. 91:184–196.

Lusk, J. L., and J. A. Fox. 2003. Value elicitation in retail and laboratory environments. Econ. Lett. 79:27–34.

Morgan, D.L. 1997. Focus Groups as Qualitative Research. SAGE Publications. Thousand Oaks, London, New Delhi, pp. 1–88.

Onyeka, T. J., D. Petro, G. Ano, S. Etienne, and S. Rubens. 2006. Resistance in water yam (*Dioscorea alata*) cultivars in the French West Indies to anthracnose disease based on tissue culture-derived whole-plant assay. Plant. Pathol. 55:671–678.

Rastoin, J.-L., and G. Ghersi. 2010. Le système alimentaire mondial. Editions Quae, Versailles.

Scott, G. J., M. W. Rosegrant, and C. Ringler. 2000. Global projections for root and tuber crops to the year 2020. Food Policy 25:561–597.

Selfa, T., R. A. Jussaume, and M. Winter. 2008. Envisioning agricultural sustainability from field to plate: comparing producer and consumer attitudes and practices toward 'environmentally friendly' food and farming in Washington State, USA. J. Rural Stud. 24:262–276.

Tsolakis, N. K., C. A. Keramydas, A. K. Toka, D. A. Aidonis, and E. T. Iakovou. 2014. Agrifood supply chain management: A comprehensive hierarchical decision-making framework and a critical taxonomy. Biosyst. Eng. 120:47–64.

Wan, V. C.-H., C. M. Lee, and S.-Y. Lee. 2007. Understanding consumer attitudes on edible films and coatings: focus group findings. J. Sens. Stud. 22:353–366.

18

Effects of pretreatments of banana (*Musa AAA*, Omini) on the composition, rheological properties, and baking quality of its flour and composite blends with wheat flour

Adegoke H. Bakare[1], Olukemi D. Ogunbowale[2], Mojisola O. Adegunwa[1] & Joseph O. Olusanya[3]

[1]Department of Hospitality and Tourism Federal University of Agriculture, Abeokuta, Nigeria
[2]Department of Food Science and Technology, Federal University of Agriculture, Abeokuta, Nigeria
[3]Department of Home Economics and Hotel Management, Tai Solarin University of Education Nigeria, Ijebu-Ode, Nigeria

Keywords
Baking, banana, bread, pretreaments, production, rheology

Correspondence
Adegoke H. Bakare, Department of Hospitality and Tourism Federal University of Agriculture, Abeokuta, Nigeria.
E-mail:bakare65@gmail.com

Funding Information
No funding information provided.

Abstract

Effects of chemical and heat pretreatments on the protein, gluten, and alpha-amylase activity, pasting (Peak [*P*], Final [*F*] setback [*S*] viscosity, pasting temperature [*PT*] and time [*T*]) and alveogram (Energy [*E*], maximum inflation [*MI*], *P*/*L*, and elasticity index [*EI*]) properties of flour from the pretreated bananas and its composite with wheat flour (WF) were examined. The baking (water absorption [WA] and specific volume [SV]) and sensory properties of bread produced from the flour were also examined. Protein, gluten, and alpha-amylase activity ranged from 4.75 ± 0.07%, 30.25 ± 0.05%, and 4.00 ± 0.05 min to 13.75 ± 0.06%, 35.64 ± 0.06%, and 39.61 ± 1.18 min with WF:PTBF/95:05, WF:CTBF/00:100, WF:BBF/80:20, WF:100 and WF:CTBF/00:100, WF:PTBF/95:05, WF:100, WF:PTBF/00:100 having lowest and highest values, respectively. *P*, *F*, *S* viscosities, *PT* and *T* ranged from 186.17 ± 0.71, 217.08 ± 1.41, 38.92 ± 5.42 RVU, 84.70 ± 0.28°C, 5.04 ± 0.05 min to 461.0 ± 5.07, 348.5 ± 8.84, 88.83 ± 0.24 RVU, 87.20 ± 0.00°C, 6.24 ± 0.05 min, respectively. *E*, *MI*, *P*/*L*, and *EI* ranged from 141.50 ± 0.71 × 10^{-4}J, 15.35 ± 0.07, 0.59 ± 0.83 and 35.85 ± 0.07 to 325.00 ± 1.4 × 10^{-4}J, 22.55 ± 0.07, 2.75 ± 0.07, and 70.50 ± 0.71, respectively. WA and SV were 48.12 ± 0.07 to 52.60 ± 0.14 and 2.850 ± 0.07 to 5.635 ± 0.18 with the WF having significantly ($P < 0.05$) higher values than other blends and the most acceptable in terms of appearance and taste.

Introduction

Consumption of wheat-based products is not likely to decrease, considering the growth in population and urbanization (Bakare 2008; Malomo et al. 2011) and the exotic lifestyle and food habits adopted by the citizens of most of the non-wheat-producing countries (Bakare et al. 2015). Bread is a staple food consumed in different parts of the World. It was described as a fermented confectionery product produced mainly from wheat flour (WF), water, yeast, and salt by a series of process involving mixing, kneading, proofing, shaping, and baking (Dewettinck et al. 2008). Inspite of some of the nutritional disorder attributed to the consumption of bread, it is still desired by many people across various socio-demographic characteristics.

Several studies have reported the prospects of composite flour technology as a means of reducing the dependence on wheat for the production of bakery products (Mepba et al. 2007; Biljan and Bojana 2008; Manuel et al. 2008; Alex et al. 2008; Ade-Omowaye et al. 2008; Lin et al. 2009; Adeleke and Odedeji 2010; Malomo et al. 2011, 2013; Bakare et al. 2013, 2014a,b, 2015). Partial replacement of WF with flour from suitable indigenous crops remains the only viable practical option for reducing the consumption of wheat, provided that some of the challenges associated with the utilization of composite technology at industrial scale can be minimized (Bakare et al. 2015). It is also necessary to explore the possibility of using crops that are underutilized and with less competing uses, those highly prone to postharvest losses and those that possess strategic nutritional advantages that can be used to alleviate endemic malnutrtional challenges.

Bananas (*Musa* spp) are highly perishable crop produced in the tropical and subtropical countries of the world where they are mostly grown for either home consumption or for the local markets. It is the world's most popular fruit and one of the world's most important staple foods, after rice, wheat, and maize. About 107 million metric tons of bananas were produced in more than 130 countries in 2011 representing a total trade value of US$9 billion (FAO 2013). Nigeria, with an estimated population of 177.5 million people, gross domestic product per capita of US$3,203.3 (World Bank 2013) is one of the largest producer in Africa recording about 2.78 million tons of banana production (FAOSTAT 2013). Africa exported about 649 000 tons of bananas in 2012 representing 3.9 percent of global export with Côte d'Ivoire and Cameroon being the two topmost exporters (FAO 2014).

Bananas are good sources of carbohydrate, vitamins A, B, and C. It is also rich in phosphorus, potassium, magnesium, selenium, and iron. (Wall 2006). Banana contains a large amount of easily assimilable sugars, making it a good source of quick energy and an important means of recovery from fatigue (Pius 1994; Kyamuchangine et al. 2002).

Major limitations to the utilization of banana is its limited shelf life and its rapid susceptibility to postharvest losses, particularly when fully matured, which necessitate the need for processing to a more stable intermediate or ready-to-consume forms. Drying is one of the traditional methods used in the tropics for processing bananas into stable storage forms. Drying brings about a substantial reduction in weight and volume; thereby minimizing packaging, storage, and transportation cost and also enable storability of the product under ambient temperature, especially in developing countries (Senadeera et al. 2005). Dried bananas are easy to handle and can be easily incorporated during food formulation and preparation. Hot-air drying of food materials also help to control product quality, enhance hygienic handling and reduce product losses (Corzo et al. 2008). In addition, food poisoning and spoilage are minimized, because reduction in moisture content often resulted in food with low water activity which in turn enhances bacteriostatic control of the activities of microbes in food.

Common problems associated with drying of tropical fruits included shrinkage of the food cells, browning, and loss of rehydration ability, wettability, and case hardening. Browning is an important physiological disorder that degrades the qualities of fruits and vegetables. Enzymatic browning is a widespread color reaction occurring in fruits and vegetables, which involves the interaction of oxygen, phenolic compounds and polyphenol oxidases (PPO). Browning is usually initiated by the enzymatic oxidation of monophenols into o-diphenols and o-diphenols into quinones, which undergo further nonenzymatic polymerization leading to the formation of pigments. Enzymatic browning negatively affects the quality of fresh-cut fruit and vegetable (Ioannou and Ghoul 2013). Banana is susceptible to enzymatic browning during processing (Luo and Tao 2003) and storage. Browning has a negative effect on their appearance, sensory properties (taste, odor, and texture) and nutritional value (Jiang 2004; Komthong et al. 2006).

Banana is susceptible to enzymatic browning during processing (Luo Y and Tao Y, 2003) and storage. Browning has a negative effect on the appearance, sensory properties (taste, odour and texture) and nutritional value (Jiang, 2004; Komthong et al., 2006) of banana. Some of the factors that determine the rate of enzymatic browning in banana are concentrations of PPO and other phenolic compounds, pH, temperature and availability of oxygen. Techniques and mechanisms that have been explored to control the enzymatic browning are meant to eliminate one or more of these factors. According to Ioannou and Ghoul (2013) some of these techniques included chemical treatments (antioxidants, acidifying, agents of firmness, or chelating agents) and then physical methods (blanching, freezing, and the modification of product atmosphere). It has been noted that acidification may reduce or inactivate the PPO activity, particularly when pH is below 3 (Grimm et al. 2012). Citric acid may act both as acidifying (Ihl et al. 2003) as well as a chelating agent (Jiang et al. 2004). Heat treatment of up to 60°C has been used to induce heat shock which inhibit browning and also provide protection against pathogens (Loaiza-Velarde et al. 2003; Qiang and Yaguang, 2007). Blanching is a type of heat treatment given to food primarily to inactivate enzyme systems responsible for sensory and other quality alterations in food. Blanching limits the oxidation and may also enhance the colors of some vegetables. It can, however, alter the consistency of treated product and also generate loss of nutrients, particularly when done in water (Mazzeo et al. 2011) instead of steam which is also suitable for high moisture, enzyme active, and soft texture food like banana.

Protein-starch interaction catalyzed by enzyme-induced biochemical processes also affects the quality of baked products, generally, and bread in particular.

In summary, bananas are nutritive, highly perishable with limited shelf life. Nigeria is one of the largest producers of banana in Africa, its susceptibility to postharvest losses can be reduced and its utilization can be enhanced by drying and converting bananas to flour. This may increase its versatility and application for different end use, particularly in bakery products like bread. However, because banana is an enzyme active food, suitable pretreatment prior to drying is a necessity. It is therefore necessary to assess the effects of such pretreatments on the functionality of its flour before it can be recommended for use in bread making. This study, therefore, examined the effect of chemical pretreatments and blanching on the proximate and chemical composition of banana flour, their pasting properties, and the rheological and baking qualities of their composite blends with WF.

Materials and Methods

Source of materials

Mature green banana (Musa AAA group, Omini) bunches were purchased from an Agriculture produce market in Abeokuta South Local Government area of Ogun State, Nigeria. WF was obtained from the Nigeria Eagle Flour Mills Ltd, Ibadan, Oyo State while other ingredients such as sugar, iodized salt, yeast, fat, and ascorbic acid were purchased in the retail markets.

Preparation of flour

Banana was processed as described by Bakare et al. (2015) with some modifications. Mature green but unripe banana were de-fingered, washed, peeled, manually sliced into cylindrical pieces of 2-mm thickness and samples were subjected to two types of pretreatments; chemical pretreatments with 5% potassium metabisulphite and citric acid solution for 30 minutes, respectively, as well as steam blanching at 100°C for 2 min after which it was blotted dry with clean tissue paper to remove adhered surface water, making a total of three treatments.

The banana slices were placed on a foil paper placed on drying racks to avoid sticking together; it was then dried in a cross-flow Gallenkamp oven (Model OV-160 size 2 BS, Weiss Technik UK Loughborough, Leicestershire, U.K.) at 70°C for 18 h. The dried chips were milled to flour in a Disc mill (Model FFC-15, Shandong-Jimo Agricultural Machinery, Qingdao City, Shandong Province, China) at 8800 rpm and sieved through a 250 μm mesh sieve (no.60.W.S. 8570 Tyler Blvd, Mentor, OH 44060).

Analysis of flour

All analyses were performed in triplicates. Proximate, gluten, and water absorption of WF and blends were analyzed with official methods (AACC 2000) using a Partens Inframatic analyzer (Model 9140, SE-126 53, Hägersten, Sweden). Gluten content was determined according to AACC International method No. 38–12 by using the Glutomatic (Partens Glutomatic system (Model 2200, Instrumentvägen 31 SE-126 53 Hägersten, Sweden) to measure the gluten quantity and quality of the flour. Alpha-amylase activity was determined with the Hagberg falling numbers instrument (Partens model no 1500, Instrumentvägen 31 SE-126 53, Hägersten Sweden, USA), based on (AACC 2000) approved method. Crude fiber content of flour was determined by trichloroacetic acid method as described by Entwisted et al. (1949).

Viscosity characteristics of flour

Pasting characteristics of the treated flour were determined according to ICC No 162 method. Rapid visco analyser (RVA) series 4 (RVA; series 4, Newport Scientific P.T.V., Warriewood, Australia) with the aid of thermocline for Windows (version 1.1. Software, 1996) was used for the analysis. The 12-min profile was used for all the analyses. It consists of idle temp of 50°C for 1 min, then 50–95°C in 3 min 45 sec, held at 95°C for 2 min 30 sec, cooled to 50°C over 3 min 45 sec, finally, held at 50°C for 2 min. Two paddle speeds of 960 rpm for the first 10 sec followed by 150 rpm were employed for the remaining duration of the test cycle. The weight per sample used for each analysis was calculated from the formula:

$$\text{Corrected sample weight for RVA}(S) = \frac{A \times 100}{100 - M}$$

$$(W) = 25 + (A - S)$$

where A = weight of flour sample: using the RVA manual as a guide.

S = corrected sample weight.

M = actual moisture content of the sample.

W = volume of water used.

Alveogram chararcteristics

The Alveograph (Chopin NG France) was used to measure (AACC 2010) characteristics that provided insight into the fermentation tolerance of the dough as may be exhibited during proofing stage of bread making. Characteristics of interest that were measured included the average resistance to expansion indicated by the peak height (mm), extensibility indicated by length (L) of the alveogram curve, energy input (Joules) required for the mechanical deformation of the dough (W), inflation required for maximum development (G) and the elastic resistance (Ie) of the measured dough samples.

Flour sample (250 g) of known moisture content was placed into the mixer, sodium chloride solution (2.5%) was added through a buret (i.e., 129.4 mL for flour with 14% moisture) and mixed for 7 min. The dough was forced through the extrusion gate in the form of a thin strip on to a small oiled steel plate. Five extruded dough pieces of designated length were cut off, rolled with an oiled rolling pin to a uniform thinness, cut into a circular disk, transferred to an oiled steel plate and subjected to a brief rest period in a tempered compartment of the alveograph for 15 min. Each circular dough test pieces were removed from the compartment and inserted between two metal plates that held it securely in position. The air valve was opened to supply air pressure to the held dough through an orifice. The electrically driven recording manometer was simultaneously activated to record the air pressure inside the dough bubble against time.

Bread production

Bread loaves were produced according to AACC (2010) with slight modification. Formulations included: wheat/banana (100:00, 90:05, 90:10, 85:15, and 80:20) composite flour 100 g (14% moisture), 9.0 g sugar, 1.1 g iodized salt, 1.8 g yeast, 1.8 g fat, and 20 ppm of ascorbic acid as dough improver.

The bread samples were produced in the laboratory of Nigerian Eagle Flour Mills Ltd, Ibadan-Lagos Expressway, Ibadan, Oyo State, Nigeria. The dough was mixed using Chaplain spiral mixer (Model BT10C, Caplain Machines 999 rue du Tuboeuf–BP.99–77170 Brie Comte Robert–France), fermented (proofed) at initial and final fermentation time of 15 and 28 min and at ambient condition of 28 ± 2°C and 85 ± 12% relative humidity and baked in an oven (Model, Convecta U/B Macadams Baking System, Cape Town, South Africa) at 220°C for 30 min. The bread samples were cooled for 1 h, then placed in low-density polyethylene bags and kept at 24 ± 2°C.

Determination of physical quality of bread

Weights of bread loaves were measured with a Mettler Toledo (A204) digital weighing scale. Volume was measured by millet seed displacement method (AACC 2010) with minor modification.

Weight loss

The weight loss of the bread was determined as described by Kim et al. (2003). The dough was weighed before baking, and the breads were weighed after baking. The percent weight loss of the bread samples was calculated as:

$$\%\ \text{weight loss} = \frac{A - B \times 100}{A}$$

where:

A = weight of dough.

B = weight of baked bread.

Sensory analysis

Selection of panelists

Thirty people were selected from a pool of volunteers comprising of officers, lecturers, and students of tertiary institutions. The panelists were selected after an oral interview conducted on the basis of a criteria checklist that included: good health, nonsmoker, nonallergic to wheat/banana, willingness to participate, and passion/likeness for the consumption of bread.

Quantitative acceptance test was used to assess consumers' liking for the product. The thirty untrained panelists rated their liking or otherwise for the bread samples produced from the blends on a 9-point hedonic scale (1 = disliked extremely as compared to reference sample 'R', and 9 = liked extremely as compared to reference sample 'R').

Statistical analysis

All experiments and analyses were conducted in triplicates. Data obtained from different aspects of the study were subjected to analysis of variance and the Duncan multiple range test was used to separate the means (Duncan 1955). Statistical analysis package software SPSS 17 for windows was used for all the analyses.

Results and Discussion

Composition of the flours and their blends

Moisture content determination is an important index of quality for flour generally, and WF in particular. Moisture content above 14% affects the storage quality of flour and at more higher content, it may increase the microbial content and may also predispose the flour to infestation by insects. It may also cause the flour to agglomerate, become wet, and create production problem. The moisture content of the flour (Table 1) ranged from 9.27 ± 0.02% to 13.50 ± 0.11% and is thus, below the 14% safety limit.

The treated banana flour (PTBF, CTBF, and BBF) had relatively lower protein content (4.64 ± 0.06–5.46 ± 0.00%) than the WF (11.00 ± 0.14). The pretreatment appeared to have significantly ($P < 0.05$) affected the protein content (Table 1) of the flour as the PTBF had significantly higher value than the CTBF and BBF. The protein content of treated banana flour observed in this study are more than the values reported by Zuwariah and Aziah (2009) for heat-modified and nonmodified banana flour.

The protein contents of the flour blends ranged from 11.00 ± 0.14 to 13.75 ± 0.06 with the WF having the lowest and PTBF the highest. In all cases, protein content decreased as the banana flour was used to replace the WF in the blends. The 5% WF:PTBF had significantly higher value than the WF:CTBF/95 and WF:BBF/95, respectively, indicating that the effect of the pretreatment was more noticeable at this blending ratio. The PTBF blends had relatively higher protein values than the others in all the blending ratios except at 15% level. Aside from its

Table 1. Effects of pretreatments on the composition of wheat-banana composite flour.

Flour	Moisture%	Protein %	Fiber %	Fat %	Ash %	CHO %	Gluten (Wet)	Alpha-amylase min	Water absorption %
WF:100	$13.50 \pm 0.11_{h}$	$11.00 \pm 0.14_{c}$	$1.77 \pm 0.01_{k}$	$1.38 \pm 0.02_{def}$	$0.63 \pm 0.01_{ab}$	$71.73 \pm 0.02_{b}$	$35.64 \pm 0.06_{g}$	$4.0.00 \pm 0.05_{a}$	$51.80 \pm 0.14_{f}$
WF:PTBF/00:100	$9.92 \pm 0.03_{b}$	$5.46 \pm 0.00_{b}$	$1.54 \pm 0.06_{j}$	$2.05 \pm 0.07_{i}$	3.87 ± 00	$77.03 \pm 0.04_{i}$	NA	$39.61 \pm 1.18_{k}$	na
WF:CTBF/00:100	$9.27 \pm 0.02_{a}$	$4.75 \pm 0.07_{a}$	$0.34 \pm 0.01_{c}$	$1.27 \pm 0.01_{c}$	$2.69 \pm 0.01_{i}$	$81.62 \pm 0.02_{k}$	NA	$27.78 \pm 0.11_{i}$	na
WF:BBF/00:100	$10.32 \pm 0.03_{b}$	$4.64 \pm 0.06_{a}$	$1.36 \pm 0.02_{i}$	$1.71 \pm 0.01_{h}$	$3.00 \pm 0.00_{j}$	$78.75 \pm 0.21_{j}$	NA	$37.95 \pm 0.14_{k}$	na
WF:PTBF/95: 05	$11.80 \pm 0.00_{efg}$	$13.75 \pm 0.06_{k}$	$0.81 \pm 0.01_{f}$	$1.41 \pm 0.01_{efg}$	$0.88 \pm 0.00_{g}$	$71.35 \pm 0.06_{a}$	$35.12 \pm 0.14_{h}$	$5.47 \pm 0.21_{bcd}$	$53.85 \pm 0.21_{h}$
WF:CTBF/95:05	$11.10 \pm 0.14_{c}$	$12.29 \pm 0.07_{i}$	$0.58 \pm 0.01_{d}$	$1.46 \pm 0.01_{f}$	$0.69 \pm 0.01_{bc}$	$73.79 \pm 0.07_{e}$	$35.09 \pm 0.13_{f}$	$5.66 \pm 0.13_{def}$	$52.70 \pm 0.70_{fg}$
WF:BBF/95:05	$11.55 \pm 0.35_{cdef}$	$12.74 \pm 0.06_{j}$	$1.06 \pm 0.03_{h}$	$1.36 \pm 0.03_{cdef}$	$0.74 \pm 0.01_{cde}$	$72.21 \pm 0.01_{c}$	$34.07 \pm 0.08_{de}$	$5.19 \pm 0.13_{b}$	$50.75 \pm 0.07_{e}$
WF:PTBF/90:10	$11.65 \pm 0.21_{defg}$	$12.14 \pm 0.07_{hi}$	$0.67 \pm 0.03_{e}$	$1.38 \pm 0.01_{cdef}$	$0.84 \pm 0.00_{efg}$	$73.21 \pm 0.29_{d}$	$34.19 \pm 0.01_{de}$	$5.99 \pm 0.13_{fg}$	$53.55 \pm 0.63_{gh}$
WF:CTBF/90:10	$12.05 \pm 0.07_{fg}$	$11.82 \pm 0.07_{efg}$	$0.79 \pm 0.01_{f}$	$1.31 \pm 0.01_{cde}$	$0.82 \pm 0.01_{efg}$	$73.18 \pm 0.07_{d}$	$32.65 \pm 0.49_{cd}$	$5.73 \pm 0.19_{defg}$	$50.25 \pm 0.071_{de}$
WF:BBF/90:10	$11.35 \pm 0.21_{cdef}$	$12.06 \pm 0.04_{ghi}$	$0.10 \pm 00_{b}$	$1.28 \pm 0.01_{bcd}$	$0.83 \pm 0.01_{fg}$	$74.32 \pm 0.14_{f}$	$34.16 \pm 21_{e}$	$5.28 \pm 0.25_{b}$	$47.60 \pm 0.14_{c}$
WF:PTBF/85:15	$11.30 \pm 0.42_{cd}$	$11.84 \pm 0.05_{fg}$	$0.03 \pm 0.01_{a}$	$1.26 \pm 0.01_{b}$	$0.72 \pm 0.00_{bcd}$	$74.42 \pm 0.28_{f}$	$33.00 \pm 0.28_{d}$	$6.06 \pm 0.11_{cdg}$	$52.75 \pm 0.07_{fg}$
WF:CTBF/85:15	$11.10 \pm 0.00_{c}$	$11.36 \pm 0.07_{d}$	$0.83 \pm 0.01_{f}$	$1.32 \pm 0.01_{bcde}$	$0.60 \pm 0.001_{a}$	$74.92 \pm 0.07_{g}$	$32.46 \pm 0.05_{c}$	$5.87 \pm 0.31_{efg}$	$49.75 \pm 0.21_{d}$
WF:BBF/85:15	$11.50 \pm 0.28_{cdef}$	$11.92 \pm 0.03_{fgh}$	$0.92 \pm 0.01_{g}$	$1.30 \pm 0.14_{cde}$	$0.80 \pm 0.14d_{efg}$	$73.08 \pm 0.07_{d}$	$32.17 \pm 0.06_{c}$	$5.56 \pm 0.11_{e}$	$45.40 \pm 0.56_{b}$
WF:PTBF/80:20	$11.40 \pm 0.00_{cdef}$	$11.72 \pm 0.40_{efg}$	$0.32 \pm 0.02_{c}$	$1.19 \pm 0.01_{b}$	$1.22 \pm 0.00_{h}$	$74.20 \pm 0.28_{f}$	$30.25 \pm 0.05_{a}$	$6.52 \pm 0.05_{h}$	$52.60 \pm 0.85_{fg}$
WF:CTBF/80:20	$11.10 \pm 0.14_{c}$	$11.02 \pm 0.03_{c}$	$0.83 \pm 0.02_{f}$	$1.55 \pm 0.07_{g}$	$0.75 \pm 0.07_{cdef}$	$75.38 \pm 0.00_{h}$	$31.18 \pm 0.43_{b}$	$5.13 \pm 0.08_{ab}$	$48.40 \pm 0.28_{c}$
WF:BBF/80:20	$11.25 \pm 0.35_{cd}$	$11.61 \pm 0.14_{de}$	$0.05 \pm 0.007_{a}$	$1.08 \pm 0.01_{a}$	$0.72 \pm 0.01_{bcd}$	$74.88 \pm 0.07_{g}$	$30.34 \pm 0.33_{a}$	$5.41 \pm 0.15_{bcd}$	$43.10 \pm 0.14_{a}$

-d-a. Mean in same column with the same subscripts are not significantly different ($P < 0.05$). WF, wheat flour; BF, banana flour from potassium (PT)-, citric acid (CT)-treated and blanched banana (BBF); (05–100), composite blends; n a, not applicable; NA, not available.

nutritive values, protein content is an important criterion for selecting WF for use in bakery products. Generally, for WF, higher the protein content, the better the bread-making characteristics of the flour. WF having high protein content is also likely to absorb more water during mixing, may also have longer mixing time, and their dough are more tolerant to over-mixing (Bakare et al. 2015). However, this may not necessarily be applicable to composite flour with high protein content as shown in Table 1.

The fiber content of the treated banana flour ranged from 0.34 ± 0.01% to 1.54 ± 0.06% and was significantly lower than that of the WF. Crude fiber decreased as the WF was replaced by the treated flour for the various pretreatments with the PTBF and CTBF having significantly higher values at 5% and 10–20% substitution level, respectively.

The fat content of the WF was significantly ($P > 0.05$) lower than that of the treated flour, except for CTBF. The fat content of the PTBF containing blends was higher in the 5% and 10% blend, but lower at subsequent substitution levels except at 20%. In all, the fat contents of the blends ranged from 1.08 ± 0.01 to 1.46 ± 0.01 with the WF:CTBF/95:05 and WF:BBF/80:20 having the highest and lowest values, respectively.

Flour from the treated banana had significantly higher ash contents than the WF and this resulted in significant ($P < 0.05$) increase in the ash content of the blends at all levels of substitution except that of WF:CTBF/85:15.

The carbohydrate content of the pretreated flour ranged from 77.03 ± 0.04% to 81.62 ± 0.02% and was significantly ($P < 0.05$) lower than the value reported by Zuwariah and Aziah (2009), with the CTBF and PTBF the highest and lowest values, respectively. The carbohydrate content of the blends increased as WF was substituted for the treated banana flour.

The gluten content of the blends ranged from 30.25 ± 0.05% to 35.64 ± 0.06% with the WF and the PTBF/80:20 having the highest and lowest values, respectively. It also decreased in all the blends as WF was replaced with flour from the treated banana. This is to be expected since banana does not have any gluten Braganza and Tolentino 2011) and agreed with reports from previous studies (Biljan and Bojana 2008; Manuel et al. 2008; Alex et al. 2008; Ade-Omowaye et al. 2008; Lin et al. 2009; Adeleke and Odedeji 2010; Malomo et al. 2011, 2013).

Many enzymes are naturally present in flour but only few of them have active influence on bakary operation. Alpha amylase (α-amylase) is one such few enzymes. α-amylases are endoenzymes that randomly hydrolyze the a-(1,4)-linkages in the starch polymers, generating low molecular weight dextrin (Hoseney 1994; Bowles 1996). Although, maltogenic and other maltooligosaccharide-producing α-amylases also act on the a-(1,4)-bonds of starch, alpha- amylase activity in flour is measured in Falling number values. Flour from the pretreated banana had significantly ($P < 0.05$) higher Falling number values (27.78 ± 0.11–39.61 ± 1.18) than the WF (4.0.00 ± 0.05). However, the effect of this was not pronounced in the composite blends suggesting that the flour either possesses little or no endogenous alpha-amylase, the long outer amylopectin chains in banana starch (Zuwariah and Aziah 2009) may have resisted the liquefying effect of the alpha-amylase, or that the pretreatment may have either inactivated or limited the activity of the enzyme. Alpha-amylase activity in the blends ranged from 4.0.00 ± 0.05 to 6.52 ± 0.05 with the WF and the WF:PTBF/80:20 having the lowest and highest values, respectively. This implied that the extent of liquefaction and diastatic activity of the starches in the blends decreased as the proportion of the flour from the treated banana was increased (Schiller 1984; Watson 1984; Bakare et al. 2015).

Water absorption of the composite flour blends ranged from 43.10 ± 0.14 to 53.85 ± 0.21 with the WF:PTBF/95:05 and WF:BBF/80:20 having the highest and lowest values, respectively. Also, water absorption decreased as WF was replaced with flour from each of the treated bananas which was at variance with reports of earlier studies on sweet-potato flour (Malomo et al. 2011) and breadfruit flour (Olatunji and Akinrele 1978; Bakare et al. 2015).

Rheological characteristics

Rheology is the science of the deformation and flow of matter. It is the study of the manner in which materials respond to applied stress or strain (Mirsaeedghazi et al. 2008). The rheological properties of food materials measured or tested by rheometers like rapid visco analyser, and alveograph provides empirical information that correlates well with actual quality results for bakery products.

Viscosity characteristics

Banana is a high moisture starchy food, but also contains polyphenolic compounds that change the color of the fruit few hours after peeling. The pretreatments were meant to prevent enzymic browning that may negatively affect product quality. The pretreatments may also modify the properties of the banana starch in different ways.

Pasting temperature gives an indication of temperature required to cook the flour beyond its gelatinization point (BeMiller 2011). It corresponds to the temperature where viscosities first increase by at least 2 RVU over a 20 sec period (Olkku and Rha 1978; Appelqvist and Debet 1997). Changes that may occur when a starch–water system is heated, included enormous swelling, increased viscosity, translucency and solubility, and loss of anisotropy (birefringence) (Shimelis et al. 2006). Pasting temperature of the flour from the treated banana ranged from 84.70 ± 0.28 to 86.45 ± 0.00 with the WF:BBF/00:100 and the WF:PTBF/00:100 having the highest and lowest values, respectively. Flour from the chemically pretreated flour were significantly different from the blanched samples and both cooked at significantly lower temperature than the WF.

Peak viscosity is the maximum viscosity developed during or soon after the heating phase of the test. It occurred after most of the granule swelling had ceased. Hot starch paste is a mixture of swollen starch granules and granule fragments, together with colloidal and molecularly dispersed starch molecules. It gelatinizes when heated beyond 50°C. This caused a marked increase in the viscosity and further disintegration of the starch granules. The viscosity of the starch paste dropped at elevated temperature near 95°C depicting the characteristic peak in the viscosity-temperature curve of the RVA graph (Dengate 1978; Bakare et al. 2012). The peak viscosity also measures the alpha-amylase activity and other contributory factors such as the inherent susceptibility of the starch to amylase and the starch gel strength (Watson 1984; Meera 2010). Therefore, a higher value of RVU at the peak of the curve indicated a lower diastatic activity and vice versa (Schiller 1984). The peak viscosity of WF (186.17 ± 0.71 RVU) was found to be significantly lower than that of the treated flour (344.25 ± 12.74–461.0 ± 5.07) (Table 2). This showed that the WF had a relatively higher diastatic activity and lower gel strength than the flour from the treated banana.

Table 2. Effects of pretreatments on the pasting characteristics of wheat and pretreated banana flour.

Flours	Peak viscosity ([1]RVU)	Holding strength (RVU)	Breakdown viscosity (RVU)	Final viscosity (RVU)	Setback viscosity (RVU)	Peak time (min)	Pasting temp (°C)
WF: 100	186.17 ± 0.71^{a}	128.25 ± 1.18^{a}	67.92 ± 0.47^{a}	217.08 ± 1.41^{a}	88.83 ± 0.24^{c}	6.24 ± 0.05^{c}	87.20 ± 0.00^{c}
WF:PTBF/00:100	461.0 ± 5.07^{d}	308.13 ± 4.77^{c}	152.88 ± 9.84^{c}	348.5 ± 8.84^{d}	40.38 ± 4.07^{a}	5.14 ± 0.09^{ab}	84.70 ± 0.28^{a}
WF:CTBF/00:100	412.42 ± 6.13^{c}	248.79 ± 3.95^{b}	163.63 ± 2.18^{c}	287.71 ± 9.37^{b}	38.92 ± 5.42^{a}	5.04 ± .05^{a}	84.88 ± 0.035^{a}
WF:BBF/00:100	344.25 ± 12.74^{b}	245.13 ± 5.60^{b}	99.13 ± 7.13^{b}	312.88 ± 4.89^{c}	67.75 ± 0.71^{b}	5.30 ± 04^{b}	86.45 ± 0.00^{b}

-d-a. Mean in same column with the same superscripts are not significantly different ($P < 0.05$). WF, wheat flour; BF, banana flour from potassium (PT)-, citric acid (CT)-treated and blanched banana (BBF); (05–100), composite blends.

[1]1RVU is approximately 12 cP.

It also suggested that the gel strength of the composite flour and not the alpha-amylase activity was what was measured by the Hagberg falling numbers instrument (Table 1). The peak viscosity of the flour from the pretreated banana was also significantly different from each other. Peak viscosities occur at equilibrium between swelling of the granules (that increases the viscosity) and the granule rupture and alignment (that reduces viscosity). The relatively high swelling capacity exhibited by the treated flour may have resulted from a weak internal bonding in the starch granules.

Holding strength indicated the ability of the starch granules to maintain their gelatinized structure when the paste was held at 95°C for 2 min 30 sec under mechanical shearing stress. The treated flour had significantly higher holding strength value than that of WF, and were also significantly different from each other.

Breakdown viscosity is a measure of the degree of starch disintegration. It is an indication of hot paste stability of the starch. The smaller the breakdown viscosity, the higher the paste stability (Hugo et al. 2000; Bakare et al. 2012). The WF had significantly lower (67.92 ± 0.47 RVU) breakdown viscosity value than flour from the banana (99.13 ± 7.13–163.63 ± 2.18 RVU) indicating that the WF and the blanched samples have relatively better hot paste stability than the chemically treated samples (Table 2).

Final viscosity is the section of the paste gel curve where the gelatinized dispersion of starch becomes viscoelastic on cooling, resulting in the formation of a loose paste or gel. The final viscosity of flour from the treated banana ranged from 287.71 ± 9.37 to 348.5 ± 8.84 RVU; they are significantly different from each other and have significantly higher values than the WF. This indicated that the banana flour formed a firmer gel after cooking and cooling.

Setback viscosity is the phase of the pasting curve after cooling the starches to 50°C. This stage involved reassociation, retrogradation, or reordering of starch molecules. Also, the water previously bounded in the viscoelastic gel are released at this stage in a process referred to as syneresis. Higher the setback viscosity, greater is the tendency toward retrogradation. The blanched sample (WF:BBF/00:100) had more tendency toward retrogradation than the chemically treated sample, but both were better than the WF in this regard.

Peak time was the time at which the peak viscosity was attained in minutes. The WF had a significantly higher peak time than flour from the treated banana.

Alveograph

The alveograph is an important dough testing instrument used to evaluate the quality of WFs for bread and biscuit and cookie making (Bettge et al. 1989; Janssen et al. 1996). It measures the resistance to expansion and the extensibility of a dough by providing the measurement for maximum over pressure, average abscissa at rupture, index of swelling and deformation energy (Fig. 1) of dough (Indrani and Rao 2007). It impacts strain rates of 0.1–1 per second, which are about 100-fold higher than those occurring in actual baking processes (Chin and Campbell 2005).

The peak height (*P*) indicated the resistance that the dough offered to deformation and it is related to the tensile strength or stability that the dough exhibited during the proofing stage of bread making (Pyler 1988; Mepba et al. 2007). The *P* values ranged from 61.50 ± 0.71 to 128.50 ± 0.71 mm with the WF and the WF: CTBF/80:20 blend offering the least and highest resistance to expansion, respectively (Table 3). Resistance to expansion increased in the respective blends as the WF was replaced with flour from the treated banana, but samples containing the blanched samples (Figs. 1, 2) have significantly higher *P* values at each of the levels of substitution. The *P* values of the WF was, however, significantly different from that of the blends.

The length (*L*) indicated the extensibility of the dough. The *L* values ranged from 46.50 ± 0.71 to 103.00 ± 1.41 mm with the WF:PTBF/95:05 and WF:BBF/80:20 having the highest and least extensibility, respectively. The *L* values decreased significantly with substitution levels with the WF:BBF being the least extensible at 5% level while at subsequent levels the WF:CTBF was the least extensible.

The *P*/*L* (configuration ratio) ranged from 0.59 ± 0.83 to 2.75 ± 0.07 with the WF:BBF/95:05 and WF:BBF/80:20 having the lowest and highest values, respectively. The *P*/*L* values increased as the WF was replaced with flour from each of the treated banana, respectively. There were no significant ($P < 0.05$) differences between the WF and the WF:PTBF (5–20%), WF:CTBF (5%), and WF:BBF (5–10%). The curve configuration ratio (*P*/*L*) is an index of gluten behavior. However, the strength of composite flour are influenced by considerations other than gluten behavior. Obviously, the significantly higher *P*/*L* values of WF:CTBF/90:10, WF:CTBF/85:15, WF:CTBF/80:20, WF:BBF/85:15, and WF:BBF/80:20 relative to other blends and the WF could not have been due to the effect of gluten as shown in Table 1. These implied that other factors that influenced the rheological attributes of the dough were probably at play and these factors may not have been clearly/succinctly captured by the test method or the interpretation of the values.

The area under the curve represents the energy required to expand the dough and is related to the baking strength of the flour. This area is generally much larger for hard

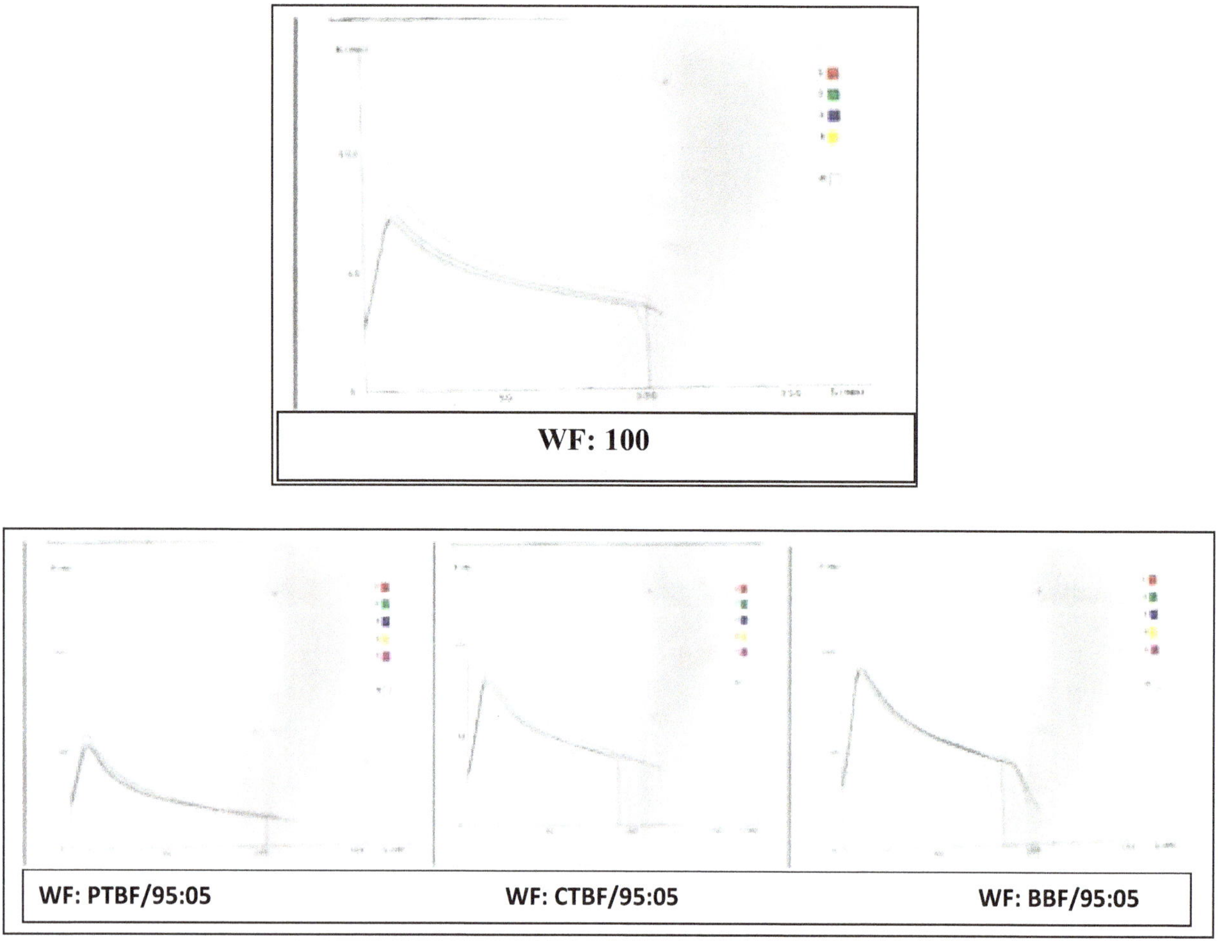

Figure 1. Alveogram characteristics of wheat flour and flour from composite containing 5% of pretreated banana.

Table 3. Effects of pretreatments on the alveogram characteristics of wheat-banana composite flour.

Flours	Peak height (mm) (*P*)	Length (mm) (*L*)	Energy (10^{-4}J) (*W*)	Curve configuration (*P/L*)	Maximum inflation (*G*)	Elasticity index (%) (*Ie*)
WF:100	$82.50 \pm 0.71_d$	$100.50 \pm 0.71_h$	$325.00 \pm 1.41_j$	$0.83 \pm 0.01_a$	$22.35 \pm 0.07_{gh}$	$70.50 \pm 0.71_l$
WF:PTBF/95: 05	$61.50 \pm 0.71_a$	$103.00 \pm 1.41_i$	$186.50 \pm 0.71_d$	$0.65 \pm 0.07_a$	$22.55 \pm 0.07_h$	$51.40 \pm 0.14_e$
WF:CTBF/95:05	$91.50 \pm 0.71_e$	$91.50 \pm 0.70_f$	$321.50 \pm 0.71_i$	$1.00 \pm 0.00_{ab}$	$21.30 \pm 0.14_{ef}$	$67.75 \pm 0.07_j$
WF:BBF/95:05	$100.50 \pm 0.71_f$	$85.50 \pm 0.71_e$	$337.50 \pm 0.71_k$	$0.59 \pm 0.83_a$	$21.00 \pm 0.70_e$	$68.70 \pm 0.14_k$
WF:PTBF/90:10	$61.00 \pm 1.41_a$	$95.00 \pm 1.41_g$	$157.00 \pm 1.41_c$	$0.65 \pm 0.01_a$	$21.75 \pm 0.21_{fg}$	$45.35 \pm 0.35_c$
WF:CTBF/90:10	$113.50 \pm 0.70_i$	$57.50 \pm 0.71_b$	$274.50 \pm 0.71_g$	$1.96 \pm 0.01_{cd}$	$17.50 \pm 0.70_c$	$62.50 \pm 0.28_h$
WF:BBF/90:10	$103.25 \pm 0.35_g$	$65.50 \pm 0.71_c$	$273.50 \pm 0.71_g$	$0.79 \pm 1.1_a$	$17.85 \pm 0.07_c$	$64.80 \pm 0.14_i$
WF:PTBF/85:15	$63.50 \pm 0.70_b$	$86.50 \pm 0.71_e$	$145.50 \pm 0.71_b$	$0.74 \pm 0.01_a$	$20.70 \pm 0.14_e$	$40.30 \pm 0.14_b$
WF:CTBF/85:15	$108.50 \pm 0.71_h$	$56.50 \pm 0.71_b$	$240.50 \pm 0.71_f$	$1.93 \pm 0.01_{cd}$	$16.80 \pm 0.14_b$	$57.35 \pm 0.07_g$
WF:BBF/85:15	$114.00 \pm 0.00_i$	$64.00 \pm 0.00_c$	$293.00 \pm 0.00_h$	$1.78 \pm 0.00_{bc}$	$17.80 \pm 0.00_c$	$62.10 \pm 0.00_h$
WF:PTBF/80:20	$69.50 \pm 0.71c$	$77.50 \pm 0.70_d$	$141.50 \pm 0.71_a$	$0.90 \pm 0.00_a$	$19.55 \pm 0.07_d$	$35.85 \pm 0.07_a$
WF:CTBF/80:20	$128.50 \pm 0.71_k$	$47.50 \pm 0.71_a$	$240.50 \pm 0.71_f$	$2.73 \pm 0.01_d$	$15.35 \pm 0.07_a$	$50.65 \pm 0.07_d$
WF:BBF/80:20	$124.50 \pm 0.71_j$	$46.50 \pm 0.71_a$	$237.50 \pm 0.71_e$	$2.75 \pm 0.07_d$	$15.40 \pm 0.42_a$	$55.75 \pm 0.21_f$

-d-a. Mean in same column with the same superscripts are not significantly different ($P < 0.05$). WF, wheat flour; BF, banana flour from potassium (PT)-, citric acid (CT)- treated and blanched banana (BBF); (05–100), composite blends.

WFs than for soft WFs. It ranged from 141.50×10^{-4}J to 337.50×10^{-4}J WF:BBF/95:05 and WF:PTBF/80:20 having the highest and lowest values, respectively. Except for WF:BBF/95:05, baking strength decreased as WF was replaced with flour from the treated banana. The energy required to expand the dough for each of the three

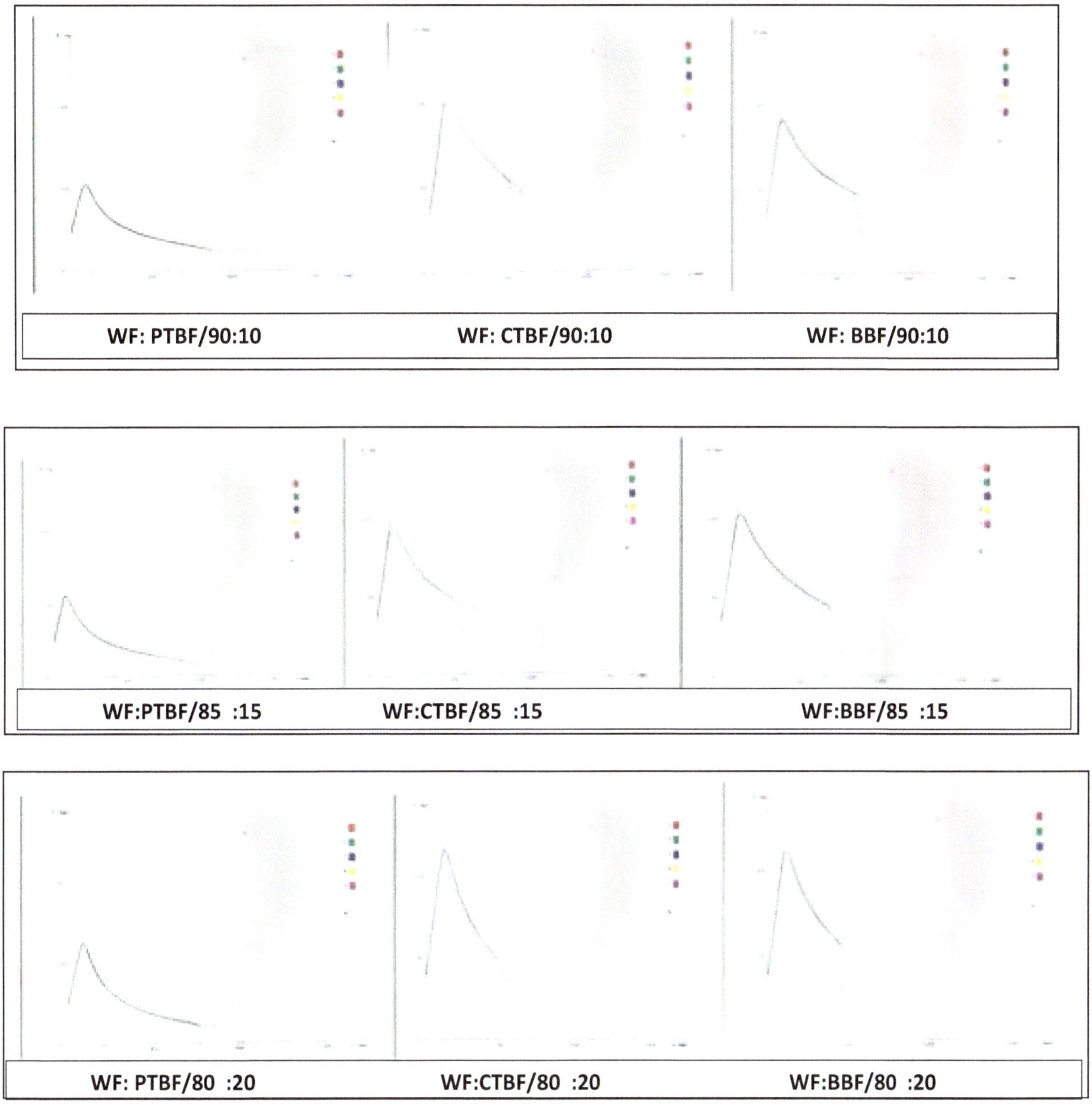

Figure 2. Alveogram characteristics of wheat flour and flour from composites containing 10, 15, and 20% of pretreated banana.

categories of blends decreased significantly with levels of substitution.

The *G* values (Table 3) depicted the relative abilities of the dough to be inflated for maximum development until they eventually burst. It is a measure of the magnitude of the total response of the dough to the biaxial stress and strain imposed on it by the instrument. It ranged from 15.35 ± 0.07 to 22.55 ± 0.07 with the WF:CTBF/80:20 and WF:PTBF/95: 05 having the lowest and highest values, respectively. It also decreased significantly as the WF was replaced with the treated flour. The WF:PTBF/95:05 and the WF had higher values than other blends but there was no significant difference between the WF and WF:PTBF (5–10%).

Elasticity index (*Ie*) may be used to characterize the dough on the basis of the elastic resistance that they offer during their biaxial deformation (Pyler 1988; Banu et al. 2011).

It also decreased with substitution levels and the WF offered significantly better elastic resistance relative to other blends. The WF:BBF had significantly higher elasticity index at each levels of substitution than the other

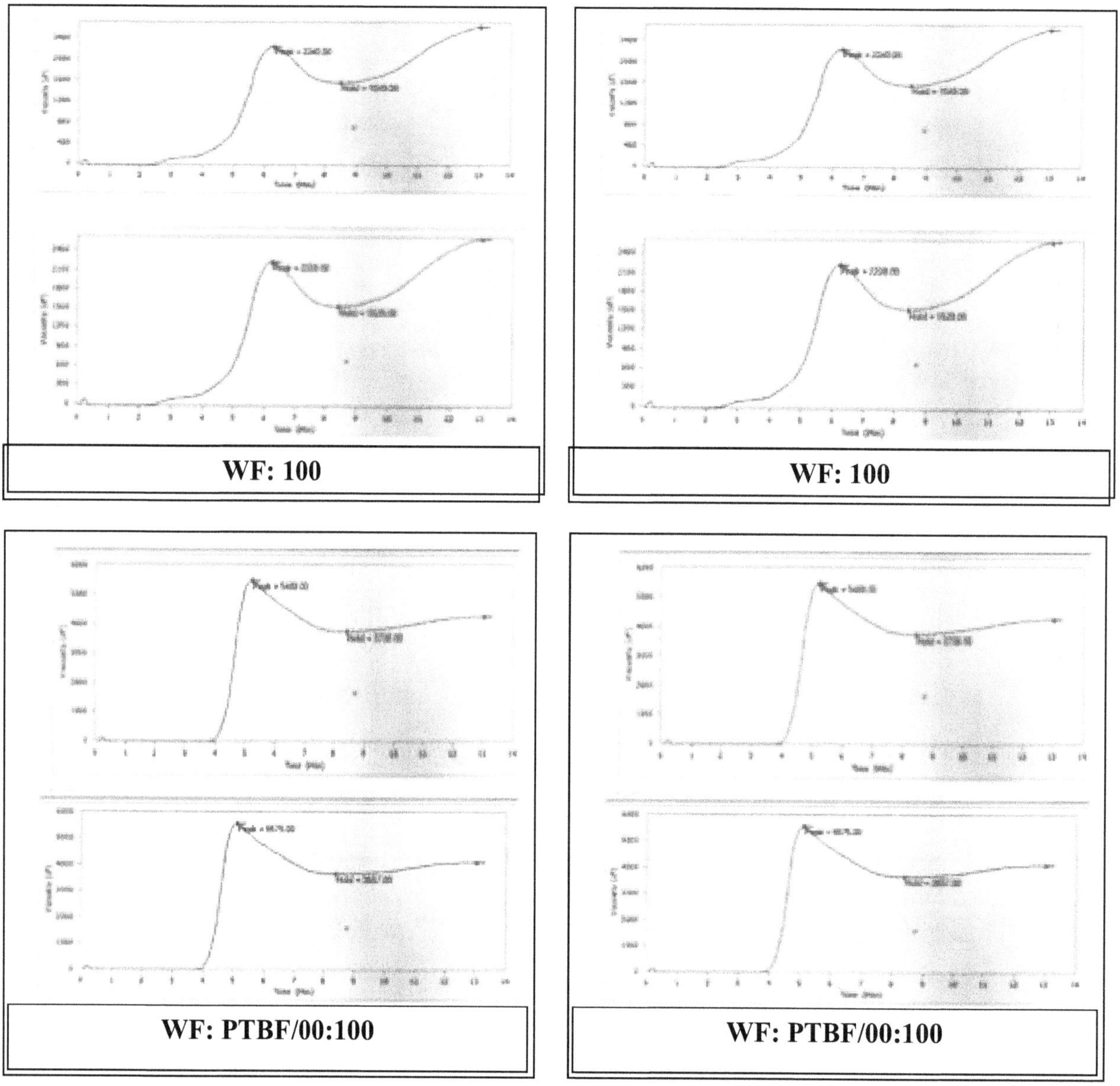

Figure 3. Pasting profile of wheat flour and flour from pretreated banana.

blends that contained flour from each of the treated bananas.

The nonlinear viscoelastic behavior of WF dough has been attributed to the continuous gluten matrix and starch granules embedded in it (Collar et al. 2007). It possesses the properties of both solid and liquid bodies, and exhibited the rheological properties that were in between that of the ideal solid and fluid bodies. The inclusion of banana flour in the blends was expected to increase the carbohydrate starch content while decreasing the quantity and quality of protein needed to sustain the viscoelastic behavior of the dough. Each of the pretreatments given to the bananas affected their composition (Table 1), pasting characteristics (Fig. 3), and the rheological characteristics of the dough made from their blends with the WF as captured by the alveograph (Figs. 1, 2).

Evaluation of bread quality

Absorbed water by dough

The quantity of water used to form the dough for baking (Table 4) ranged from 48.12 ± 0.07 to 52.60 ± 0.14% with the WF:CTBF/80:20 and WF having the lowest and highest values, respectively. The WF was significantly ($P < 0.05$) different from the blends. Actual water

Table 4. Effects of pretreatments on the physical quality characteristics of wheat-banana composite flour.

Flours	Actual water absorption (%)	Dough weight (g)	Loaf height	Loaf weight (g)	Weight loss (%)	Loaf volume (cm^3)	Loaf-specific volume (cm^3/g)
WF:100	52.60 ± 0.14^{e}	327.0 ± 0.00^{a}	10.75 ± 0.35^{f}	271.65 ± 0.21^{a}	16.93 ± 0.06^{f}	1531.70 ± 49.24^{f}	5.635 ± 0.18^{f}
WF:PTBF/95: 05	51.52 ± 0.05^{d}	327.0 ± 0.00^{a}	11.20 ± 0.14^{g}	281.05 ± 1.34^{g}	14.45 ± 0.21^{a}	1636.02 ± 7.07^{g}	5.865 ± 0.01^{g}
WF:CTBF/95:05	51.47 ± 0.03^{d}	327.0 ± 0.00^{a}	8.50 ± 0.14^{bc}	280.10 ± 0.70^{f}	14.47 ± 0.04^{a}	1144.95 ± 0.04^{c}	4.085 ± 0.01^{bc}
WF:BBF/95:05	51.51 ± 0.08^{d}	327.5 ± 0.00^{b}	9.85 ± 0.07^{e}	271.90 ± 0.70^{ab}	17.50 ± 0.71^{g}	1411.49 ± 0.21^{e}	5.250 ± 0.07^{e}
WF:PTBF/90:10	50.38 ± 0.01^{c}	327.0 ± 0.00^{a}	9.45 ± 0.07^{d}	278.00 ± 0.70^{e}	15.24 ± 0.14^{bc}	1394.85 ± 7.1^{e}	5.090 ± 0.07^{e}
WF:CTBF/90:10	50.33 ± 0.02^{c}	327.0 ± 0.00^{a}	8.25 ± 0.07^{b}	277.85 ± 0.07^{e}	15.06 ± 0.01^{b}	1157.68 ± 0.71^{c}	4.175 ± 0.01^{bc}
WF:BBF/90:10	50.34 ± 0.04^{c}	327.0 ± 0.00^{a}	6.35 ± 0.07^{a}	276.70 ± 0.14^{cde}	15.43 ± 0.03^{bcd}	774.77 ± 0.01^{a}	2.850 ± 0.07^{a}
WF:PTBF/85:15	49.34 ± 0.14^{b}	327.0 ± 0.00^{a}	8.45 ± 0.21^{bc}	278.50 ± 1.41^{e}	15.24 ± 0.14^{bc}	1223.82 ± 0.14^{d}	4.415 ± 0.01^{d}
WF:CTBF/85:15	49.28 ± 0.09^{b}	327.0 ± 0.71^{a}	8.26 ± 0.01^{b}	275.75 ± 0.071^{cd}	15.70 ± 0.01^{cd}	1164.25 ± 0.01^{cd}	4.225 ± 0.01^{c}
WF:BBF/85:15	49.27 ± 0.07^{b}	327.0 ± 0.00^{a}	8.65 ± 0.07^{c}	273.50 ± 0.14^{b}	16.39 ± 0.01^{e}	1222.07 ± 0.01^{d}	4.475 ± 0.01^{d}
WF:PTBF/80:20	48.18 ± 0.09^{a}	327.0 ± 0.00^{a}	8.35 ± 0.21^{bc}	277.40 ± 1.55^{de}	15.46 ± 0.06^{bcd}	1226.55 ± 24.57^{d}	4.495 ± 0.16^{d}
WF:CTBF/80:20	48.12 ± 0.07^{a}	327.0 ± 0.00^{a}	8.15 ± 0.07^{b}	277.25 ± 0.071^{cde}	15.24 ± 0.01^{bc}	1131.43 ± 0.03^{bc}	4.185 ± 0.01^{bc}
WF:BBF/80:20	48.14 ± 0.06^{a}	327.0 ± 0.00^{a}	8.26 ± 0.01^{b}	275.55 ± 0.21^{c}	15.79 ± 0.01^{d}	1104.85 ± 0.01^{b}	4.020 ± 0.01^{b}

-d-a. Mean in same column with the same superscripts are not significantly different ($P < 0.05$). WF, wheat flour; BF, banana flour from potassium (PT)-, citric acid (CT)-treated and blanched banana (BBF); (05–100), composite blends.

absorption decreased as the WF was replaced by each of the flour from the treated bananas and there was no significant difference between the blends at each of the substitution ratios.

Specific volume

Loaf volume is used as a criterion to measure the quality of fresh bread in research quality control in industry and by consumers (Penfield and Campbell 1990; Zuwariah and Aziah 2009). Specific volume of loaves of bread provide a uniform basis for comparing results of various studies (Oyeku et al. 2008; Bakare et al. 2015). It ranged from 2.850 ± 0.07 to 5.865 ± 0.01 cm^3/g with the WF:PTBF/95: 05 having significantly higher specific volume than other blends. The values decreased as flour from the treated banana replaces the WF in the blends but the 5% WF:PTBF was significantly ($P > 0.05$) better than the WF.

In WF, specific volume is an indication of the gluten content of the bread (Van Hall 2000; Abang Zaidel et al. 2010) but other constituents such as starch and fiber also contribute to the specific volume of bread. Gluten or more precisely glutenin, is the main structure-forming protein in WF that is responsible for the elastic and extensible properties needed to produce good quality wheat bread (Bloksma 1990b; Gallagher et al. 2003). Bread made from soft WF usually yield lower loaf volumes. It has also been shown that the difference between weak and strong flours can be explained by differences in the molecular mass distribution of their proteins (MacRitchie 1973). Abundance of glutenin molecules with long chain was

Table 5. Effects of pretreatments on the sensory quality characteristics of wheat-banana composite flour.

Flours	Appearance	Flavor	Aroma	Texture	Taste
WF: 100	8.27 ± 0.64 ^{g}	7.83 ± 1.05^{c}	7.30 ± 1.24^{d}	8.03 ± 1.03^{c}	7.87 ± 0.93^{e}
WF:PTBF/95: 05	6.30 ± 1.56^{ef}	5.83 ± 1.63^{ab}	5.53 ± 1.81^{abc}	6.70 ± 1.51^{b}	6.33 ± 1.35^{cd}
WF:CTPT/95:05	6.63 ± 1.03^{f}	6.26 ± 1.57^{b}	5.77 ± 1.65^{bc}	6.40 ± 1.33^{b}	6.53 ± 1.46^{d}
WF:BPT/95:05	5.83 ± 1.76^{def}	5.87 ± 1.43^{ab}	5.70 ± 1.21^{bc}	5.83 ± 1.80^{ab}	6.03 ± 1.40^{cd}
WF:PTBF/90:10	5.63 ± 1.65^{cde}	5.90 ± 1.45^{ab}	5.63 ± 1.69^{abc}	5.40 ± 2.13^{a}	6.13 ± 1.68^{cd}
WF:CTPT/90:10	5.53 ± 1.33^{cde}	5.67 ± 1.83^{ab}	5.97 ± 1.27^{c}	5.77 ± 1.79^{ab}	6.50 ± 1.38^{d}
WF:BPT/90:10	5.47 ± 1.96^{bcde}	6.00 ± 1.11^{ab}	5.77 ± 1.43^{bc}	6.10 ± 2.01^{ab}	6.13 ± 1.61^{cd}
WF:PTBF/85:15	4.67 ± 1.92^{abc}	5.57 ± 1.38^{ab}	5.33 ± 1.56^{abc}	5.27 ± 1.66^{a}	5.47 ± 1.63^{abc}
WF:CTPT/85:15	5.17 ± 1.72^{bcd}	5.90 ± 1.56^{ab}	5.57 ± 1.55^{abc}	5.93 ± 1.51^{ab}	5.63 ± 1.61^{bcd}
WF:BPT/85:15	4.50 ± 2.21^{ab}	5.33 ± 1.71^{ab}	5.03 ± 1.83^{ab}	5.87 ± 1.89^{ab}	5.47 ± 1.66^{abc}
WF:PTBF/80:20	4.80 ± 1.94^{abc}	5.33 ± 1.75^{ab}	4.93 ± 1.57^{ab}	5.13 ± 1.69^{a}	5.03 ± 1.92^{ab}
WF:CTPT/80:20	4.50 ± 1.66^{ab}	5.16 ± 1.42^{a}	4.93 ± 1.53^{ab}	5.17 ± 1.68^{a}	4.70 ± 1.68^{a}
WF:BPT/80:20	3.87 ± 1.81^{a}	5.33 ± 1.92^{ab}	4.77 ± 1.76^{a}	5.33 ± 1.88^{a}	5.47 ± 2.17^{abc}

-d-a. Mean in same column with the same superscripts are not significantly different ($P < 0.05$). WF, wheat flour; BF, banana flour from potassium (PT)-, citric acid (CT)-treated and blanched banana (BBF); (05–100), composite blends.

observed to have made the protein phase, and consequently the dough, highly extensible (Bloksma 1990a). Differences in the pasting temperature and peak viscosity of composite starches have also been suspected to influence extensibility (Greene and Bovell-Benjamin 2004).

Weight loss

Cut-out dough losses weight during the proofing and baking stages of bread processing. This may be due to both fermentation losses brought about by amylases of starch and utilization of soluble sugar by yeast, and also by evaporation of moisture during baking. Weight loss ranged from 14.45 ± 0.21 to 17.50 ± 0.71%. The WF:PTBF/95:05 lost the most weight while the WF:BBF/95:05 lost the least weight. Except for the blends that contain the blanched sample, weight loss increased as the flour from the treated bananas replaces the WF in the blends (Table 4).

Sensory evaluation

Sensory scores ranged from 3.87 ± 1.81, 5.16 ± 1.42, 4.77 ± 1.76, 5.13 ± 1.69, and 4.70 ± 1.68 to 8.27 ± 0.64, 7.83 ± 1.05, 7.30 ± 1.24, 8.03 ± 1.03, and 7.87 ± 0.93 for appearance, flavor, aroma, texture, and taste, respectively (Table 5). Bread samples prepared from the WF had significantly higher scores for all the sensory attributes while the WF:BPT/80:20 scored the lowest in appearance, aroma, texture, and the WF:CTPT/80:20, the lowest score for flavor and taste, respectively.

In the blends containing flour from the treated samples, the WF:PTBF/95:05 had better scores for appearance, texture, and taste while the WF:CTPT/95:05 had better scores for flavor and aroma, respectively.

Conclusion

The main aim of this study was to produce bread from composite flour comprising of banana and wheat flour without having to alter considerably, the rheological attributes of the dough and the quality attributes associated with bread from wheat flour. These necessarily involve the conversion of the banana to flour while controlling the undesirable enzyme induced discoloration associated with the use of banana flour. That was why it was necessary to evaluate how the pretreatments that were primarily meant to mitigate the discoloration effect of the enzyme activities modified the composition, rheology, and baking qualities of the flour.

The study concluded that the pretreatments have significant effects on the composition of the banana flour and also have varying effects on the composition and pasting properties of their composite flour with WF. For instance, the PTBF had significantly higher protein value than the CTBF and BBF, while the PTBF containing blends had relatively higher protein values than other blends except at 15% level. Crude fiber of the blends decreased as the WF was replaced by the treated flour for the various pretreatments with the PTBF and CTBF having significantly higher values at 5% and 10–20% substitution level, respectively.

Flour from the pretreated banana had significantly ($P < 0.05$) higher Falling number values implying that the pretreatments may have (since the study design did not include untreated banana flour) reduced the alpha-amylase activity of the treated flour thereby decreasing the extent of liquefaction and diastatic activity of their starches. This observation reflected in the blends as the proportion of the flour from the treated banana was increased.

Also, contrary to reports of earlier studies on sweet-potato and breadfruit flour, water absorption decreased as WF was replaced with flour from each of the treated bananas. This indicated that the pretreatments modified the pasting properties of the banana starch in several ways. For instance, the pasting temperature of the chemically pretreated flour was significantly different from the blanched samples and both cooked at significantly lower temperature than the WF. Similarly, the peak viscosity of the flour from the pretreated banana were also significantly different from each other.

The rheological attributes of the composite flour in which they were included was also affected in different ways at various levels of inclusion in their composite with WF. For instance, the curve configuration ratio (P/L), which is an index of the rheological attributes of the dough, showed that composite flour containing the potassium-treated flour (WF:PTBF) was not significantly different from the WF at all the levels of inclusion (5–20%) in this study, while those containing the blanched sample (WF:BBF) and the citric acid-treated (CTBF) sample were only comparable to the WF at 5% and up to 10% levels of inclusions, respectively. The specific volume of WF:PTBF bread was significantly ($P > 0.05$) better than the bread produced from the WF and had better scores for appearance, texture, and taste than bread samples from other blends.

Conflict of Interest

None declared.

References

AACC. 2000. American association of cereal chemists approved methods of analysis. St. AACC International, St. Paul, MN. Available at: http://dx.doi.org/10.1094/AACCIntMethod (accessed 19 November 2013)

AACC. 2010. American Association of Cereal Chemists International. Approved methods of analysis, 11th ed. Method 54-30.02. Physical dough tests: alveograph method for soft and hard wheat flour. AACC International, St. Paul, MN. Available at: http://dx.doi.org/10.1094/AACCIntMethod (Accessed 19 November 2013).

Abang Zaidel, D. N., N. L. Chin, and Y. A. Yusof. 2010. A review on rheological properties and measurements of dough and gluten. J. Appl. Sci. 10:2478–2490.

Adeleke, R. O., and J. O. Odedeji. 2010. Functional properties of wheat sweet potato flour blend. Pak. J. Nutr. 9:535–538.

Ade-Omowaye, B. I. O., B. A. Bolarinwa, and A. O. Adebiyi. 2008. Evaluation of tigernut (*Cyperus esculentus*) - wheat composite flour and bread. Afr. J. Food Sci. 2:87–89.

Alex, A. A., A. R. Kelly, M. L. Odean, R. G. Fulcher, and D. A. Susan. 2008. Influence of added bean flour (*Phaseolus vulgaris* L.) on some physical and nutritional properties of wheat flour tortillas. Food Chem. 109:33–41.

Appelqvist, I. A. M., and M. R. M. Debet. 1997. Starch – biopolymer interactions – A review. Food Rev. Int. 13:163–224.

Bakare, H. A. 2008. Evaluation of the rheological properties and baking performance of wheat composite flour produced from lye-peeled breadfruit (*Artocarpus communis* Forst) and cassava (*Manihot esculenta* crantz). Ph. D Thesis in Food Science and Technology Department, University of Ibadan, Ibadan.

Bakare, H. A., M. O. Adegunwa, O. F. Osundahunsi, and J. O. Olusanya. 2012. Composition and pasting properties of breadfruit (*Artocarpus communis* Forst) from South West States of Nigeria. Niger. Food J. 30:11–17.

Bakare, H. A., O. F. Osundahunsi, M. O. Adegunwa, and J. O. Olusanya. 2013. Batter rheology, baking, and sensory qualities of cake from blends of breadfruit and wheat flours. J. Culinary Sci. Technol. 11:203–221.

Bakare, H. A., O. F. Osundahunsi, M. O. Adegunwa, and J. O. Olusanya. 2014a. Pasting characteristics, baking and sensory qualities of cakes from blends of cassava and wheat flours. J. Culinary Sci. Technol. 12:109–127.

Bakare, H. A., M. O. Adegunwa, O. M. Akinribido, and O. A. Obadina. 2014b. Proximate, baking, and sensory qualities of biscuits from wheat and fermented breadfruit (*Artocarpus communis* Frost) flour. J. Culinary Sci. Technol. 12:316–325.

Bakare, H. A., O. F. Osundahunsi, and J. O. Olusanya. 2015. Rheological, baking, and sensory properties of composite bread dough with breadfruit (*Artocarpus communis* Forst) and wheat flours. J. Food Sci. Nutr. doi: 10.1002/fsn3.321

Banu, J., G. Stoenescu, V. Ionescu, and J. Aprodu. 2011. Estimation of the baking quality of wheat flours based on rheological parameters of the mixolab curve. Czech J. Food Sci. 29:35–44.

BeMiller, J. N. 2011. Pasting, paste, and gel properties of starch-hydrocolloid combinations. Carbohydr. Polym. 86:386–423.

Bettge, A., G. L. Rubenthaler, and Y. Pomeranz. 1989. Alveograph algorithms to predict functional properties of in bread and cookie baking. Cereal Chem. 66:81–86.

Biljan, S., and F. Bojana. 2008. Nutritional and sensory evaluation of wheat bread supplemented with oleic-rich sunflower seed. Food Chem. 108:119–129.

Bloksma, A. H. 1990a. Rheology of the bread making process. Cereal Food World 35:232–236.

Bloksma, A. H. 1990b. Dough structure, dough rheology and baking quality. Cereal Food World 35:237–243.

Bowles, L. K. 1996. Amylolytic enzymes. Pp. 105–129 *in* R. E. Hebeda and H. F. Zobel, eds. Baked goods freshness: technology, evaluation, and inhibition of staling. Marcel Dekker, Inc., New York.

Braganza, M. L. T., and E. H. Tolentino. 2011. Banana (*Musa sapientum var. Cavendish*) Flour as wheat flour extender in selected bakery products. Pp. 1–6 *in* A paper presented at the 12th ASEAN Food conference held on the 16th to 18th of June, 2011 at BITEC Bangna, Thailand.

Chin, N. L., and G. M. Campbell. 2005. Dough aeration and rheology: part 2. Effects of flour type, mixing speed and total work input on aeration and rheology of bread dough. J. Sci. Food Agric. 85:2194–2202.

Collar, C., C. Bollain, and C. M. Rosell. 2007. Rheological behaviour of formulated bread doughs during mixing and heating. Food Sci. Technol. Int. 13:99–106.

Corzo, O. N., A. V. Brancho, and A. Pureira. 2008. Energy and Energy amylases of thin layer drying of coroba slices. J. Food Eng. 86:151–161.

Dengate, H. N. 1978. Swelling, pasting and gelling of wheat starch. Pp. 49–82 *in* Y. Pomeranz,ed. Advances in cereal science and technology. Am Assoc. Cereal Chem, inc. St. Paul, MN.

Dewettinck, K., F. Van Bockstaele, B. Kühne, D. Van de Walle, T. M. Courtens, and X. Gellynck. 2008. Nutritional value of bread: influence of processing, food interaction and consumer perception- review. J. Cereal Sci. 48:243–257.

Duncan, D. B. 1955. Multiple range and multiple F-tests. Biometrics 11:1–5. doi:10.2307/3001478 CrossRef, Web of Science® Times Cited: 13957.

Entwistle, P. V., and W. L. Hunter. 1949. Report on crude fiber. J. AOAC 32:65–656.

FAO. 2013. FAOStat. Available at: http://faostat.fao.org/default.aspx?lang=en (accessed 14 March 2013).

FAO. 2014. Banana market review and banana statistics 2012–2013: market and policy analyses of raw materials, horticulture and tropical (RAMHOT) products team. Pp. 1–39. Food and Agriculture Organization of the United Nations, Rome.

FAOSTAT. 2013. Production/Crop. Food and Agriculture Organisation of the United nations, Rome. Available at: http://faostat3.fao.org/download/Q/QC/E (accessed 05 February 2013).

Gallagher, E., T. R. Gormley, and E. M. Arendt. 2003. Crust and crumb characteristics of gluten free breads. J. Food Eng. 56:153–161.

Greene, J. L., and A. C. Bovell-Benjamin. 2004. Macroscopic and sensory evaluation of bread supplemented with sweet potato flour. J. Food Sci. 69:167–173.

Grimm, E., B. P. Khanal, A. Winkler, M. Knoche, and D. Koepcke. 2012. Structural and physiological changes associated with the skin spot disorder in apple. Postharvest Biol. Technol. 64:111–118.

Hoseney, R. C. 1994. Gas retention in bread doughs. Cereal Foods World 29:305–306.

Hugo, L. F., L. W. Rooney, and J. R. N. Taylor. 2000. Malted sorghum as a functional ingredient in composite bread. Cereal Chem. 77:428–432.

Ihl, M., L. Aravena, E. Scheuermann, E. Uquiche, and V. Bifani. 2003. Effect of immersion solutions on shelf life of minimally processed lettuce. Lebensmittel- Wissenschaft und-Technologie 36:591–599.

Indrani, D., and G. V. Rao. 2007. Rheological characteristics of wheat flour dough as influenced by ingredients of parotta. J. Food Eng. 79:100–105.

Ioannou, I., and M. Ghoul. 2013. Prevention of enzymatic browning in fruit and vegetables. Eur. Sci. J. 9:1857–7881.

Janssen, A. M., T. van Vliet, and J. M. Vereijken. 1996. Fundamental and empirical rheological behaviour of wheat flour doughs and comparison with bread making performance. J. Cereal Sci. 23:43–54.

Jiang, Y. 2004. Advances in understanding of enzymatic browning in harvested litchi fruit. Food Chem. 88:443–446.

Jiang, Y. M., L. Pen, and J. Li. 2004. Use of citric acid for shelf life and quality maintenance of fresh-cut Chinese water chestnut. J. Food Eng. 63:325–328.

Kim, H. J., N. Morita, S. H. Lee, and K. D. Moon. 2003. Scanning electron microscopic observations of dough and bread supplemented with Gastrodia elata Blume powder. Food Res. Int. 36:387–389.

Komthong, P., T. Katoh, N. Igura, and M. Shimoda. 2006. Changes in odours of apple juice during enzymatic browning. Food Qual. Ref. 17:497–504.

Kyamuchangine, W., H. Myhre, H. T. Sorensen, and R. Rehrson. 2002. Yield, characteristics and composition and banana juice extracted by the enzymatic and mechanical methods. J. Sci. Food Agric. 82:478–482.

Lin, L., H. Liu, Y. Yu, S. Lin, and J. Mau. 2009. Quality and antioxidant property of buckwheat enhanced wheat bread. Food Chem. 37:461–467.

Loaiza-Velarde, J. G., M. E. Mangrich, R. Campos-Vargas, and M. E. Saltveit. 2003. Heat shock reduces browning of fresh-cut celery petioles. Postharvest Biol. Technol. 27:305–311.

Luo, Y., and Y. Tao. 2003. Determining tissue damage of fresh-cut vegetables using imaging technology. Acta Hortic. Proc. 628:97–102.

MacRitchie, F. 1973. Conversion of a weal flour to a strong one by increasing the proportion of its high molecular weight gluten protein. J. Sci. Food Agric. 24:1325.

Malomo, S. A., A. F. Eleyinmi, and J. B. Fashakin. 2011. Chemical composition, rheological properties and bread making potentials of composite flours from breadfruit, breadnut and wheat. Afr. J. Food Sci. 5:400–410.

Malomo, O., M. O. Jimoh, O. O. Adekoyeni, O. E. Soyebi, and E. A. Alamu. 2013. Effect of blanching and unblanching on rheological properties of sweet-potato bread. Acad. Res. J. 1:24–41.

Manuel, G., O. Bonastre, M. R. Cristina, P. Valentin, and F. Encarnacion. 2008. Studies on cake quality made of wheat- chickpea flour blends. LWT Food Sci. Technol. 41:1701–1709.

Mazzeo, T., D. N'Dri, E. Chiavaro, A. Visconti, V. Fogliano, and N. Pellegrini. 2011. Effect of two cooking procedures on phytochemical compounds, total antioxidant capacity and colour of selected frozen vegetables. Food Chem. 128:627–633.

Meera, K. 2010. Falling number in wheat-how is it calculated and what does it mean to producers? USDA, ARS, Soft wheat Quality Lab, USA. Alpha amylase mkweon-FN-012810 [1], pdf (accessed 19 May 2011).

Mepba, H. D., L. Eboh, and S. U. Nwaojigwa. 2007. Chemical composition, functional and baking properties of wheat- plantain composite flours. Afr. J. Food Nutr. Dev. 7:1–22.

Mirsaeedghazi, H., Z. Emam-Djomeh, and S. M. A. Mousavi. 2008. Rheometric measurement of dough rheological characteristics and factors affecting it. Int. J. Agric. Biol. 10:112–119.

Olatunji, O., and I. A. Akinrele. 1978. Comparative rheological properties and bread qualities of wheat flour diluted with tropical tuber and breadfruit flour. Cereal Chem. 55:1–6.

Olkku, T., and C. Rha. 1978. Gelatinisation of starch and wheat flour starch – A review. Food Chem. 3:293–317.

Oyeku, M. O., C. F. Kupoluyi, H. A. Osibanjo, C. U. Orji, F. N. Ajuebor, I. O. Ajiboshin, et al. 2008. An economic assessment of commercial production of 10% cassava-wheat composite flour bread. J. Ind. Res. Technol. 2:13–20.

Penfield, M. P., and A. M. Campbell. 1990. Experimental food science. 3rd ed. Pp. 519–520. San Diego, California: Academic Press, Inc.

Pius, B. N. 1994. Banana and their management. 1st ed. Mc Graw-Hill Publuishing co Ltd., New Delhi, India.

Pyler, E. J. 1988. Baking science and technology. 3rd ed. 1 and II Sosland Publishing Company, USA.

Qiang, He, Yaguang Luo. 2007. Enzymatic browning and its control in fresh-cut produce Stewart Postharvest Review. 6:3.

Schiller, G. W. 1984. Bakery flour specifications. Cereal Foods World 29:647–651.

Senadeera, W., B. R. Bhandari, G. Young, and B. Wijesinghe. 2005. Modelling dimensional shrinkage of shaped foods in fluidized bed drying. J. Food Process. Preserv. 29:109–119.

Shimelis, E., M. Meaza, and S. Raskshit. 2006. Physico-chemical properties, pasting behaviour and functional characteristics of flour and starches from improved bean (*Phaseoulus vulgaris* L.) varieties grown in East Africa. Agric. Eng. Int. CIGR J. VIII:05-015.

Van Hall, M. V. 2000. Quality of sweet potato flour during processing and storage. Food Rev. Int. 16:1–37.

Wall, M. M. 2006. Ascorbic acid, pro vitamin A, and mineral composition of banana (*Musa sp*) and papaya (*Carica papaya*) cultivars grown in Hawaii. J. Food Compos. Anal. 19:434–455.

Watson, C. A. 1984. An instrument for determining alpha – amylase activity. Cereal Foods World 29:507–509.

World Bank. 2013. Data- Nigeria. The World Bank Group, NW, Washington, DC. Available at: http://data.worldbank.org/indicator/NY.GDP.PCAP.CD (accessed 22 April 2016).

Zuwariah, I., and A. N. Aziah. 2009. Physicochemical properties of wheat breads substituted with banana flour and modified banana flour. J. Trop. Agric. Food Sci. 37:33–42.

PERMISSIONS

All chapters in this book were first published in FSN, by John Wiley & Sons Ltd.; hereby published with permission under the Creative Commons Attribution License or equivalent. Every chapter published in this book has been scrutinized by our experts. Their significance has been extensively debated. The topics covered herein carry significant findings which will fuel the growth of the discipline. They may even be implemented as practical applications or may be referred to as a beginning point for another development.

The contributors of this book come from diverse backgrounds, making this book a truly international effort. This book will bring forth new frontiers with its revolutionizing research information and detailed analysis of the nascent developments around the world.

We would like to thank all the contributing authors for lending their expertise to make the book truly unique. They have played a crucial role in the development of this book. Without their invaluable contributions this book wouldn't have been possible. They have made vital efforts to compile up to date information on the varied aspects of this subject to make this book a valuable addition to the collection of many professionals and students.

This book was conceptualized with the vision of imparting up-to-date information and advanced data in this field. To ensure the same, a matchless editorial board was set up. Every individual on the board went through rigorous rounds of assessment to prove their worth. After which they invested a large part of their time researching and compiling the most relevant data for our readers.

The editorial board has been involved in producing this book since its inception. They have spent rigorous hours researching and exploring the diverse topics which have resulted in the successful publishing of this book. They have passed on their knowledge of decades through this book. To expedite this challenging task, the publisher supported the team at every step. A small team of assistant editors was also appointed to further simplify the editing procedure and attain best results for the readers.

Apart from the editorial board, the designing team has also invested a significant amount of their time in understanding the subject and creating the most relevant covers. They scrutinized every image to scout for the most suitable representation of the subject and create an appropriate cover for the book.

The publishing team has been an ardent support to the editorial, designing and production team. Their endless efforts to recruit the best for this project, has resulted in the accomplishment of this book. They are a veteran in the field of academics and their pool of knowledge is as vast as their experience in printing. Their expertise and guidance has proved useful at every step. Their uncompromising quality standards have made this book an exceptional effort. Their encouragement from time to time has been an inspiration for everyone.

The publisher and the editorial board hope that this book will prove to be a valuable piece of knowledge for researchers, students, practitioners and scholars across the globe.

LIST OF CONTRIBUTORS

Olugbenga O. Awolu, Olufunmilayo S. Omoba and Olumide Olawoye
Department of Food Science and Technology, Federal University of Technology, Akure, Nigeria

Modupe Dairo
Quintas Renewable Energy Solutions Ltd, Akure, Nigeria

Daniel B. Hannon and Jerry T. Thompson
Department of Veterinary and Biomedical Sciences and Center for Molecular Toxicology and Carcinogenesis, Penn State University, 325 Life Sciences Building, University Park, Pennsylvania 16802

Christina Khoo
Ocean Spray Cranberries, Inc., One Ocean Spray Drive, Lakeville-Middleboro, Massachusetts 02349

Vijaya Juturu
UnitedBio-Med Inc., 102 Hunters Run, Dobbs Ferry, New York 10502

John P. Vanden Heuvel
Department of Veterinary and Biomedical Sciences and Center for Molecular Toxicology and Carcinogenesis, Penn State University, 325 Life Sciences Building, University Park, Pennsylvania 16802
INDIGO Biosciences Inc., 1981 Pine Hall Road, State College, Pennsylvania 16801

Emmanuel A. Irondi and Jacob K. Akintunde
Biochemistry Unit, Department of Biosciences and Biotechnology, Kwara State University, Malete, P.M.B. 1530, Ilorin, Nigeria

Samson O. Agboola
Department of Veterinary Physiology, Biochemistry and Pharmacology, University of Ibadan, Ibadan, Nigeria

Aline A. Boligon and Margareth L. Athayde
Phytochemical Research Laboratory, Department of Industrial Pharmacy, Federal University of Santa Maria, Building 26, room 1115, Santa Maria, CEP 97105-900, Brazil

Roslizawati Ab Lah
Marine Ecology Research Centre, School of Environment, Science and Engineering, University of Southern Cross, Lismore 2480, New South Wales, Australia
University Malaysia Terengganu, Kuala 21030, Terengganu, Malaysia

Joshua Smith
Marine Ecology Research Centre, School of Environment, Science and Engineering, University of Southern Cross, Lismore 2480, New South Wales, Australia
Southern Cross Plant Science, University of Southern Cross, Lismore 2480, New South Wales, Australia

Dale Savins and Ashley Dowell
Southern Cross Plant Science, University of Southern Cross, Lismore 2480, New South Wales, Australia

Daniel Bucher and Kirsten Benkendorff
Marine Ecology Research Centre, School of Environment, Science and Engineering, University of Southern Cross, Lismore 2480, New South Wales, Australia

Patricia Martorell, Silvia Llopis, Nuria Gonzalez, Daniel Ramón and Salvador Genovés
Cell Biology Laboratory, Food Biotechnology Department, Biópolis SL, Paterna, Valencia 46980, Spain

Gabriel Serrano, Ana Torrens, Juan M. Serrano and Maria Navarro
Research and Development Department, Sesderma Laboratories, Rafelbuñol, Valencia 46138, Spain

Elias K. Mibei, Arnold N. Onyango and Willis O. Owino
Department of Food Science and Technology, Jomo Kenyatta University of Agriculture and Technology, Nairobi, Kenya

Jane Ambuko
Department of Plant Science and Crop Protection, University of Nairobi, Nairobi, Kenya

James J. Giovannoni
Boyce Thompson Institute for Plant Research, Cornell University Campus, Ithaca, New York 14853

Florence K. M'Kaibi
Stellenbosch University, Cape Town, South Africa

Nelia P. Steyn
Division of Human Nutrition, Department of Human Biology, University of Cape Town, Anzio Road, Cape Town, South Africa

Sophie A. Ochola
Department of Foods, Nutrition and Dietetics, Kenyatta University, Nairobi, Kenya

Lissane Du Plessis
Division of Human Nutrition, Stellenbosch University, Cape Town, South Africa

Earle R. Nestmann
Health Science Consultants Inc., Mississauga, Ontario L5N 7S2, Canada

Judith Kanensi Okoth and Anselimo Makokha
Department of Food Science and Technology, Jomo Kenyatta University of Agriculture and Technology, P.O. Box 62000-00200, Nairobi, Kenya

Sophie Atieno Ochola
Department of Foods, Nutrition and Dietetics, Kenyatta University, P.O. Box 43844-00100, Nairobi, Kenya

Nicholas K. Gikonyo
Department of Pharmacy and Complementary/ Alternative Medicine, Kenyatta University, P.O. Box 43844-00100, Nairobi, Kenya

Gideon O. Oladipo and Emmanuel O. Ibukun
Department of Biochemistry, Federal University of Technology Akure, Akure, Ondo State, Nigeria

Ajda Ota, Rajko Vidrih, Janez Hribar and Sonja Smole Možina
Biotechnical Faculty, University of Ljubljana, Jamnikarjeva 101, Ljubljana SI-1000, Slovenia

Ana Miklavčič Višnjevec and Milena Bučar-Miklavčič
Science and Research Centre of Koper, University of Primorska, Zelena ulica 8, Izola SI-6310, Slovenia

Željko Prgomet
Agricultural Department in Poreč, University of Rijeka, Carla Huguesa 6, Porecˇ, Croatia

Marijan Nečemer
Institute Jožef Stefan, Jamova cesta 39, Ljubljana SI-1000, Slovenia

Nina Gunde Cimerman and Nataša Poklar Ulrih
Biotechnical Faculty, University of Ljubljana, Jamnikarjeva 101, Ljubljana SI-1000, Slovenia
Centre of Excellence for Integrated Approaches in Chemistry and Biology of Proteins (CIPKeBiP), Jamova cesta 39, Ljubljana SI-1000, Slovenia

Lateefah A. Oyinlola, Adewale O. Obadina and Olusola B. Oyewole
Department of Food Science and Technology, Federal University of Agriculture, Abeokuta, Nigeria

Adebukunola M. Omemu
Department of Hospitality and Tourism Management, Federal University of Agriculture, Abeokuta, Nigeria

Zahra Sayyari
Department of Food Science and Technology, Savadkooh branch, Islamic Azad University, Savadkooh, Iran

Reza Farahmandfar
Department of Food Science and Technology, Sari Agricultural Sciences and Natural Resources University (SANRU), Sari, Iran

Geoffrey Ssepuuya, Ivan Muzira Mukisa and Dorothy Nakimbugwe
Department of Food Technology and Nutrition, School of Food Technology, Nutrition and Bio-Engineering, College of Agricultural and Environmental Sciences, Makerere University, P.O. Box, 7062 Kampala, Uganda

Yi Wang, Chen Wang, Wei Cheng and Peng Guo
Hubei Academy of Agricultural Sciences, Institute of Agricultural Products Processing and Nuclear Agriculture Technology Research, Wuhan 430064, China

Yinbing Bian
Institute of Applied Mycology, Huazhong Agricultural University, Wuhan 430070, China

Obse Fikiru
Department of Food Science and Postharvest Technology, Ambo University, Ambo, Ethiopia

Geremew Bultosa
Department of Food Science and Technology, Botswana College of Agriculture, Private Bag 0027, Gaborone, Botswana

Sirawdink Fikreyesus Forsido
Department of Postharvest Management, Jimma University, Jimma, Ethiopia

Mathewos Temesgen
Department of Biology, Ambo University, Ambo, Ethiopia

Carla Barlagne, Jean-Marc Blazy, Jean-Louis Diman and Harry Ozier-Lafontaine
UR1321 ASTRO Agrosystèmes tropicaux, INRA, Petit-Bourg (Guadeloupe) F-97170, France

Denis Cornet
UMR AGAP, CIRAD, Petit-Bourg (Guadeloupe) F-97170, France

Adegoke H. Bakare and Mojisola O. Adegunwa
Department of Hospitality and Tourism Federal University of Agriculture, Abeokuta, Nigeria

Olukemi D. Ogunbowale
Department of Food Science and Technology, Federal University of Agriculture, Abeokuta, Nigeria

Joseph O. Olusanya
Department of Home Economics and Hotel Management, Tai Solarin University of Education Nigeria, Ijebu-Ode, Nigeria

Index